total parenteral nutrition

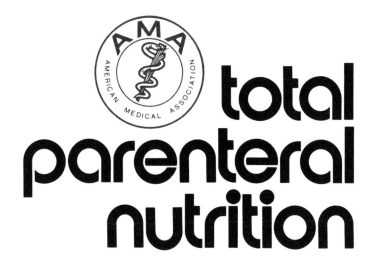

total parenteral nutrition

edited by Philip L. White, Sc.D.
and Margarita E. Nagy, M.S.

PUBLISHING SCIENCES GROUP, INC.

Acton, Massachusetts

a subsidiary of CHC Corporation

This book is based upon the proceedings of the SYMPOSIUM ON TOTAL PARENTERAL NUTRITION sponsored by the *Food Science Committee, Council on Foods and Nutrition* of the American Medical Association held in Nashville, Tennessee in 1972.

Distributed in

Canada
   McAinsh & Company, Ltd.
   1835 Yonge Street
   Toronto, Ontario M4S 1L6
   Canada

Europe
   Verlag Urban and Schwarzenberg
   8 Muenchen 2
   Pettenkoferstrasse 18
   Germany

Printed in the United States of America.

International Standard Book Number: 0-88416-005-X

Library of Congress Catalog Card Number: 73-84169

iv

Contents

FOREWORD
INTRODUCTION

PART ONE   **EVALUATION OF THE PATIENT**

   1 Criteria for Measurement of Efficacy   3
    Stanley J. Dudrick, M.D.

    Colloquium: Evaluation of the Patient   9
    Digest of Colloquium   50
    Robert W. Winters, M.D., and Douglas W. Wilmore, M.D.

PART TWO   **NUTRITIONAL COMPOSITION**

Section One   **Protein Hydrolysates and Amino Acids**
                Calories: Nitrogen: Disease and Injury Relationships

   2 Protein Hydrolysates and Amino Acids   59
    Hamish N. Munro, M.B., D.Sc.
   3 Calories: Nitrogen: Disease and Injury Relationships   81
    John M. Kinney, M.D.

    Colloquium: Protein Hydrolysates and Amino Acids
                 Calories: Nitrogen: Disease and Injury
                 Relationships   92
    Digest of Colloquium   139
    Stanley M. Levenson, M.D., and Hans Fisher, Ph.D.

Section Two   **Carbohydrates and Fats**

   4 Carbohydrates   147
    George F. Cahill, M.D.
   5 Fats   155
    H. C. Meng, M.D., Ph.D.

    Colloquium: Carbohydrates and Fats   186
    Digest of Colloquium   235
    Arvid Wretlind, Ph.D., and William Schumer, M.D.

Section Three   Vitamins and Minerals

6 Vitamins 241
Harry L. Greene, M.D.
7 Minerals 257
Maurice E. Shils, M.D., Sc.D.

Colloquium: Vitamins and Minerals 276
Digest of Colloquium 309
Theodore B. Van Itallie, M.D., and Harold H. Sandstead, M.D.

PART THREE   SAFETY AND DELIVERY OF SOLUTIONS

Section One   A. Microbiological Safety

8 Problems in Preparation and Handling of Solutions 313
William F. Schaffner, M.D.
9 The Problem of Sepsis 319
Donald A. Goldmann, M.D., and Dennis G. Maki, M.D.
10 Preparation and Guidelines to Utilization of Solutions 329
W. Arthur Burke, Pharm.D.
11 Hospital Practice of Total Parenteral Nutrition 349
Robert L. Ruberg, M.D.

B. Chemical and Physical Safety

12 Migration of Phthalate Ester Plasticizers 359
Robert J. Rubin, Ph.D., and Rudolph J. Jaeger, Ph.D.
13 Chemicals and Particulate Matter 365
Kenneth E. Avis, D.Sc.

Colloquium: Safety 377
Digest of Colloquium 403
P. William Curreri, M.D., and Robert H. Henry, M.S.

Section Two   Delivery

14 The Problem of Circulatory Access 409
John W. Broviac, M.D., and Belding H. Scribner, M.D.
15 Pumps and Filters 419
Jay W. Cooke

Colloquium: Delivery 423
Digest of Colloquium 436
James A. O'Neill, Jr., M.D., and Charles W. Van Way III, M.D.

**PART FOUR   FDA REGULATORY PRACTICES
AND PHILOSOPHY**

16 FDA Regulatory Practices and Philosophy   443
Leon J. DeMerre, Ph.D.

APPENDIX A

Vitamin Preparations for Parenteral Use   457
Nutrition Advisory Group on Total Parenteral Nutrition,
    Department of Nutrition, American Medical Association

APPENDIX B

Recommended Daily Dietary Allowances   466

APPENDIX C

Participants   471

FOREWORD

Total parenteral nutrition (TPN) is a lifesaving art. Pre- and post-surgical management of the emaciated or difficult-to-nourish patient has been greatly facilitated by the ability to feed this patient completely while bypassing the gastrointestinal tract. But the technique is relatively new and much remains to be learned about the availability and efficacy of nutrients delivered by vein, about the safety of solutions and their delivery systems, and about the care of catheters.

The Council on Foods and Nutrition of the American Medical Association has been studying all aspects of TPN with the counsel of an expert Nutrition Advisory Group on Total Parenteral Nutrition. The first formal effort of the advisory group was the organization of a symposium that afforded its participants an opportunity to review current knowledge and the research in progress to ascertain nutritional needs of patients receiving total parenteral nutrition. Their discussions exposed areas where research still is needed to individualize supportive nutritional care of patients and to assure optimal composition and safety of nutrient solutions, safe delivery systems, and efficient hospital practices. The symposium was held in January 1972 in Nashville, Tennessee. This volume constitutes an updated record of that conference.

In addition to formal papers and discussions during the conference, six workshops or colloquia were held to explore further the more current developments in the field of TPN and to prepare recommendations for research and practice. The colloquia provided opportunities for all participants to freely express their concerns and ideas. This thorough treatment of complex subjects is unique; perhaps of greater originality was the mix of participating specialists. The organizing committee obtained an optimum blend of experts in all aspects of TPN including regulatory agencies and the supportive industries from here and abroad. Participating in the discussions were nutrition scientists, surgeons and clinicians, toxicologists, hospital pharmacists, representatives of governmental regulatory agencies, engineers, and scientists in industry. It is the interaction among the users, providers, and the regulators that supplies the sparkle to this report.

At the time of the Nashville symposium, less was known about what to do than about what not to do in the application of intravenous alimentation. The challenge was to avoid exposing patients to metabolic and toxemic side effects while providing needed nourishment. While this may be a slight over-statement, it illustrates the "state of the art." The symposium pulled together many of the loose ends that must be woven to help TPN progress to a science.

Dr. Stanley Dudrick illustrated some of these challenges during his introductory statement at the symposium:

> We can probably make a great deal of progress in determining nutrient utilization simply by performing rather tedious but meticulous long-term studies to determine to what extent the nutrient moieties in an intravenous regimen can be effectively used by patients. Nutrient toxicology is also of utmost importance, involving a vast amount of information on the myriad biochemical reactions of the various substances we refer to as nutrients, although it is difficult now to separate what is a nutrient from what is really an essential biochemical substrate. We are going to have to think of total intravenous nutrient regimens, chemically-formulated oral diets, or any types of diets which are synthesized *de novo* as mixtures of biochemical substrates with which the body can react either to its benefit or to its detriment. Thus we may be administering substances in the future—in addition to the basic amino acids, simple carbohydrates, electrolytes, and vitamins—that we had not thought of as nutrients, but as metabolic intermediaries.

> We are going to require a tremendous amount of help from industry and our regulatory agencies to get products that are reasonably safely tested in simple, less expensive and effective experiments. Otherwise, I submit to you that none of us is ever going to live long enough to see an ideal intravenous diet developed. We simply cannot afford the time, cost, or energy to do all of the various experiments that will have to be done if one spins off the permutations, combinations, and probabilities of all of the various dosages of all of the required dietary components. We must be realistic if we really want to improve parenteral nutrition.

> I believe that we must press ahead with reasonable attempts at clinical investigation of total parenteral nutrition, balancing the risks against potential therapeutic benefits, as we do in our practice of medicine every day. As we are all aware, the use of potent treatment regimens is sometimes accompanied by serious complications. Occasionally it seems as though some otherwise fine physicians have a "death wish," in that they appear to want to be the first to do the most to show how much trouble they can get into by violating the established principles in applying total intravenous feeding techniques.

> It is easier to be a critic than to be an investigator. I sincerely believe that if we can encourage our colleagues and each other to try to do things as well as possible, and direct our efforts towards improving what we all recognize as the

inadequacies, we may end up with something of real therapeutic merit. If we remain satisfied with the current "routine"
or "standard" methods of providing nourishment because
they ostensibly are "safe," we can "safe" our patients to death.
I am not sure that it is any better to die "safe" as a result of
inadequate nutrition than it is to die from sepsis associated
with parenteral nutrition.

The work of the AMA advisory group on TPN continues. Late in 1973
another conference was held on intravascular catheters and related devices.
This was an interdisciplinary conference that should lead to the development
of useful standards for catheter performance.

Included as an addendum in this book is a report that illustrates yet
another phase of AMA involvement in TPN, "Vitamin Preparations for Parenteral Use," a statement of the Nutrition Advisory Group.

Nutrient requirements of healthy individuals are rather well understood and are represented as the Recommended Dietary Allowances, published in a report of the Food and Nutrition Board of the National Research
Council by the National Academy of Sciences. Requirements in states of
trauma and disease are not well established, nor are requirements for nutrients delivered solely by vein well understood. But a start has been made. The
Food and Drug Administration wishes to establish appropriate regulations
for use of nutrients in large-volume parenteral solutions. As of now, no regulations exist. Largely as a result of deliberations of the colloquium on vitamins
and minerals of the 1972 Symposium, a report has been prepared on a concept for the vitamin composition of large volume parenterals and presented
to the FDA.

A recommendation of this nature represents scientific judgment more
than scientific fact and it is for this reason that the advisory group carefully
labeled the table as a "working draft of suggested composition." The recommendations require careful evaluation and clinical confirmation before they
become locked into regulations. Thus the American Medical Association with
other interested agencies sponsored another working conference to develop
protocols for evaluation of nutrient solutions.

The purpose of this book is to open up areas in which knowledge is
lacking and stimulate research in these areas. The continued development of
TPN depends upon this. These needs are well expressed in the foreword of the
book, *General Principles of Blood Transfusion*, written about ten years ago:

> It is inevitable that new discoveries contributing to
> human welfare will not always be exploited with full under-
> standing and good judgment. There will always be examples
> of abuse, which will arouse criticism, that tends to bring some
> disrepute to the new practice. So it has been with the trans-
> fusion of blood, which, as with any procedure that affects the
> integrity of the human body, is accompanied by some hazards.
> Year by year, however, the increasing power of medical sci-
> ence is progressively refining procedures toward maximizing
> the benefits and minimizing the risks. In this situation, the
> proper purpose of criticism of current inadequacies should

be to emphasize the need for speeding up the incorporation into general medical practice of the fruits of contemporary experiments and experience.

We wish to express our sincere gratitude to Parker Vanamee, M.D. His vision and guidance from the conception of the 1972 Symposium through the completion of this book were of the utmost importance. We are grateful to Mr. James L. Breeling whose organizational skills were reflected in the Symposium and early drafts of this manuscript. Special thanks are due to the participants and contributors of the 1972 Symposium for their generous donations of time to the conference and to the preparation of this book. Our thanks too, for the hard work and vision of the members of the organizing committee for the Symposium who developed a conference of a large-scale nature, encompassing so many of the problems—from choosing the nutrient, to choosing the delivery system, to all things the concerned physician must think about.

Assistance of this committee and the guidance of Dr. Dean C. Fletcher, Secretary of the Council's Committee on Food Science, were invaluable in bringing this book into being. Miss Mary Ellis was technical editor; without her efforts the book might never have been produced.

The Symposium organizing committee included these members:

Parker Vanamee, MD, Chairman
Maurice E. Shils, MD, ScD
H. C. Meng, MD, PhD
Stanley J. Dudrick, MD
Theodore B. Van Itallie, MD
James L. Breeling, Secretary

Our warm thanks go also to our publisher, Publishing Sciences Group, Inc., and to the patience and unwavering assistance of its editorial staff.

Philip L. White, Sc.D.
Secretary
Council on Foods and Nutrition
The American Medical Association

INTRODUCTION

What is total parenteral nutrition? Total parenteral nutrition (TPN) ideally includes the intravenous administration of nutrients in amounts sufficient to achieve tissue synthesis and an anabolic state in the severely ill when oral ingestion is not possible or is not adequate alone. TPN is a lifesaving procedure through which delivery of food by vein is physiologically effective, sustaining and even improving normal nutritional status during short-term needs or over long periods of time while the patient is recovering from massive trauma (eg, burns), from drastic surgical procedures, or while underlying disease is being treated, and in medical emergencies. It is of value in maintenance of noningesting patients preparatory to surgery or others with debility or dysfunction of the gastrointestinal tract.

Table 1.—General Indications for Total Parenteral Nutrition

Malnutrition	Diverticulitis
Malabsorption	Alimentary tract fistula
Chronic diarrhea	Alimentary tract anomalies
Chronic vomiting	Reversible liver failure
Failure to thrive	Acute and chronic renal failure
Gastrointestinal obstruction	Major full thickness burns
Ulcer disease	Hypermetabolic state
Granulomatous enterocolitis	Complicated trauma
Ulcerative colitis	Malignant disease (adjunctive therapy)
Pancreatitis (acute or chronic)	Short-bowel syndrome
Severe anorexia nervosa	Protein-losing gastroenteropathy
Indolent wounds and decubitus ulcers	Nonterminal coma

"The basic problem associated with conventional intravenous feeding (ie, 5% glucose or 10% glucose solutions with electrolytes) is the inability to provide sufficient calories to permit utilization of administered amino acids unless very large volumes of water are infused," writes Dr. Maurice E. Shils, in the *Journal of the American Medical Association* (**220**:1721, 1972). "Persistent negative caloric and nitrogen balances result in gradual loss of tissue and, if protracted, in debilitation with its multiple problems. Conventional parenteral feeding is incapable of improving the condition of the already malnourished individual for the same reasons."

Studies of fat as a calorie source (fat has more than twice the energy value of carbohydrate or protein) continue, but a fat emulsion ideal for intravenous use still is not available for general use in the United States. Combinations of carbohydrate (dextrose) and protein (amino acids or hydrolysates) with minerals and vitamins form the basis of the usual IV solution. Although 5% dextrose solutions (approximately isotonic) can be given by peripheral vein, more concentrated hypertonic solutions irritate the blood vessel intima. Phlebitis may result. A few drops of a hypertonic solution introduced into a peripheral vein will produce pain and spasm of the blood vessel. For this reason, hypertonic nutritional solutions must be delivered into a large-diameter vein, such as the superior vena cava. In such a high-flow system rapid dilution occurs, lessening the danger of irritation of the intima and of phlebitis.

Use of parenteral nutrition in the practice of medicine is not new. Its history has been reviewed by various authors. Although intravenous administration of glucose was attempted in the latter half of the 19th century, Dr. Stanley J. Dudrick and associates provided "the first demonstration that growth, development, and positive nitrogen balance can be achieved by long-term total parenteral nutrition in animals and man." (*Surgery* **64:**134, 1968). Much earlier—in the 17th century—Harvey's discovery of the circulation of blood labeled it as the means through which water, oxygen, and other nutrients required by cells are circulated to them and through which end products of cell metabolism are carried away and excreted. Subsequently attempts by Sir Christopher Wren and others to introduce substances intravenously and to transfuse blood into animals were followed by transfusion of blood into a human being. In the early 19th century infusion of saline solutions was used successfully in treating patients with cholera, and the possibility of successful use of parenteral therapy was increased with the discoveries in microbiology of Louis Pasteur and application of principles of asepsis introduced by Joseph Lister.

In the early part of the 20th century, Wilder and his associates (*JAMA* **65:**2067, 1915) were able to estimate—through studies of the disappearance of intravenously administered glucose—the glucose utilization of different individuals. They also reported on the work of Kausch (1911) who introduced glucose intravenously in treating hyperemesis gravidarum, surgical conditions, and gastrointestinal disorders. Although attempts had been made to give other nutrients by injection, it was not until 1915 that intravenous utilization of fat emulsions was successful. Later, in 1935, Holt and his associates established intravenous infusion of fat as a practical therapeutic measure. Elman and Weiner in 1939 reported on the use of intravenous alimentation of amino acids, believing that they were the first to succeed in this procedure. Use of intravenous alimentation increased during World War II and continued actively thereafter as recognition and knowledge of nutrient interrelationships heightened. Dr. Dudrick and Dr. Jonathan E. Rhoads have given more complete and detailed historical information—and it is an exciting history—in *JAMA* **215:**939, 1971.

Watkins and Steinfeld, in their study of intravenous administration of fat (*Am J Clin Nutr* **16:**182, 1965), spoke of the procedure as hyperalimentation.

Although hyperalimentation could well refer to extra caloric alimentation by any means, the term has been used rather generally in reference to intravenous provision of nutrients; it is not synonymous with total parenteral nutrition.

As Dr. Shils points out (*JAMA* **220**:1721, 1972):

> It is my opinion that the term hyperalimentation may be mistakenly interpreted as meaning that *all* patients being maintained in adequate nutritional status solely by intravenous means require solutions providing calories, amino acids, and other nutrients in amounts much larger than those indicated for maintenance of normal body weight. To the contrary, patients who are overweight will actually benefit from a calorie deficit in situations where wound healing is normal and other nutrient intakes are adequate. Many other patients in an acceptable weight range will do well at maintenance caloric levels. Patients with prior significant weight loss or with serious hypermetabolic problems will require calories and certain other nutrients in excess of usual basal requirements. The aim of parenteral nutrition, like that of diet therapy by other routes, is the provision of calories and nutrients required by the specific patient. The terms "total parenteral nutrition" or "total parenteral alimentation" appear to be more accurate and inclusive than the term "hyperalimentation." The latter, if used, should refer to the administration of calories appreciably in excess of those usually required.

It is in this sense—in reference to administration of calories appreciably in excess of those usually required—that the term hyperalimentation is used throughout this book. Total parenteral nutrition refers to delivery of hypertonic solutions into a large-diameter vein.

Mary Ellis

PART ONE

1 Criteria for Measurement of Efficacy
Stanley J. Dudrick, M.D.

Colloquium: Evaluation of the Patient
Digest of the Colloquium
Robert W. Winters, M.D., and Douglas W. Wilmore, M.D.

EVALUATION
OF THE
PATIENT

1

Chapter 1

Criteria for Measurement of Efficacy

Stanley J. Dudrick, M.D.

> *Criteria for measurement of efficacy of parenteral nutrition regimens cannot be applied regularly to all patients requiring parenteral nutrition support. Individual differences, concurrent disorders of health, and many other considerations dictate which criteria can be evaluated and be helpful in determining the overall impact of TPN on the patient's clinical course. No single criterion nor set of criteria will be uniformly useful or infallible in predicting or actually measuring the efficacy of a nutrient regimen in all patients at all times during a prolonged therapeutic and convalescent course of a single patient.*

Criteria for measuring efficacy of parenteral nutrition regimens cannot be applied uniformly to all patients because of the differences which exist among those requiring parenteral nutrition support. Among these differences are age, sex, size, pathological condition, previous nutritional status, current metabolic status, ambulatory capability, and concurrent disorders of health. The criteria we use are not entirely black or white but fall into a wide gray area vaguely defined as a normal or acceptable range. Many are subjective on the part of the patient, the physician, or attending personnel, rather than being scientifically objective measurements.

These facts of life can make the accumulation of data on the efficacy of nutrient regimens a difficult, if not impossible, task.

STUDIES OF EFFICACY OF NUTRIENT SOLUTIONS

Studies Under Normal Conditions

Most TPN regimens are based on or modified from recommendations for enteral nutrient requirements. Nutrients infused by vein must be in forms compatible with each other in solution for direct delivery into the blood stream. After the theoretical and practical problems of solution formulation have been overcome, a solution formulated for patient use must be tested initially for safety and efficacy in experimental models.

Toxicity studies are carried out by administering new diets by mouth, by vein, or intraperitoneally. At least two or three species of animals are involved. In addition to close observations of the animals' behavior and general health, fairly complete hematological and biochemical studies are carried out. To ascertain lethal dosage (LD), LD_{50} and LD_{100} are determined, and histological studies of virtually every tissue are performed.

Efficacy studies follow, after it has been shown that the nutrient regimen can be administered safely by vein in animals. Infusion of the diet into an immature or adolescent animal helps to show whether the diet is capable of supporting normal growth and development. It is important to determine:

whether the animal can gain weight at the normal rate,
whether the body composition remains normal,
whether the animal synthesizes new tissue in a normal fashion, and
whether any abnormalities can be detected in the various organ and system functions during periods of crucial growth and development.

In long-term studies such criteria as the normal development and eruption of teeth, appearance and fusion of the epiphyses and diaphyses of the long bones, weight of the brain and other organs, cerebral cell counts and DNA determinations, and many other criteria can be studied. The advantage of working with immature animals is that their body stores of nutrients are limited, and their metabolic demands for exogenous nutrient substrates are relatively greater than in adulthood. Any deficiencies in the diet will be aggravated or magnified in this model, although the comparatively small size of the subject may create some technical difficulties for the investigator.

Among the easiest criteria to estimate in adult animals maintained on long-term total parenteral nutrition are maintenance of normal weight, vigor, and health. Simple but tedious *balance studies* of the nutrient components infused are compared with the levels of the same constituents or their metabolites in the urine, stool, or other excrement and provide answers on how the animal is metabolizing the diet.

Another valuable system of investigation involves total intravenous support of dogs or other animals throughout *pregnancy and lactation*. The nutrient requirements of a pregnant or lactating animal place demands on intravenous feeding regimens and may unmask deficiencies or imbalances in the diet, either in the mother, the offspring, or both.

Nitrogen balance studies can be used as a gross yardstick of protein-calorie metabolism. Determination of levels of all of the components in the diet—including individual amino acids—should be determined in the serum in order to insure that significant imbalances are not induced by the diet.

Biochemical studies must include frequent liver function tests, kidney function tests, and the usual biological ion concentrations. Serum profiles of fat-soluble and water-soluble vitamins, serum lipids (including phospholipids), fatty acids, cholesterol and lipoproteins, and tests of hematopoietic function must be obtained at regular intervals throughout the study. Determination of the creatine-creatinine ratio, blood urea nitrogen, and blood ammonia are useful expedient parameters for monitoring nitrogen metabolism. Acid-base balance must be assessed frequently initially, and at regular intervals thereafter.

More sophisticated *studies of body composition* are obtained by use of biological isotopes to study total body water, various water spaces, the fate and distribution of tagged nitrogen, and the fate of tagged nonprotein caloric sources. From biopsy or autopsy specimens, tissues should be examined histologically and histochemically to rule out microscopic or ultramicroscopic abnormalities. In smaller animals (eg, rats) autoradiographs and carcass composition studies yield valuable information.

It is virtually impossible to obtain this information on only one animal because of the mutually exclusive nature of many of the tests, the unavailability of sufficient serum and other body fluids and tissues to study, and the enormous amounts of time, energy, and expense involved in such investigations. Using many animals and distributing work among several laboratories is a solution to this problem.

Studies under conditions of stress determine to what extent diets can be efficacious in maintaining nutritional integrity of animals under stressful conditions usually associated with a catabolic response.

To conduct these studies we simulate critical clinical situations under controlled conditions which are either unethical or impractical or impossible in human beings and are possible only with the use of animals. Investigations are under way in our laboratory and in others on strength of healing surgical wounds, strength of colon anastomoses, regeneration of serum protein, deposition of collagen and hydroxyproline at operative sites, and restoration of normal liver morphology in previously fatty livers. Additional data are being gathered to document the efficacy of IV solutions in reducing the magnitude of the catabolic response or reversing it in animals subjected to major burns, significant soft tissue injury, or multiple major fractures.

In one study, we are serially reducing the dose of each amino acid in a so-called complete amino acid regimen to the level at which nitrogen balance is significantly impaired. Our aim is to determine the minimum quantities of essential, and eventually of nonessential, amino acids that are required for adequate nutrition.

CLINICAL CRITERIA FOR EFFICACY

Most or all of these techniques can be used comparably or in a modified form to gather data clinically in man. Indeed, only those nutritional data gathered in man will be truly significant for man. Animal data can be a useful wind sock in helping us to determine direction but cannot replace the necessity for good clinical nutritional research. From a practical standpoint, clinical criteria for efficacy of intravenous nutrient regimens fall into two broad categories:

> gathering data which will help a clinician to determine whether the nutrient regimen he has chosen for his patient is accomplishing the goals he seeks;
> gathering basic clinical nutritional data from selected patients who lend themselves to the study of specific aspects of the overall determination of nutrient efficacy and safety.

The *clinician* is primarily interested in knowing whether the nutrient regimen will help to reduce morbidity, reduce mortality, speed recovery, accelerate and increase the extent of rehabilitation, and improve the quality

6

of life. The *neonatologist* is interested in increasing the salvage rate and physiologic quality of low-birth-weight premature infants and in the degree and rate to which he can restore the infant to normal growth and development. The *pediatrician* and *pediatric surgeon* are interested in maintaining normal growth, weight gain, and development during periods when an infant or child is subjected to malabsorption states, diarrheal syndromes, sepsis, trauma, major operative procedures, and congenital catastrophes.

In these patients, care is exerted to maintain TPN regimens that do not adversely affect serum osmolarity and acid-base balance, do not impair or overwhelm liver function (especially ammonia metabolism), do not impair or overwhelm renal function, do not interfere with central nervous system development or function, and are neither excessive nor deficient in any dietary requirement for normal growth and development.

In the management of adult patients, particularly, the *clinician* wants to know whether the diet is successful in helping the patient subjectively by improving his energy, mental acuity, sense of well-being, and morale. He may note:

- a qualitative increase in muscular strength or may actually quantitate it by studies with an ergometer or treadmill;
- improvement in strength and effectiveness of ventilation, with concomitant reduction in the problems of pulmonary toilet and respiration;
- a patient who is more eager, willing, and able to ambulate and to care for himself and his personal hygiene and so, in effect, further improves his nutritional status;
- a patient who becomes more interested in engaging in social activities about him and in physical and occupational therapy;
- increase in skin thickness and thickness of subcutaneous fat;
- previously infected indolent wounds or decubitus ulcers that show signs of healing for the first time or begin to heal at an accelerated rate;
- enterocutaneous fistulas healing completely without operation;
- inflammatory diseases of the bowel, such as regional enteritis, granulomatous colitis, or ulcerative colitis, that undergo remission or resolve during a few weeks of therapy, after months or years of unsuccessful medical treatment; and
- patients with multiple, severe trauma, or major burns complicated by multiple abscesses or sepsis, who might not have survived previously, supported through the serial crises that usually accompany their clinical courses without the added risk of severe malnutrition.

These are general, indefinite, impressionistic, and rather unscientific observations, too nonspecific and indefinite to be of true objective value. They are certainly not discriminating enough to provide the reproducible control data necessary to compare the efficacy of different nutrient regimens. But such data do have potential value. Over the period of a decade or more of studying several thousand patients, it may be possible to show that morbidity and mortality figures are improved, that length of hospital stay is shortened, duration of convalescence and rehabilitation is shortened, and the cost of hospitalization is ultimately reduced.

NUTRITION EXPERIMENTS IN MAN

One difficulty in clinical investigation of the efficacy of nutrient regimens is standardization of the patient and conditions under which the study is to be done. There appear to be an infinite number of variables in control in each patient studied. These variables change during the course of therapy of the patient as his condition improves or deteriorates. It is almost impossible to have another patient of approximately the same age, the same sex, at approximately the same time, with the same biological process, similar nutritional status, and common clinical condition to serve as a control. And it might be unethical to use that patient as a control.

Despite the difficulty in performing ideal nutrition experiments in man, data have been, and are being, collected to determine efficacy of parenteral nutrition regimens. Weight gain and nitrogen balance remain two of the best—though not the ideal—criteria we have in adult man. Measurements of all of the biochemical and hematological parameters mentioned previously in the animal experiments can be performed in man, although such studies are impractical for any length of time—if not impossible—in one human being because of the quantity of blood which would be required for the many determinations.

Thus, most studies are fractionated among a series of patients, and the pieces of the puzzle are eventually fitted together to give the whole picture. Studies of the efficacy of intravenous nutrient regimens will have to include the regular measurement of intake-output balances, serum levels, and tissue levels of the components of parenteral diets. These studies will have to be done under defined conditions, and consideration must be given to the metabolic interrelationships of the individual constituents of the diets.

Utilization of amino acids or other sources of nitrogen cannot be determined validly without reference to the nonprotein calories in the diet. Requirements for calcium may vary with the level of phosphorus or magnesium in the mixture. Requirements for thiamine and other B vitamins and magnesium may be influenced by the quantity of glucose or carbohydrate in the formula.

Acid-base balance, liver function tests, and kidney function tests are basic parameters of measurement which must not be adversely affected by parenteral solutions. Normal hematopoietic function, serum electrolyte levels, and vitamin levels must be maintained. The serum lipid profile—including cholesterol, fatty acids, phospholipids, lipoproteins—should remain within normal limits. Normal levels of blood urea nitrogen and blood ammonia should also be maintained throughout the parenteral therapy.

Sophisticated studies of body composition and energy expenditure provide valuable guideline information. More complete studies of serum amino acid profiles will provide us with information to formulate "ideal diets" for the vast majority of patients. Investigations of intracellular metabolism of various nutrient regimens have been undertaken by studying the electrolyte flux in the erythrocytes of patients with burns and through studies of intermediary metabolism of red cells, white cells, liver, and muscle as affected by various intravenous nutrient regimens.

It is inevitable that, as our technology, expertise, and experience increase, so, too, will our ability to determine the efficacy of the potent biochemical substrates that we call nutrients in the management of the complex "test tubes" of biochemical reactions that we refer to as patients.

Evaluation of the Patient

Colloquium

Robert W. Winters, M.D., chairman
Douglas W. Wilmore, M.D., rapporteur

Dr. Winters: To determine what kind of information we can accumulate to stimulate or accelerate progress toward our goal of making parenteral nutrition safe and efficacious for our patients, our exploration into all avenues of research followed this sequence:

I. Indications for the use of total intravenous nutrition
  A. Infants and children
    1. The low-birth-weight infant
    2. The surgical neonate
    3. The infant with chronic diarrhea
    4. Summary
  B. Adults
    1. The surgical patient with gastrointestinal disease
    2. The chronically cachetic patient
    3. The hypermetabolic patient
    4. Promotion of anabolism in the surgical patient
    5. The patient with cancer
    6. The patient with kidney disease
II. Metabolic studies and complications
  A. Introduction
  B. Hyperglycemia and azotemia
  C. Plasma electrolytes
  D. Quality of growth
  E. Acid-base disorders
  F. Calcium and phosphorus metabolism
  G. Changes in hepatic function and structure
III. Suggested guidelines for the use of total intravenous nutrition
  A. Introduction
  B. The team approach
  C. Guidelines for variables to be monitored

Dr. Winters: In October 1971, I was chairman of a meeting on intravenous nutrition in the high-risk infant, held under the auspices of the National Institute of Child Health and Human Development.[1]

In the course of that interdisciplinary conference, the participants identified specific groups of patients in the pediatric age range for whom this technique was indicated and developed guidelines for use of the technique (see p 43).

INDICATIONS FOR USE OF TPN

Infants and Children

In general, there are three groups of pediatric patients in whom intra-venous alimentation is used. In one of these three, the indications are quite uncertain; in the other two, they are reasonably well established.

The first group consists of low-birth-weight babies (under 1,200 gm birth weight). It usually takes these infants several weeks to regain their birth weight with conventional management, hence the IV technique appeals to neonatologists. An appropriate-for-dates infant with a birth weight of 1,200 to 1,500 gm usually has a gestational age of about 24 to 26 weeks. His brain growth *in utero* during that period of time is literally in an exponential phase. Animal data and some inferential human data suggest that the brain, once it is de-prived during a critical period of growth, suffers a nonrecoupable deficit in cell number.[2] The challenge to the neonatologist is to feed these infants promptly in the hope that neither brain growth nor somatic growth will be delayed.

The technique is being evaluated in these patients in a number of institutions, although poorly for the most part. All participants at the NIH conference[1] regarded this group as *strictly* experimental. The technique is emphatically *not* part of accepted routine neonatal care and probably will not be for a long time, if ever. It should not be used in these babies unless the physician has all of the necessary backup support and is trying to answer a research question or questions in a controlled fashion.

Our group has accumulated data on nine very low-birth-weight infants fed parenterally beginning shortly after birth.[3] These preliminary results look promising. The babies gain weight, and the weight gained is tissue, not simply edema. The survival rate probably is increased versus controls. To prove it we need larger numbers. The infants seem to regain birth weight faster. Clearly, what is needed here is not only a larger group of patients with appropriate controls to assess the short-term effects but, more importantly, a critical psychological and neurological long-term follow-up as well.

In contrast to this first group, the other two groups of patients for whom there is a legitimate and demonstrated indication for the use of this technique are *surgical neonates* and *infants with chronic malabsorption and diarrhea.* The surgical neonates are infants born with catastrophic gastrointestinal anomalies of one sort or another, the most common of which is omphalocele or gastroschisis. Prior to the technique of parenteral alimentation, mortality of these infants following the extensive but necessary surgery was probably 60% to 80%. Now most of these patients live because they can be tided over nutritionally by the use of parenteral alimentation. Another group of surgical neonates are those with long atretic segments of the gastrointestinal tract. Mortality in these patients prior to parenteral alimentation was equally high.

The surgical neonate (ie, an infant who is deprived of a significant fraction of his intestinal tract, which in some cases may be 70% to 80%) should receive parenteral nutrition postoperatively. It unquestionably helps in healing defects in the abdominal wall in the cases of omphalocele and gastroschisis and is useful in tiding over the infants with atresia of the small intestine who often develop postoperative gastrointestinal obstruction for significant periods of time.

While there is no serious question about this group of patients, there is one problem—fortunately rare—and this is the patient who has essentially no small intestine remaining. Most pediatric institutions involved in parenteral alimentation of surgical neonates have experienced one or two such babies, who simply have an insufficient amount of small intestine remaining ever to survive. One example is reported by Dudrick and Wilmore,[4] an infant who did not have enough intestine to be compatible with life.

I am not aware of firm guidelines on the minimal amount of small bowel compatible with survival. My surgical colleagues tell me that this minimal amount is about 10% of the small intestine past the ligament of Treitz. The length of the small intestine in a newborn infant varies widely according to how it is measured, but it is roughly 250 to 300 cm. This places 25 cm as the minimal amount. Yet, I know of a few instances of successful management of patients with less than that. Clearly some systematically collected data are needed. Data collected by the American Pediatric Surgical Association would assure a firmer basis for decisions about these patients.

Fortunately such surgical neonates are rare, but they are important. First, it costs about two and one-half times the basic bed rate to hyperaliment an infant under the conditions which we employ. If the bed rate is $100, the total cost is $350 per day. This figure, multiplied by a year of hospitalization, amounts to a substantial sum of money. Prolongation of a hopeless situation is wrong, but I do not know how to define hopeless. Finally, such patients occupy beds and divert services from other patients for whom the outlook is far better.

Dr. Wilmore: Data in the literature help to clarify the question of the minimum amount of small intestine compatible with life. Survival following small bowel resection in 50 infants was related to the length of the remaining bowel, presence of the ileocecal valve, normal birth weight, successful operative therapy, and lack of associated anomalies. All but one infant survived resection which left 38 to 75 cm; 7 of 14 lived with 15 to 38 cm of small bowel and an intact ileocecal valve, and none survived with less than 15 cm jejunum or ileum. Death occurred in all infants with ileocecal resection and small intestinal segments measuring less than 40 cm (Fig 1). Body weights were within the normal range after the first year of life (Fig 2).

This group of patients has not had good neurological follow-up examinations. Several were reported to be mentally retarded. The relationship between undernutrition, brain growth, and intellectual development in these infants is unknown. Reports reemphasize the need to maintain adequate nutrition throughout the entire postenterectomy period if successful salvage and development of a full genetic potential are to be achieved.

Dr. McGill: Do you think the small intestine elongates and is proportional to body growth? Two hundred fifty cm is a bit short for the normal adult small bowel.

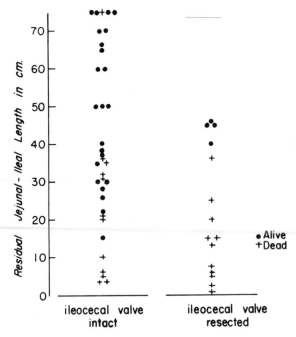

Fig 1. Survival in infants following massive intestinal resection as related to the length of the residual segment and presence of the ileocecal valve (from Wilmore DW, *J. Pediatr* **80**:88, 1972).

Dr. Wilmore: Yes, it does grow and get longer.

Dr. Winters: The surface area also increases. The increase in length, judged crudely by x-ray, is not all that impressive, but the surface area is enormous. X-rays of the first patient reported on by Dudrick and Wilmore showed a stomach and then another very dilated segment which was about as big as the stomach.[4] This was the residual small intestine. I believe that at autopsy there was an enormous hypertrophy of the villi, therefore a substantial increase in the surface area.

Dr. McGill: But the normal adult small bowel is 350 to 400 cm or a bit more. It is difficult to measure because of telescopic effects, but it is quite a bit longer than 250 cm. How are you measuring it?

Dr. Wilmore: Most measurements are done along the antimesenteric border from the ligament of Treitz to the ileocecal valve.

Dr. Winters: Let me interject a highly experimental development which involves the surgical neonate. This concerns an infant with a birth weight of 1,700 gm and a tracheoesophageal fistula. Rather than doing a two-stage repair, we alimented the child parenterally until she achieved a weight of about 2,300 gm. The defect could then be repaired in a single procedure, thus avoiding one major surgical procedure. I cannot recommend this as routine as yet. It is still experimental and should be examined more carefully.

In summary, surgical patients are a gratifying group to deal with. The end results, at least from the physical outcome, are usually rewarding.

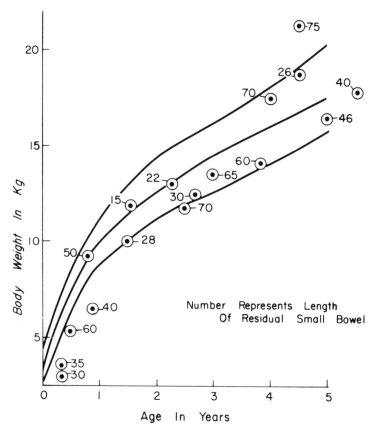

Fig 2. Body weight following massive intestinal resection demonstrates an initial lag in the first year of life, followed by accelerated weight gain and normal distribution. The three lines represent the 10th, 50th, and 90th percentile of body weight (as adapted from the anthropometric charts, The Children's Medical Center, Boston, MA).

The third group of pediatric patients in whom the technique of parenteral alimentation is of proved value consists of infants with chronic undiagnosed malabsorptive defects presenting as chronic diarrhea. Of course, diarrhea is a common disease in infants. Usually a previously healthy infant gets what we call infectious diarrhea, characterized by an episode of acute dehydration and accompanied by metabolic acidosis. If the diarrhea is severe enough, peripheral vascular collapse may occur. Most of those patients—80% to 90%—can be treated adequately by conventional fluid therapy with nothing orally (NPO) for a few days, then cautiously tried on oral feedings with a nonlactose-containing formula gradually increasing to full strength. They usually make an uneventful recovery and are switched back to cow's milk. But roughly 10% of these infants will relapse when oral feedings are reintroduced. Out of this group we can identify some who have disaccharide intolerance or other identifiable etiology. There remains a small subgroup with chronic diarrhea, usually starting the first few months of life. Despite any formula fed, they cannot be controlled. Every diagnostic test fails to uncover a specific etiology. This small group of patients eventually dies in what I call a thermodynamic death. The terminal episode is characterized by failure to maintain body temperature, a slow pulse, and a slow respiratory rate. They simply seem to "run out of steam." At autopsy there is absolutely no depot fat anywhere. Their total body stores of energy have been completely exhausted.

This group of patients with chronic undiagnosed malabsorptive disorders deserves total parenteral alimentation. At the St. Louis Children's Hospital, Keating treated 16 such infants with intravenous hyperalimentation.[1] One died of septicemia and was found on autopsy to have thymic alymphoplasia and profound immunological defect. In the 15 surviving infants there were no major significant complications except for two episodes of the superior vena cava syndrome and one instance of accidental displacement of the catheter. The patients were alimented from two to six weeks. Then the cycle of malnutrition leading to further malabsorption and to further malnutrition apparently was broken. All 15 of the surviving infants eventually received oral alimentation. They usually started with a nonlactose-containing, medium-chain triglyceride formula which was slowly increased as intravenous intake was reduced. After catheter removal, the children did well.

In this group of patients total parenteral nutrition is indicated following:

a history of chronic diarrhea for (arbitrarily) at least 21 days,
evidence of a significant degree of malnutrition,
trial of a nonlactose-containing, semisynthetic formula with
    a medium-chain triglyceride, and
a complete gastrointestinal workup to rule out all known
    etiologies of chronic diarrhea.

While it is possible to err in the direction of being overly zealous, it is also possible to err in the direction of letting malnutrition go on too long. It takes mature clinical judgment to decide when one should institute the technique. Our present inclination is to start earlier than we formerly did, since we do not want the patient to approach thermodynamic death.

In summary, the technique of parenteral alimentation in the pediatric age group has an accepted place in surgical neonates with major gastrointestinal anomalies and in infants with chronic undiagnosed malabsorption with malnutrition. It is strictly experimental in the low-birth-weight infant.

Adults

Dr. Wilmore: *The first group of adult patients* requiring parenteral nutrition includes those with a weight loss of about 10% who require a gastrointestinal operation. The 10% weight loss figure is somewhat arbitrary but is supported by a large body of data on starvation which demonstrates that only minimal physiologic dysfunction occurs with a 10% loss of body weight. These starvation studies are of normal individuals during controlled starvation and not of the acutely ill or injured patient; consequently, extrapolation of these data should be done with care. Erosion of the lean body mass follows weight loss of more than 8% to 12%, resulting in altered physiologic function. Aggressive attempts to limit loss of the body mass beyond this point should be made. Patients in this group will require an operation, and a decision should be made about the timing of the operative procedure. In some cases, restoration of blood volume, electrolyte concentration, and colloid osmotic pressure can be achieved over several days followed by the operative procedure.

In other patients, however, two to three weeks of parenteral nutrition may be necessary before surgical reconstruction and resolution of the gastrointestinal disorder should be attempted. The decision to operate immediately versus the decision to operate only after two to three weeks of parenteral nutrition requires surgical judgment, which is modified in part by the safety with which long-term parenteral feeding can be delivered. As techniques of parenteral nutrition improve, safe delivery of preoperative nutrition can be achieved by the busiest general surgeon. This will be of tremendous value to patients with chronic recurrent gastrointestinal disease, such as a patient with recurrent small bowel obstruction or the individual with marked weight loss secondary to pyloric stenosis.

The second group of adult patients requiring parenteral nutrition includes those who are chronically cachetic and malnourished, whether they be admitted to a medical or surgical service. Usually, these individuals have a gastrointestinal disease which precludes adequate enteral nutrition (eg, an enterocutaneous fistula, regional enteritis, ulcerative colitis, or one of the many malabsorption syndromes). These individuals should be started on a parenteral diet if they demonstrate a loss of more than 10%. Often these patients are admitted to a medical service to undergo diagnostic evaluation. Parenteral nutrition can be carried out during the most vigorous diagnostic evaluation.

Dr. Krumdieck: Is this 10% below ideal weight?

Dr. Wilmore: Yes.

Dr. Krumdieck: Then I would require parenteral feedings as I exist today.

Dr. Wilmore: If you are sick with a chronic disease, you represent more of a nutritional risk than the gentleman who is a few pounds overweight and has body stores that can be utilized during stress or starvation. You would represent more of a nutritional risk in thermal injury because you simply don't have the energy reserves to withstand the hypermetabolic response to burn trauma. Another point which your question emphasizes is that we are talking about ideal body weight. The obese patient may represent a starving lean tissue mass in a sea of plenty, and interpretations need to be made concerning the body composition in these individuals.

Dr. McGill: Do you have data relating operative mortality and morbidity to body weight?

Dr. Wilmore: If you examine a population of patients with burns—an injury which represents the maximum stress sustained by man—the extent of the injury correlates well with body weight loss (Fig 3). These weight-loss curves can be greatly altered by an active feeding program using combined enteral-parenteral feedings; loss of body weight with a burn greater than 40% of total body surface can be greatly reduced or even abolished.[5]

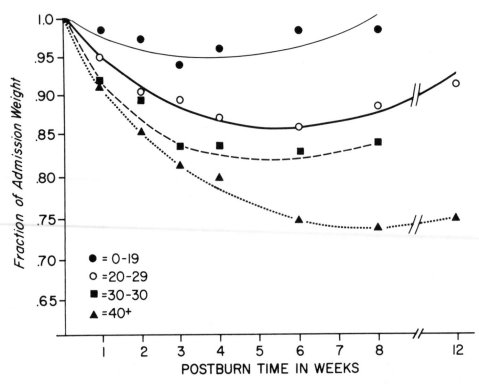

Fig 3. Weight change following burn injury (from Wilmore DW, in Cowan G Jr, Scheetz W (eds): *Intravenous Hyperalimentation*, Philadelphia, Lea and Febiger, 1972, p 105).

Finally, there is evidence suggesting that people who are 10% to 15% over their ideal weight can withstand major thermal trauma better than a comparable group who are underweight and have sustained the same intensity of injury. The overweight group of people appear to have a lower morbidity and mortality than do patients with a lesser quantity of nutritional stores on board. This certainly does not mean that the obese patient will withstand major trauma better because he has a large store of basic nutrients. This is not the case. However, the individual who is 10% overweight (not obese) can withstand the ravage of long-term starvation and long-term hypercatabolism and the long-term hypercatabolic response to injury better than his normal-weight or underweight counterpart.

Dr. McGill: How about the patient who needs an ileostomy, let us say, who has had his electrolyte problems corrected over a two- to three-day period? Will he stand to benefit by two weeks of parenteral nutrition if he is 10% less than ideal weight? Is it worth the effort? The risk of the operation is less than 10%. What difference does it make in the end result?

Dr. Wilmore: One has to rely on surgical judgment and individualize each case. Certainly, for the uncomplicated procedure which results in prompt restoration of gastrointestinal function, parenteral nutrition is not necessary. If the patient has had a previous operation and complications, I would provide nutrients by the parenteral route, restore body stores, then plan the next operative procedure. This requires surgical judgment. The key to care of the patient requiring a gastrointestinal operation is restoration of blood volume and colloid osmotic pressure, correction of electrolyte imbalance, prevention or drainage of intra-abdominal infection and, finally, restoration of adequate nutrition. In those patients with chronic recurrent gastrointestinal disease, we now are not forced to perform surgery—which usually has been performed earlier under better circumstances—but can "buy time" by providing long-term parenteral nutrition and can prepare the patient for corrective surgical procedure.

The third group of patients requiring parenteral nutrition includes the hypermetabolic patient who has sustained thermal injury, undergone multiple trauma, or in whom septicemia appears. These patients may have a daily caloric expenditure which exceeds 5,000 kcal/day. When enteral feedings are possible, they should be utilized. However, gastrointestinal dysfunction is not uncommon in these patients. Ileus often occurs with repeated episodes of sepsis. Facial and pharyngeal burns and injuries to the upper extremities preclude adequate enteral intake. Tube feedings are possible but often result in diarrhea, so while the gastrointestinal tract frequently is available for feeding, it is often impossible to provide the quantity of calories necessary to prevent weight loss in the hypermetabolic patient.

The quantity of food taken by the patient following major injury can be estimated by determining his preinjury dietary intake. As a rule, the daily intake of the injured individual will be about 10% to 15% less than his preinjury caloric intake. The lumberman who was accustomed to eating 5,000 kcal/day before injury can maintain a large caloric intake of 4,000 kilocalories or more. On the other hand, the individual who has sustained his body weight by eating hot dogs and potato chips isn't going to change his dietary habits after injury. This presents a problem, because the caloric needs of this patient following injury are one and one-half to two times basal. The caloric deficit is provided in part by parenteral nutrition and in part by oral supplements. At the US Army Institute of Surgical Research we use an oral dietary supplement (Provomalt*), which tastes like malted milk. Provomalt is provided between meals and at bedtime and will often supplement the oral diet with 2,000 to 3,000 additional kilocalories.

Dr. Winters: Suppose they won't take it? Would you next move to an elemental diet by tube?

Dr. Wilmore: We would rely on tube feedings. We generally do not use the elemental diet but prefer one of the commercially prepared tube feeding preparations. In some cases we perform a feeding gastrostomy. We rely on the gastrointestinal tract as our main route for caloric intake, realizing that it is often difficult to achieve more than a 2,500- to 3,000-kilocalorie input per day by this route.

The hypermetabolic patient who starts to lose weight may require parenteral support. He may require supplemental nutrients parenterally, or, if

*Use of trade names is for identification only and does not imply endorsement by the American Medical Association.

the gastrointestinal tract will not tolerate enteral feedings, he will require total parenteral nutrition. We are now utilizing an intravenous fat emulsion as a caloric source and can provide between 3,000 to 4,000 kcal/day by peripheral vein.

Dr. Winters: Do you ever use 5% amino acids and 5% glucose by peripheral vein as a supplement to what the patient takes orally? We have had a small experience with this approach.[6]

Dr. Wilmore: One of the problems with the parenteral diet is that the dextrose seems to depress the patient's appetite, probably by causing hyperglycemia or, secondary to the infusion of amino acids, may cause nausea and vomiting. Our initial impression is that this degree of appetite suppression does not occur with the intravenous fat emulsion, and we are using that to provide approximately 2,000 kcal/day using fat and nitrogen infusions nightly.

Dr. Winters: Your patients can talk and mine can't. This matter of suppression of appetite is an interesting question. As I understand it, a lot of your patients claim they are hungry, but when you actually offer them something, they really don't take very much. Is that true?

Dr. Wilmore: That is correct.

Dr. McGill: Are you speaking about patients with burns or other types of patients?

Dr. Winters: Any kind of an adult patient who is receiving hyperosmolar alimentation tends to show this phenomenon, I believe. Dr. Ruberg has further data on this point.

Dr. Ruberg: We have been studying this question extensively in our series at the University of Pennsylvania. Although it is a difficult study to control, it has led to the observation that those patients who are fairly near their normal weight or patients who are below their normal weight will claim to have a good deal of hunger while being fed intravenously. We used to think they were not hungry if they *said* they were not hungry, but apparently they were rather sick patients who—even if they were not being fed intravenously—would not be thinking about eating. Once over their acute problems and recuperating on intravenous nutrition, they will say they are very hungry. But when they eat, their caloric intake is remarkably small. We have seen this now in a large series of cases. Clearly, caloric intake is not the factor that tells them they are not hungry; it is something else.

We are evaluating dietary intake in normal individuals receiving glucose, amino acid solutions, and intravenous fat preparations. We have no "hard" data on this group as yet, but we have the impression that intravenous fat administered at night depresses the appetite of the patients less than does infusion of glucose and/or amino acids. In our patients, it would be a great advantage to be able to administer a couple of thousand kilocalories of fat and nitrogen by peripheral intravenous route at night and then stop the intravenous route in the morning, let them eat, get up, walk around, go to physical therapy.

Dr. McGill: Practically speaking, do you provide intravenous alimentation to all of your patients who have more than 10% body surface burns, third degree, or do you wait until they start to lose weight?

Dr. Wilmore: We will follow the patient as he loses weight from 8% to 10% of his ideal body weight, then evaluate his clinical course to see how long he will remain in the catabolic phase of injury. Because the restoration of body weight is usually associated with coverage of the burn wound, we determine the duration of the hypercatabolic phase of injury by how close the patient is to skin grafting. If we are just a week or so away from satisfactory wound coverage, we will support the patient until the grafting is accomplished. But if we are 10 to 14 days away from adequate wound coverage—and predictably the patient will continue to lose weight during this time—then more vigorous nutritional support is required. This may take the form of additional oral feedings or tube feedings. This supplementation may require nighttime intravenous feedings. We have now studied a series of patients, however, who have received combined enteral-parenteral feedings. Some extremely depleted patients take up to 9,000 kcal/day.

In these hypermetabolic patients we must break the cycle of ongoing weight loss secondary to hypermetabolism which results in poor granulation tissue and does not allow adequate wound coverage to be achieved. This cycle can be broken by supranormal nutritional support.

Dr. Winters: With a 9,000 kilocalorie intake, aren't you putting fat on them? They are not expending 9,000 kilocalories are they?

Dr. Wilmore: No. These fellows expend about 5,000 to 6,000 kcal/day.

Dr. Winters: Is that intake good for them?

Dr. Wilmore: For the uncomplicated patient with a burn of less than 35% to 40% of the total body surface, parenteral nutritional support is usually not required. For the big burns or for the burns with multiple complications and associated injuries, parenteral nutrition is often lifesaving.

Dr. Winters: I have the impression—perhaps mistakenly—that clinically the grafts take better, the infections are a little less troublesome, and the overall morbidity—maybe even the mortality—is better with the patients who are "buttered up." Is that true?

Dr. Wilmore: Interestingly, in a comparable group of patients with burns greater than 40% of total body surface, those who did not lose any weight because of the supranormal caloric support were compared with those who lost a predicted amount of weight. No significant difference in mortality or morbidity was found. There were some notable differences in these two groups of patients, however. Differences in red cell cation concentrations were found, with the group of patients receiving supranormal caloric support having near normal intracellular sodium and potassium levels compared with the other patients.[7] Probably if we took the same group of patients and started them a month after their initial burn injury, we could demonstrate significant differences in mortality and morbidity. This emphasizes the difficulty we have in measuring the clinical efficacy of this type of treatment.

Another group of patients to benefit from total parenteral nutrition consists of those individuals in whom anabolism will aid restoration of a disease process. An example is the individual who has undergone massive bowel resection and needs basic nutrients to allow villus hypertrophy and intestinal compensation of his remnant small bowel. We have demonstrated in the animal laboratory that providing nutrients allows greater growth of the small section and greater villus height, in these animals at least. We have collected evidence in a group of patients indicating that this may, in fact, be true. Otherwise, these patients have diarrhea, malabsorption, then get into a malnourished state. It becomes an endless cycle where they have malnutrition and malabsorption and more malnutrition.[8]

Another example would be one who has lost his entire anterior abdominal wall and needs nutrition to granulate and heal this wound.

Finally, I want to mention the practice of giving a larger dose of chemotherapy to *patients with cancer* who are in the anabolic state. None of the studies I have seen is controlled, and I am worried about the documentation of this impression. Patients with cancer receiving chemotherapy are being hyperalimented in certain centers. These individuals are prime candidates for complications, particularly septic complications. But the physician may see no alternative. Has anyone had experience in this area?

Dr. Kark: The protein binding of drugs is important in terms of their transport and activity. In a person whose tissue mass is decreased, transport of drugs will likely be interfered with, and the patient is readily poisoned. That patients who have protein deficiencies do not handle drugs well is affirmed through increasing evidence.

Dr. Wilmore: Claims are that patients do better and respond to chemotherapy better if their tissue mass is restored.

Dr. Kark: I suspect they do. Whether or not they need intravenous hyperalimentation is something else.

Dr. Bernard: I don't have controlled studies on this, but by accident I found myself in a situation in which I was asked to give chemotherapy to a patient who had massive metastases from an ovarian carcinoma and a partial bowel obstruction. I elected total parenteral nutrition for this high-risk patient for a period of 10 days before chemotherapy. She tolerated the drug beautifully.

Dr. Wilmore: Shils reported on evidence from New York's Memorial Hospital that feeding the cancer patient may accelerate tumor growth.

Dr. Ruberg: I would be fearful of simply feeding a patient with a tumor. Evidence from animal studies reveals that forced feeding of animals with tumors increases the tumor weight, but not the animal carcass weight. We don't have definitive evidence, but we have been looking at the responses of tumor-bearing animals to dosage of chemotherapeutic agents. We have been doing this in a clinical setting also. The clinical impression is that the patients tolerate the therapy better. Also, the dosage of the agent which can be given is greater than would have been possible without the intravenous hyperalimentation.

But the real question is: Are we cancelling effects and at the same time feeding the tumor? Our initial impressions are that this is not the case, but we would like to document it in the laboratory.

Dr. Bernard: It was demonstrated in the late forties and fifties with Sprague-Dawley rats (that can't vomit) that, if one fed them by a stomach tube, the tumors grew well.

When you have a situation in which the patient is not able to tolerate food intake at all, something must be done to replete these individuals.

Dr. Wilmore: I agree with you. The judgment of the physician to support or not to support terminal patients is a highly individualized decision. Before we conclude that patients can be treated better with chemotherapy plus parenteral nutrition, controlled studies should be done.

Dr. Kark: I want to correct an impression. In my earlier comments, I did not mean to talk primarily about chemotherapeutic agents. I was speaking about the general effects of drugs in people who are malnourished. For example, patients who are really malnourished don't respond well to diuretics. When you replete them, some of them do not respond.

Dr. Winters: Dr. Wilmore, where do the patients with medical gastrointestinal disease fit, patients with regional ileitis or ulcerative colitis, for example?

Dr. Wilmore: They fit pretty much with the second group of individuals, patients with a weight loss of approximately 10% who have gastrointestinal dysfunction which precludes adequate feeding. The patient with regional ileitis falls into this category. If the disorder appears to be self-limiting, and adequate restoration of enteral feedings will be possible in a week or so, then there is no need for vigorous parenteral support. If, however, a patient has a weight loss of 10% below ideal weight, and it looks as if we are going to go for two weeks or more without oral feeding, this patient should receive parenteral nutritional support.

Mr. Grant: Dr. Kark, is there a place for intravenous hyperalimentation in *patients with kidney disease?* Is a special alimentation mixture required?

Dr. Kark: At the present time, Dr. Oyama and I are working on hyperalimenting patients who need acute dialysis, giving both intravenous hyperalimentation and dialysis repetitively. We do not have enough data as yet. Even with the best of schemes we have had a 50% mortality. Our patients come from other hospitals after everyone else has failed. We have taken the long-term view, but our general opinion at the present time is that such patients are doing well with this kind of regimen.

Dr. Winters: A report from the group at the Massachusetts General Hospital should back that up. They are conducting a systematic, well-designed study in which one group of patients with acute renal failure is receiving high concentrations of glucose and small volumes of fluid by a central venous line [9] The other group is receiving glucose plus the essential amino acids only, the theory being that the nonessential nitrogen can be provided by urea which is recycled in the gut to produce ammonia.

In these patients the preliminary data seem to warrant several conclusions. First, the electrolyte abnormalities were much easier to control in the group receiving the essential amino acids. The patients were in positive nitrogen balance and, in a sense, were growing or, more properly, regrowing. As a result, they took up inorganic phosphate and potassium as new tissue was synthesized. In fact, some of these patients had to be given potassium. It is truly remarkable to give potassium to a patient who is not making any urine! Second, the frequency with which dialysis was needed, judged by clinical and chemical indications, was probably less. Finally—and most important—the survival rate was significantly higher. Relevant data from studies of dogs are available on this point from the group at the University of Pennsylvania.

Dr. Ruberg: These data were collected primarily by one of our medical students, who measured the blood urea nitrogen (BUN) and creatinine levels in nephrectomized dogs. The animals were divided into several groups: one received a standard kennel diet; the second received what might be termed "standard intravenous therapy" with 5% glucose solution; the third group was fed a regimen which consisted of hypertonic (70%) glucose plus essential amino acids; and the fourth group received 70% glucose alone.

The dogs in all groups had a uniform rise in the creatinine level, but significant differences in the levels of BUN. In three of the groups, the BUN level rose rapidly to levels of perhaps 150 mg/100 ml, whereas the animals which received the hypertonic dextrose plus essential amino acids in solution evidenced an early rise of the BUN, followed by a leveling off in the 30 to 40 mg/100 ml range. It appeared evident from these data that the animals could utilize nitrogen as present in BUN for protein synthesis, thus preventing the rapid rise to very highly toxic levels of BUN. Significant differences were observed in the survival times of the animals also. The total range of time was on the order of 10 days, so that the differences were subtle.

Dr. Winters: I have seen these data before, and the survival time is not as good as one would like to see in the group receiving essential amino acids. The real question is whether or not one can recycle the "uremic toxins," whatever they are. This raises the question of what killed the dogs receiving essential amino acids. They were not grossly azotemic. Presumably they were neither hyperkalemic nor severely acidotic. But they did die only a day or two after the other groups. Am I correct?

Dr. Ruberg: Actually, it was several days. The animals that had "routine" intravenous therapy or were allowed to eat a standard diet died in four to five days; the other animals died in eight to ten days. These data supplement Dr. Bernard's comments concerning the quality of survival. In the control groups, the animals had a higher incidence of diarrhea and vomiting than in the experimental group with the lower BUN levels. In addition to altering the metabolic pattern by lowering BUN, maybe—and even more significantly—we have altered the quality for survival for the animals in this experimental group even though the duration of survival is not significantly extended.

Dr. Winters: This approach looks promising but still, obviously, experimental. It may, however, help us in the medical management of the patient with acute renal failure.

Mr. Grant: Do you see the need for special formulations of essential amino acids?

Dr. Winters: There is the question, first, of whether histidine should be added. Second, there is the interesting observation made by Walser that feeding the keto acid analogues of the essential amino acids is as effective as using the essential amino acids alone.[10] This is a sophisticated Gilvannetti-Giordano approach minus the nitrogen. It is a nice observation. The whole problem of renal failure demands more work. We need to know what the "uremic toxins" are in renal failure, and we need to know whether they can be recycled by any amino acid mixture.

METABOLIC STUDIES AND COMPLICATIONS

Dr. Winters: Among metabolic complications which we and others have seen are:

> electrolyte disturbance (hypernatremia, hyponatremia, hyperkalemia, and hypokalemia);
> hyperglycemia, hyperosmolarity, glycosuria, and osmotic diuresis;
> hypoglycemia due to sudden cessation of the infusate;
> dehydration, edema, pulmonary edema;
> hypercalcemia, hypophosphatemia, hyperammonemia, hyperchloremic metabolic acidosis;
> deficiencies of vitamins K, B_{12}, folic acid, and copper; and
> abnormalities in the hepatic structure and in some of the liver enzymes.

A rather formidable list, and it probably is still incomplete!

I have collected data on infants receiving total parenteral nutrition.[3] The infant is a particularly labile subject and in many ways bears a close resemblance to the unstable adult surgical patient. Some of what we have learned from these pediatric patients can probably be applied to complex surgical adult patients. The infants that we have studied intensively are all of low birth weight. We start them out with an umbilical catheter on the first or second day of life and switch to a central venous catheter after several days. We monitor these infants chemically very closely.

We do not use any standard mixture. Each day the data are obtained from the infant, and a new fluid prescription order is written and given to the pharmacist. He is a valuable member of the team, and we could not get along without him. It is only by his kind of day-to-day feedback that we have been able to achieve a low complication rate. I am convinced that this approach is necessary in the pediatric patient; and I am sure that the same approach is necessary in the unstable adult surgical patient. But in the stable surgical or pediatric patient, one can probably use a standard mixture. It is nonsense to

24

talk about a single constant value for sodium or potassium or any other constituent in metabolically unstable patients. One has to have a team responsible enough so that the composition of a fluid can be changed daily.

Hyperglycemia and Azotemia

Figure 4 is scattergram of blood glucose values on eight infants.[3] The eight episodes of hyperglycemia are shown by the peaks. Generally, these occurred early in the course. From this, we learned that we must go more slowly in increasing the glucose concentration. More recently, we used insulin in some of these infants, particularly those with significant glycosuria and hyperglycemia (above 250 mg/100 ml). These babies weigh about 1 kg and receive about 0.5 and 1.0 IU of regular insulin. We believe that this tiny dose of insulin minimizes the occurrence of hyperglycemia. We monitor every urine that is voided for glucose. Most of the patients show some slight glycosuria. We monitor blood glucose several times a day during the initial period and every day or every other day when the patient is stable.

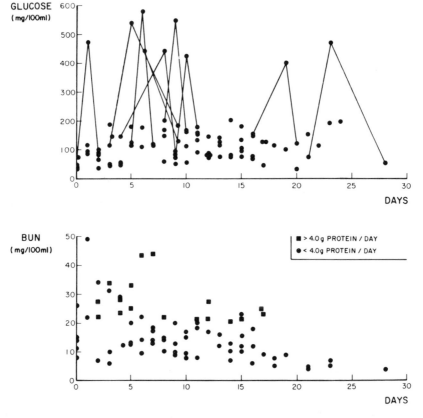

Fig 4. Changes in blood glucose concentration (top) and blood urea-nitrogen concentration (bottom). Episodes of marked hyperglycemia are indicated by the lines (from Driscoll JM Jr, et al[3]).

The appearance of unexpected hyperglycemia should always raise the possibility of sepsis. It is often the first sign that septicemia is present. Two of the peaks observed later in the course of our study occurred in patients in whom septicemia had not developed. We have no ready explanation for them. These babies were stable at that point and were not being stressed; they were simply growing. The fact that unexplained episodes of hyperglycemia occur emphasizes the need for continuous monitoring of every urine that is voided and daily blood glucose measurements.

Some pediatricians who have not adopted this rigorous policy of monitoring blood sugar have been rewarded with some horrendous consequences. I know of four patients who had blood glucose levels as high as 1,800 to 2,000 mg/100 ml. These patients developed the syndrome of hyperglycemic hyperosmolar coma; two of the four died.

With any significant degree of glycosuria, one gets a concomitant osmotic diuresis, and the osmotic diuresis in turn brings out relatively large amounts of water and salt. Hyperglycemia, then, is a double-edged sword; not only is one raising the osmolarity of the extracellular fluid and presumably dehydrating the brain, but one is also producing a secondary dehydration and salt depletion. This complication has to be looked for carefully. It is probably one of the most common metabolic complications encountered. It can be minimized, but probably not avoided completely, by the kind of monitoring I have described.

Mr. Grant: What concentration of glucose do you start with?

Dr. Winters: Initially we started with 10% glucose and went up stepwise. Now we evaluate each patient individually instead of following any standard routine. I am coming more and more to the view that insulin really does have a role in getting the calories in without significant hyperglycemia.

Mr. Grant: What final concentration do you achieve?

Dr. Winters: About 20%, which at 120 to 130 ml/kg/day amounts to a glucose load of about 25 gm/kg/day.

The postoperative patient has a glucose intolerance. If one administers TPN to intra- or postoperative patients, one has to watch for hyperglycemia and glycosuria. We have seen it in older children as we carried them on high glucose concentrations intra- and postoperatively.

Dr. Hoshal: How do you give your insulin when you are using such small doses?

Dr. Winters: We have given it intramuscularly (IM) in most cases; in one or two, however, we have added it directly to the bottle.

Dr. Hoshal: But it would be adsorbed by the glass.

Dr. Winters: I, too, thought it would stick to the glass, but I can only say that we get a nice effect, so it does not *all* stick to the glass.

Dr. McLeod: Studies have shown that a good deal of insulin can be lost on glass. It depends upon how much insulin is added. It may be that there are only a limited number of binding sites.

Dr. Ruberg: All of the information on the binding of insulin to glass comes out of a study of standard solutions. If one puts albumin in the solution, the insulin does not stick. I don't know whether anyone knows what happens to insulin binding when there are amino acids or hydrolysates in the solution.

Dr. Wilmore: It would be easy to study. This points up the fact that we often follow mythology and not hard data that could be obtained easily.

Dr. Winters: Shown in Figure 4 is a scattergram of BUN levels on these infants. Initially we started feeding these babies 4 gm or more protein equivalent per kilogram per day, and we were rewarded with a moderate degree of azotemia. For that reason, we have reduced the protein equivalent of the intake to less than 2.5 gm/kg/day. With careful monitoring, the BUN can be kept in the normal range.

A further reduction in protein concentration followed the report of Johnson et al on asymptomatic hyperammonemia in premature and full-term infants receiving hydrolysates.[11] It is known that both casein and fibrin hydrolysates contain high levels of ammonia, with values of 20 to 40 mg/100 ml or even more. With the infusion of any hydrolysate, particularly in a patient with a possible immature hepatic function or in an adult with liver disease, one gets hyperammonemia.[12] The values reported by Johnson and his associates were in excess of 200 μg/100 ml in a group of premature and full-term infants. None of these patients had any symptoms. Since that time, Walker has reported a serious degree of hyperammonemia (1,100 μg/100 ml) with CNS abnormalities.[13]

Our decision on ways to avoid the problem in the premature infant was to reduce the load of protein going in or switch to pure synthetic amino acid preparations containing no preformed ammonia.

Our group discovered a serious degree of hyperammonemia (400 to 800 μg/100 ml) occurring in three infants, premature and full term, who received a synthetic amino acid mixture (FreAmine) at a level of 2.5 gm/kg/day. Two infants had convulsions. The hyperammonemia could be corrected promptly by administration of 3 millimol/kg of arginine glutamate, arginine hydrochloride, or ornithine. It could be prevented by supplementation of FreAmine with 0.5 to 1.0 millimol of arginine. These observations raise questions about the possible deficiency of arginine in this particular mixture, also whether the hyperammonemia observed with hydrolysates may be due to a similar mechanism and not to the load of preformed ammonia as such.[14]

Plasma Electrolytes

Figure 5 is a scattergram of the plasma sodium and potassium concentrations of the low-birth-weight infants mentioned earlier (see p 24). Although we observed a few instances of hypo- or hypernatremia, we were able to correct them within 24 hours because of the flexibility of our team. We also observed cases of hypokalemia and few of hyperkalemia. The latter usually is associated with acidosis, which is fairly typical in the neonatal period in infants who have respiratory insufficiency. The plasma potassium of normal premature infants is probably in the range of 4.0 to 6.5 mEq/liter.

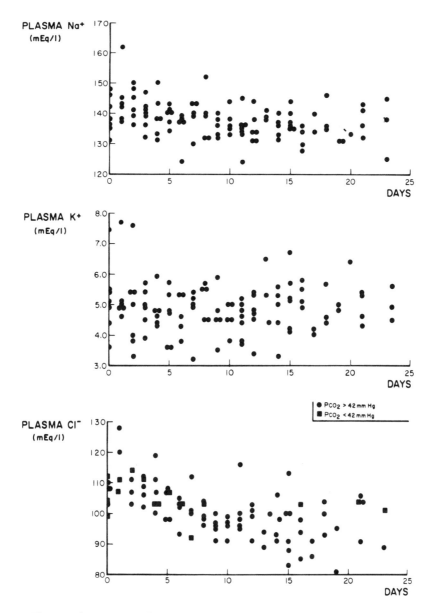

Fig 5. Changes in plasma concentration of sodium, potassium, and chloride in low-birth-weight infants receiving total parenteral nutrition. Open circles represent chloride values observed in patients with hypercapnia. X represents values obtained in one patient who received Neoaminosol (from data of Driscoll JM Jr, et al).

These data emphasize the fact that disorders of sodium and potassium metabolism in the direction of excess or deficiency have been reported in many patients. For that reason, one cannot recommend any standard electrolyte recipe to meet requirements of all patients in unsteady metabolic states.

The incidence of hypokalemia in the literature probably exceeds that of hyperkalemia. Obviously, if one does not add enough potassium and is achieving a positive nitrogen balance, potassium will enter the anabolic process in the usual ratio of 3 mEq K/gm N. Hypokalemia may result, therefore, if sufficient exogenous potassium is not available. A sensible way to approach this problem is to monitor the serum potassium and to adjust the concentration of potassium in the infusate accordingly.

It may be possible to get a standard electrolyte mixture for adults and for children who are in a steady state and who do not have extraneous losses or unpredictable stresses imposed upon them. The figures cited by Shils (see p 256) seem reasonable for pediatric patients and for adult patients, but only when serial monitoring confirms the normalcy of these electrolytes in plasma.

Dr. Winters: Figure 5 shows that in nearly all of our low-birth-weight infants the plasma chloride concentration fell. This occurred because nearly all of the patients developed a respiratory acidosis due to pulmonary immaturity. The fall in chloride concentration is secondary to the renal compensation because of the hypercapnia.

Acid-base data on this group of patients are shown in Figure 6. Blood pH tended to be low early in the course and to return toward normal later. Plasma pCO_2 was elevated in nearly all patients (the upper limit of normal for pCO_2 of infants is about 42 mm Hg with a mean value of 33 mm Hg). The values for blood base excess were initially low but rose slightly as the kidney compensated for the respiratory acidosis. Some of these patients had low values for blood pH early and high values for plasma pCO_2.

Conventional teaching holds that acidosis or hypercapnia exerts a catabolic influence upon metabolism. To examine this we plotted the nitrogen balances of these babies against the blood pH and plasma pCO_2 values (Fig 7). The data demonstrate that there is no clear relationship between the degree of positive nitrogen balance and the degree of either acidemia or hypercapnia. Even with a pCO_2 value as high as 85 mm Hg or a blood pH value as low as 7.15, one can get positive nitrogen balances.

It would appear, then, that neither acidosis nor hypercapnia constitutes any significant catabolic or anabolic influence, at least in infants. (Perhaps a similar situation obtains in adults.) These findings go counter to the conventional concept that these two chemical abnormalities inhibit growth. It may be that they do so basically by inhibiting appetite. By getting around the appetite problem—using total parenteral nutrition with a central venous catheter—one does get positive nitrogen balances.

Quality of Growth

Dr. Winters: Figure 8 provides a summary of balance data collected on these infants to illustrate the quality of growth. The total weight gain of the average infant over the entire period (average 17.4 days) was 270 gm. From the nitrogen balance, which averaged about 0.23 gm/day, one can calculate the amount of lean body mass (LBM) which was laid down. The unexplained difference between the total weight and the weight accounted for by the LBM

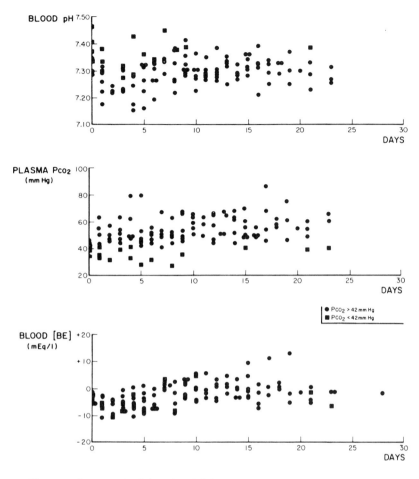

Fig 6. Changes in blood acid-base status in patients shown in Figure 5. Closed and open circles represent data obtained on patients without or with hypercapnia, respectively. X represents values obtained in one patient who received Neoaminosol (data of Driscoll JM Jr, et al).

represents fat largely. It could not be *all* water since it would amount to about 15% of the final weight and would, therefore, show itself as massive edema. These children do show signs of fat deposition clinically. In fact, most patients who have received intravenous hyperalimentation for any appreciable period of time, and who are not stressed, do show clinical evidence of fat deposition. If one visits a number of pediatric services, one can pick out the child who has received intravenous hyperalimentation for a significant period of time because they all begin to look alike. The fat which they put down is not normally distributed. They tend to look cushingoid. Dudrick points to the same trend in adults.

The data shown in Figure 8 strongly suggest that the weight gain we are observing is not simply edema. The patients are gaining lean tissue, and they are gaining fat.

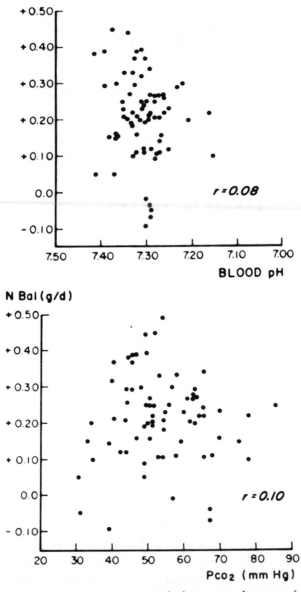

Fig 7. Relationships of nitrogen balance to degree of hyper-capnia and to the degree of acidemia in patients shown in Figure 6. There was no correlation in either case (adapted from Driscoll JM Jr, et al[3]).

Dr. Wilmore: While not minimizing the importance of gross clinical observations, should we not be doing serial body composition measurements to get a firm hold on these impressions?

Dr. Winters: Unquestionably that would be valuable. We can dismiss the idea that *all* of the weight gain in the pediatric patient is water. The same is probably true of adult patients. Suppose, for example, that an adult receiving parenteral nutrition was gaining about 0.5 kg/day and that all of that gain was water. The accumulated edema fluid over a 30- to 40-day period would be grossly apparent. Since such patients usually do not become edematous, the total weight gain must be distributed between lean tissue and fat. One crude way to get at this problem is to calculate from nitrogen balances the lean tissue deposited.

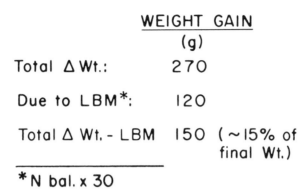

$$\text{WEIGHT GAIN}$$
$$(g)$$

Total Δ Wt.:	270
Due to LBM*:	120
Total Δ Wt. - LBM	150 (~15% of final Wt.)

—————————

*N bal. x 30

Fig 8. Summary of quality of growth achieved in 5 low-birth-weight infants receiving total intravenous nutrition. The average N balance was +0.23 gm/day and the average duration of alimentation was 17.4 days (from data of Driscoll JM Jr, et al).

Of course, this carries the inherent error of any protracted balance, namely, that the errors are always in a positive direction. Wallace wrote—in a paper which ought to be read and reread by everyone who investigates nitrogen balances—that the errors of the balance will always result in a positive number because they accumulate in the same direction.[15] This applies to long-term nitrogen balances particularly. Dr. Kark, you and your colleagues have published an ingenious and interesting new technique for nitrogen balance. Would you comment on it?

Dr. Kark: We had problems with the metabolic unit. It was closed, and we wanted to do some balance studies. Dr. Oyama suggested that if we couldn't do three-day studies we should try one-day investigations. So we did two 12-hour balances daily with excellent results. We then tried 8-hour studies. Again, nitrogen shifted between negative and positive balances. We were giving intravenous amino acids for one period, followed by glucose intravenously without any amino acids, then amino acids and glucose. We kept switching, finally reaching the point of switching every two hours.

We had some patients with diabetes insipidus. We stopped their treatment with an antidiuretic hormone (Pitressin). They put out 250 ml of urine every 10 or 15 minutes. Every time they would urinate, we would switch from intravenous glucose to glucose and amino acids intravenously, and they would switch from negative to positive balance.

In this way we can get positive and negative balance data rapidly. We don't know exactly what happens to the pools of amino acids in the body when we inject amino acids, but we are studying it.

Dr. Wilmore: Do you think it safe to recommend, Dr. Kark, that from the standpoint of general routine care we do two-hour collections and carry out total urinary nitrogen tests on urinary urea?

Dr. Kark: Although it would be interesting to do them on an experimental basis only, I would not recommend anything until we really know what is happening. Is tissue being laid down? We certainly know that you can take isolated livers and infuse them with radioactively labeled amino acids, and within 20 minutes the radioactive amino acid is incorporated into protein in cells. So it certainly could happen in the general tissues of the body when amino acids are infused. Probably it does.

Acid-Base Disorders

Dr. Winters: It is fascinating to observe that the nitrogen balance can appear to shift in such a short time. Conceivably, if this were explored clinically, it might produce a useful, simple way of assessing efficacy of nutrition short of needing a whole metabolic unit. This technique should be known and examined in some systematic way.

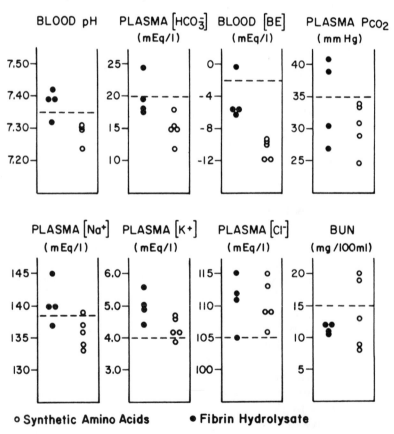

○ Synthetic Amino Acids   ● Fibrin Hydrolysate

Fig 9. Blood acid-base changes in infants receiving Neo-aminosol (open circles) and Aminosol (adapted from data of Heird WC, et al, *New Eng J Med* **287**:944, 1972).

Prior to the introduction of crystalline amino acid mixtures, few specific acid-base disturbances could be attributed to intravenous alimentation. The occasional instances reported could usually be explained by the underlying disease. But, when an experimental crystalline amino acid preparation (Neo-Aminosol) was introduced (which has the same amino acid composition as the free amino acid composition of Aminosol) we began to encounter a consistent metabolic acidosis.

Figure 9 yields data on five patients who received NeoAminosol compared with four patients who had received fibrin hydrolysate over comparable periods of time. The patients receiving NeoAminosol developed a lowered plasma bicarbonate, a lowering of blood pH, a lowering of blood base excess, and some tendency toward respiratory compensation. In addition, the plasma concentrations of chloride were high relative to those of sodium. The mild hyperchloremia observed in several patients receiving Aminosol was consistently associated with a higher than normal sodium level.

The hyperchloremic acidosis in infants receiving NeoAminosol fascinated us because they were receiving the same amino acid composition that was present in the hydrolysate. Yet the hydrolysate did not produce any significant fall in plasma bicarbonate or blood base excess. We did not allow the acidosis in our patients to progress. Once it was definite, we treated it with sodium lactate or by a reduction in the rate of administration of synthetic amino acids.

Figure 10 delineates our approach to the search for the mechanism of this acidosis. In general, when one deals with a hyperchloremic metabolic acidosis, four possibilities have to be entertained.

First, there may be an excessive stool loss of bicarbonate. This is characteristic of babies with diarrheal acidosis or of adults losing large volumes of small-intestinal juices. One can study this possibility by collecting stools and measuring the undetermined anion (UA), which is simply the sum of the

POSSIBLE ETIOLOGIES	INVESTIGATIVE TECHNIQUE
Excessive Stool Base Loss	Stool Undetermined Anion Content
Excessive Renal Base Loss	Renal Net Acid Excretion
Exogenous Load of Preformed Acid	Titratable Acidity of Infusate
Exogenous Load of Potential Acid	Cation - Anion Pattern of Infusate

Fig 10. Possible mechanisms of hyperchloremic metabolic acidosis.

inorganic cations minus the inorganic anions. This difference, the stool UA, must be bicarbonate or some other base. This possibility can be excluded almost immediately in the patients receiving NeoAminosol, because the stool volumes in such children are small. They could not possibly be losing large amounts of bicarbonate with such very low stool volumes.

Second, the general possibility of excessive renal loss of base. In effect, one could suggest that something about the fluid was producing some kind of renal tubular inhibition of bicarbonate reabsorption. This possibility is easy to examine; one simply measures the daily renal net acid excretion. Patients with renal tubular acidosis tend to make alkaline or weakly acid urines, while normal subjects will acidify the urine appropriately, and the urine will contain large amounts of titratable acid and ammonium.

Third, the fluid may contain a large amount of preformed acid. All of these alimentation fluids have acid pH values; this is desirable from the point of view of the stability and solubility of amino acids. But pH per se is not really important; rather, it is the titratable acidity of the infusate that is important in evaluating the amount of preformed acid present. Recognizing that this is a complicated physical-chemical problem, we can get a first glance at it by titrating the fluid from its original acid pH to a pH of 7.4.

The fourth possibility, the fluids themselves may contain potential acid rather than preformed acid, with the potential acid being released upon metabolism. One can approach this problem, at least initially, by looking at the cation and anion pattern of the infusate.

These, then, are the four possibilities. The first can be dismissed out of hand (see above). Data relevant to the second possibility are shown in Figure 11. The ordinate shows the daily net acid excretion, which is the urinary excretion of titratable acid plus ammonium minus bicarbonate, expressed as $mEq/m^2/day$. The abscissa shows the blood base excess, which is a measure of the intensity of the acidosis (ie, a negative base excess being associated with metabolic acidosis and a positive base excess with metabolic alkalosis). The shade zone in Figure 11 represents the performance of the normal kidney, taken from the extensive studies of Kildeberg, who investigated the net acid excretion in infants with intact kidneys with some nonrenal types of metabolic acidosis or alkalosis.[16] The distorted hexagon in the normal zone represents the performance of the normal infant and young child having no significant acid-base disturbance.

The points show 24-hour net acid measurements of our hyperalimented patients. It is evident that they are either normal or supernormal. The supernormal values suggest that more ammonium was excreted in these urines than one would have predicted. One wonders whether or not introducing the precursors of renal ammonia synthesis (ie, the amino acids), considering that the renal blood flow is about one quarter of the total cardiac output, is not priming the urinary acidification mechanism.

To digress to a practical, but perhaps a relevant, level, we have noted that many of our infants receiving alimentation develop an ammoniacal dermatitis. One wonders whether this dermatitis is due to these facts: the infants produce a lot of ammonia; they excrete a fair amount of urea as well as some amino acids, and the flora of the hyperalimented unused gut contains gram

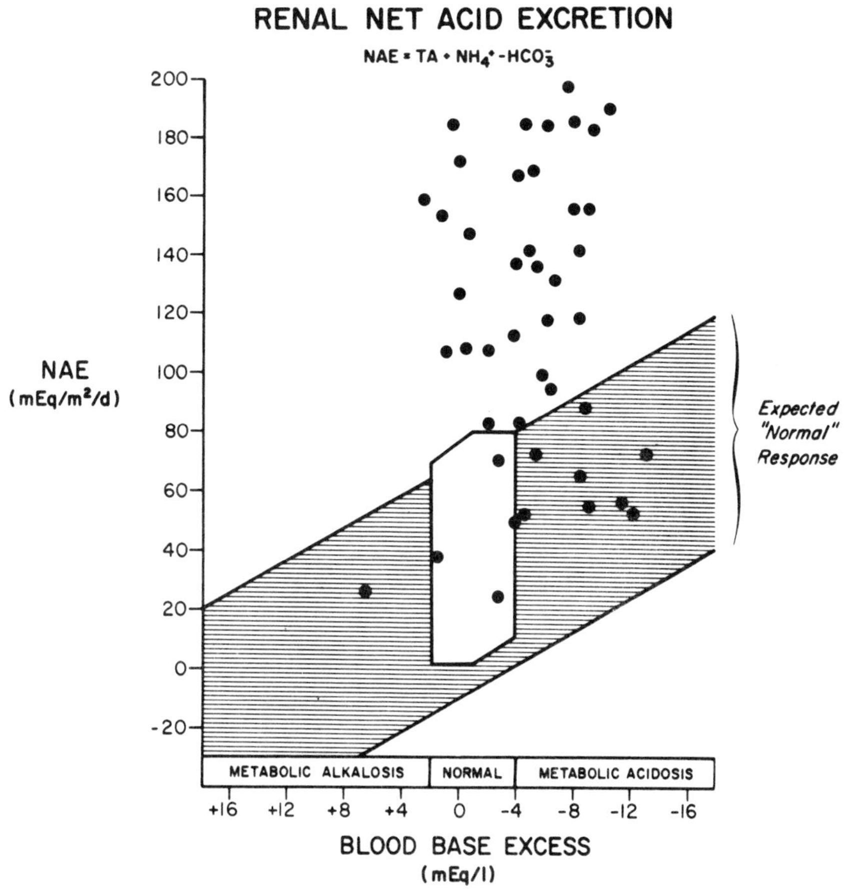

RENAL NET ACID EXCRETION

$$NAE = TA + NH_4^+ - HCO_3^-$$

Fig 11. Net acid excretion in infants and children receiving complete intravenous alimentation with Neoaminosol as the nitrogen source. The hatched area indicates the expected range of infants having intact renal function (adapted data of Heird WC, et al, *N Eng J Med* **287**:945, 1972).

negative urea splitters. This may sound like a sophisticated dissertation on the biochemistry of diaper rash, but it is an important practical point since the ammoniacal dermatitis makes urine collection difficult.

From the data in Figure 11 we can conclude that the kidney is not at fault in producing the acidosis. Rather, it is doing a supernormal job. This, then, leaves us with the two possibilities remaining.

Figure 12 shows data pertaining to one of these. The titratable acidity of the crystalline amino acid mixture NeoAminosol is only 11 mEq/per liter. Since we are administering about 130 ml/kg of this fluid, this is not a large acid load. Interestingly enough, the titratable acidity of the fibrin hydrolysate is about five times greater and is almost certainly due largely to peptides, many of which are probably metabolizable—so that this titratable acid cannot have any significant impact on blood acid-base status except in a transient way. Since the titratable acidity, or preformed acid, is not the explanation, we turned to the

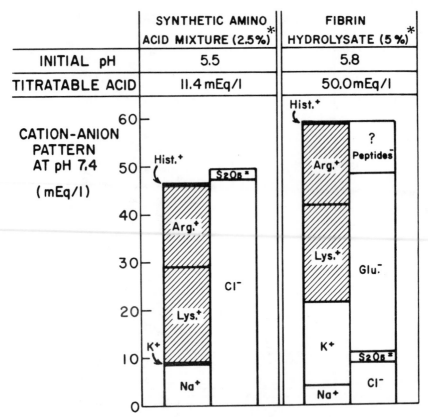

	SYNTHETIC AMINO ACID MIXTURE (2.5%)*	FIBRIN HYDROLYSATE (5%)*
INITIAL pH	5.5	5.8
TITRATABLE ACID	11.4 mEq/l	50.0 mEq/l

CATION-ANION PATTERN AT pH 7.4 (mEq/l)

*Concentration in final infusate
$S_2O_5^=$ is the preservative

Fig 12. Comparison of titratable acidity (preformed acid) and cation-anion pattern of Neoaminosol and Aminosol. Note that Neoaminosol has a cation gap which represents potential acid while Aminosol has an anion gap which is probably potential base (adapted from data of Heird WC, et al, *N Eng J Med* **287:** 946, 1972).

fourth possibility. Data on this are also shown in Figure 12. In NeoAminosol the arginine and lysine are present as hydrochloride salts. These are known to be acidifying agents. In the hydrolysates, on the other hand, the positive charges of lysine are metabolizable and upon metabolism generate base, which offsets the acid radicals generated from metabolism of arginine and lysine. But in the crystalline mixture, the arginine and lysine hydrochlorides are tantamount to infusing hydrochloric acid.

Subsequent to this work, we studied FreAmine. Initially, FreAmine had a reputation of not producing acidosis. In general, this may be true in adults, but a number of infants receiving FreAmine developed a mild to moderate metabolic acidosis of the type seen with NeoAminosol. FreAmine should not produce as much acidosis as NeoAminosol since some of the chloride salt was replaced by acetate, which is, of course, a metabolizable base.

As I indicated earlier, the treatment of the acidosis is not difficult as long as the patient can tolerate extra sodium. The sodium has to be added to the infusate as sodium lactate because of the presence of calcium.

The problem is that the amounts of sodium that have to be given may be substantial. If a patient has edema, heart failure, or some other reason for withholding sodium, one has the problem of giving the base in the face of this acidifying influence. Potassium lactate or potassium acetate could be used unless, of course, there is a concomitant problem in potassium metabolism.

The thrust of this discussion is not to make a case against any crystalline amino acid mixture on the basis of the acidosis, although this problem must be considered in future formulations. The point is that if acidosis does occur, one has to operate with sufficient flexibility to readjust the composition of the mixture by appropriate means. In general, there are two options. One would be to reduce the rate of the administration of the nitrogen source; the other, to add an appropriate amount of base. In patients in whom there are concomitant abnormal gastrointestinal losses and/or some degree of renal insufficiency, there may be additional cause for acidosis which augments the basic-acidifying character of the infusate. It may be unpredictable from patient to patient. Therefore each patient has to be monitored, particularly if he is in an unstable state.

Calcium and Phosphorus Metabolism

Dr. Winters: I can add only a few remarks to Shils' discussion of the problem of calcium and phosphorus requirements (see p 260). First, the distinction must be made between the growing and nongrowing patient, since there ought to be a considerable difference in the amount of calcium and phosphorus required for a growing skeleton versus the nongrowing skeleton. Shils correctly pointed out the additional problem of immobilization of the adult patient whose skeleton is nongrowing or, if anything, is "ungrowing itself." Presumably, that is an obligatory phenomenon of immobilization in adults.

Figure 13 shows data on plasma total calcium and inorganic phosphorus concentrations in small infants. These data were taken from an infant in whom phosphate was inadvertently omitted from the infusate. His plasma inorganic phosphate fell markedly, but his total calcium rose; he was receiving calcium in the infusion. The total plasma calcium reached a level of about 15 mg/100 ml. At this point we omitted calcium from the infusate, and the plasma calcium remained quite elevated. We then added inorganic phosphate to the infusate, and the plasma calcium came down to normal.

Note that the plasma inorganic phosphorus fell not only because phosphorus was being anabolized to make new tissue, but also (as shown in the first two balance periods) because the patient had a phosphaturia despite his developing hypophosphatemia. In other words, he was excreting phosphate despite the fact that he was becoming hypophosphatemic. I would have expected that his kidneys should have been removing phosphorus promptly and completely from the urine at this point, but they did not. One wonders—in view of the minimal amino aciduria and glucosuria that these patients show—if

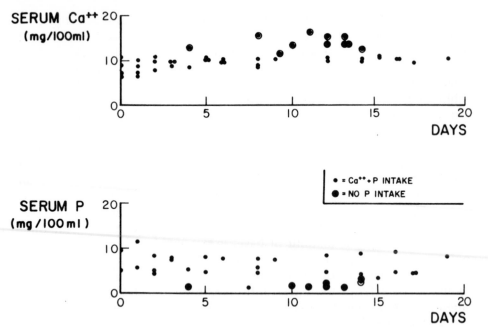

Fig 13. Changes in plasma total calcium and inorganic phosphorus. The circled points represent data on two patients who did not receive inorganic phosphate in the infusate (from Driscoll JM Jr, et al[3]).

glucose and some amino acids are not competitively inhibiting the reabsorption of phosphate in the renal tubule. This would be an additional influence in exaggerating phosphate excretion until the filtered load of phosphate became so low that all of the now almost nonexistent filtered load of phosphate could be reabsorbed.

Our babies with hypophosphatemia did not develop any symptoms as far as we could see, but the chemical evidence of abnormalities, particularly with regard to erythrocyte 2,3-diphosphoglyceride (DPG)[17] is impressive. One does not like to see this sort of abnormality. After empirically adjusting phosphate intake and calcium intake, we now give about 1 mEq/kg of body weight of calcium and 2 millimol/kg of inorganic phosphate per day to maintain normal serum calcium and phosphorus concentrations. I am reasonably sure that these amounts are too high for an adult with a nongrowing skeleton, but they seem to be appropriate for infants to produce normal skeletal growth.

The vitamin D intake, following Dudrick, is 100 IU of vitamin D per day in infants, added to the infusate as the multivitamin preparation (MVI). It is interesting that one can actually heal rickets with such small amounts of vitamin D. We have observed one patient with chronic malabsorption and celiac rickets. It usually takes large amounts of vitamin D to heal celiac rickets using oral vitamin D, but in this child celiac rickets healed with 100 IU of vitamin D parenterally along with our recommended calcium and phosphorus intakes. This is another demonstration that vitamin D exerts most of its effect on the gastrointestinal tract.

Dr. Wilmore: Because of a medication error, an adult patient being treated for a burn received an ampule of multiple vitamin infusion per bottle of solution, so that in fact he got about four times the required dose of vitamin D per day for a period extending over about two and one-half weeks. He developed symptoms of hypercalcemia. On chemical analysis, his serum calcium was found to be 16 mg/100 ml. In addition, he developed extraskeletal calcifications. The error was discovered and the whole biochemical sequence subsequently resolved. However, the man did have burns across one of his elbows, which later became completely calcified, requiring surgery. Calcium and phosphorus, then, must be monitored closely and one must be acutely aware of shifts and changes as the patient progresses.

Dr. Winters: Didn't rickets occur in a baby that you reported?

Dr. Wilmore: Yes. This was not so much a clerical error as a hesitancy on our part to load her with calcium. She developed a fracture of the humerus at about four or five months of age. X-ray demonstrated rickets.

Dr. Winters: That is another demonstration of Howland's Law: "no growth, no rickets." But if you grow infants without calcium and phosphorus you are going to get rickets.

Dr. Wilmore: One other comment about phosphorus. We are working with different solutions, and the composition of these solutions varies. Some are high in phosphorus and require no added phosphorus. If you continue to give vitamin D each day, you may in fact produce hyperphosphatemia.

Changes In Hepatic Function and Structure

Dr. Winters: We have evidence of another metabolic complication—rises in SGOT and SGPT—when we infuse the crystalline amino acid mixture NeoAminosol and with the infusion of hydrolysates.

In Figure 14 are data on several patients who received NeoAminosol. All showed elevations, often considerable, in SGOT and SGPT (our normal values being about 25 IU). We have also noticed hepatomegaly in some patients; usually it is transient. These changes do not occur in every patient, but we have seen a fair number, as have others.[1] It has been our experience that they are more likely to occur in patients who were previously malnourished.

There are two general interpretations of these phenomena. One is that what we are doing, in effect, is allowing the liver enzymatically to "flex its muscles" by supplying substrates that we have not previously provided, and we are seeing an overflow of these enzymes in the blood. The alternative interpretation is that we are seeing some form of hepatocellular damage. This problem has not been fully resolved as yet, but we now have additional information. First, we know that patients with elevations of liver enzymes have been biopsied, and the typical lesion seen is some patchy damage to the hepatocytes as well as cholestasis.[1] These have been rather consistent findings in postmortem material of premature infants who have received parenteral alimentation and have died of respiratory insufficiency. This, coupled with the biopsy data of others, suggests that we may be producing some kind of liver damage inadvertently.[1]

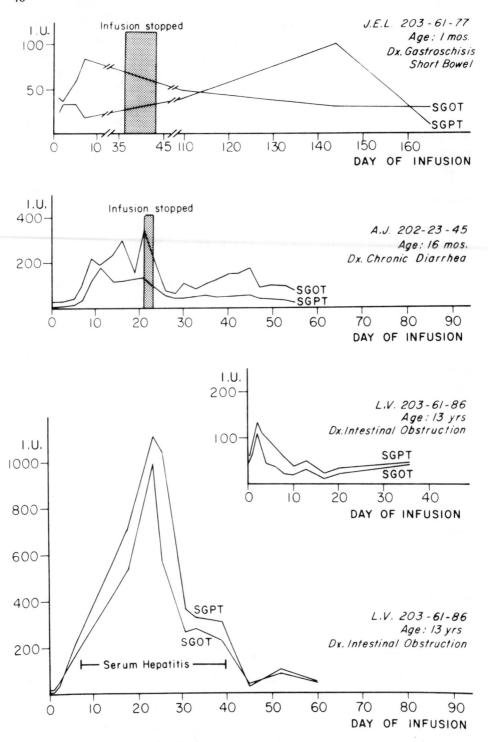

Fig 14. Changes in SGOT and SGPT in four patients receiving Neoaminosol (from Heird WC, et al[6]).

Second, Cohen took minced surviving explants of mouse liver and incubated them *in vitro* with various kinds of media.[1] When the explants were incubated with various amino acid mixtures of the type we use for intravenous hyperalimentation (at roughly one part of hyperalimentation fluid to three parts of medium), he found substantial rises in the enzymes, although they were not as high as observed when carbon tetrachloride was added.

Cohen interpreted these experiments as indicating hepatocellular damage. As alternative interpretations are possible, much further work is required. But it is possible that some of these patients are developing liver disease and that sometimes it becomes clinically apparent.

Dr. Kark: About 15 years ago in our study of hyperalimentation and attempts to produce large positive caloric balances, we observed three patients who were given between 5,000 and 9,000 kilocalories by mouth by continuous drip. All of these patients showed marked hepatomegaly to the point where we dared not biopsy the livers. We stopped the infusions and the livers returned to normal size in about two to three days. We thought it must be fluid accumulation. At that time, of course, we were not doing plasma enzyme studies. We had no evidence, therefore, of any kind of hepatic dysfunction by the tests that were available at that time. It was a reversible phenomenon. How many calories were your babies receiving?

Dr. Winters: About 100 kcal/kg.

Dr. Kark: Did their livers shrink immediately when you stopped or did they continue to be large?

Dr. Winters: It does not happen in every patient, but when it happens it tends to occur early. Subsequently, the liver recedes. The phenomenon is somewhat reminiscent of the patient who comes out of diabetic acidosis. In that case we have always assumed that the transient hepatic enlargement was somehow related to glycogen deposition. Maybe that is what is occurring in the hyperalimented patient. But there is a need to look at this problem in both patients and experimental animals.

Dr. McGill: Is methionine considered to be toxic?

Dr. Winters: Yes, but we do not quite know what to do about it, because at this point we cannot adjust the methionine content of the infusate separately.

Dr. McGill: Was there any fat in the biopsies?

Dr. Winters: Yes, some.

Dr. McGill: Were biopsies done after improvement was apparent?

Dr. Winters: Cohen biopsied several of his patients and saw improvement over protracted periods of time.

Dr. McGill: What about alkaline phosphatase?

Dr. Winters: Sometimes it shows rises; occasionally bilirubin goes up also.

Dr. McGill: I assume that the patients are all negative with respect to Australian antigen?

Dr. Winters: Yes, although we had one case of hepatitis in an adolescent surgical patient who received 16 pints of blood.

Dr. McGill: Can you tell us a little more about this group of patients with undiagnosed malabsorptive disorders?

Dr. Winters: Fanconi once characterized the whole problem of malabsorption and steatorrhea in pediatrics as a big tree: some of the branches of the tree are known (eg, celiac disease, cystic fibrosis, disaccharide intolerance, gluten intolerance); but, after excluding all of these by a thorough diagnostic workup, one is still left with branches of the tree that have not been identified.

Dr. McGill: From what you have said earlier, it seems that some of them get better with intravenous hyperalimentation.

Dr. Winters: If you take them off of everything by mouth, most of them seem to improve more or less permanently with TPN. This is why I feel that this technique should be routine therapy for this small group of patients. Prior to use of TPN, about 80% of them died of malnutrition. These seem to get into a cycle which, once malabsorption is well established, leads to malnutrition which further impairs the function of the gastrointestinal tract and leads to further malabsorption. The only way to break the cycle is to put the gut at rest. If one can do that for several weeks, most of these children will improve, and they do not appear to relapse. This technique represents a major advance in the treatment of children who fail to thrive and grow.

Dr. McGill: It may not be so much putting the gut at rest as it is allowing it to restore its enzyme complement.

Dr. Winters: That is a possibility.

Dr. Carter: The question of elevated liver enzymes brought to mind some of our experiences in treating children with protein and calorie malnutrition during the so-called recovery syndrome. In the Vanderbilt Nutrition Unit, we tried to study this recovery syndrome. During the periods of recovery we observed enlargement of the liver and, in some cases, some splenomegaly, as well as mild elevations of the liver enzymes. We tried to show that this was due to an overloading of calories or an overloading of protein, but neither seemed to be the case. Rather, it appeared to be due to a transient portal hypertension, but we could never pin it down because we did not have the facilities.

Dr. Winters: I have no clear interpretation of why it happens, but I am well aware of the fact that it does happen. We thought at first that we were dealing with a problem analogous to yours. I don't know now if we are or not. Furthermore, I am not sure whether the morphologic lesions we have observed in the liver are related to the enzyme elevations. It could be that if one doesn't use the biliary system one gets cholestasis.

We know that infants with pyloric stenosis have lesions in the liver that look much like the ones we have observed.[18] In fact, some babies with pyloric stenosis are also jaundiced.

Dr. McGill: This matter of hepatic enlargement reminds me of what happens after a patient undergoes a bypass operation for massive obesity. In the immediate postoperative period, the SGOT is normal, but the bromsulphalein excretion test of hepatic function (BSP) becomes abnormal. If the patient survives, the abnormalities return to normal over the next few months. It seems in some way to be associated with arrival to the liver of peripheral fat stores which are now being mobilized. It is a very distinctive sort of lesion. In fact, a few of these patients develop cirrhosis.

Dr. Van Way: In our experience in 30 or so adults using the intestinal bypass for obesity, we have found that the enzyme elevations tend to be transient, but the liver eventually enlarges and becomes fatty in a fair number, as demonstrated by liver biopsy. This is not associated with cholestasis particularly, but it suggests that either something is being mobilized from the periphery or else something is not being absorbed by the gut.

GUIDELINES FOR USE

Dr. Winters: The guidelines which follow, drawn up for the use of total intravenous alimentation in high-risk infants, are equally applicable to the high-risk patient of any age.[1] A review of the pediatric literature reveals this incidence of major complications of intravenous nutrition in pediatrics: 105 reported cases in which 44 experienced some type of major complication.[6] Of these the largest number had to do with complications related to the catheter, but there were a significant number of metabolic complications as well. Although these are all pediatric patients, I doubt that this is an unrepresentative sample.

One reason for this high complication rate is obvious. Some people are carrying out the technique competently while others appear to be carrying it out poorly. Thus, this promising, potentially lifesaving technique is currently obtaining a mixed reputation, particularly in view of a report in the *New England Journal of Medicine*[19] of a high incidence of fungemias, also the editorial accompanying that paper,[20] and the subsequent publication of a summary of these data and opinions in the *New York Times*.

This, in my opinion, is the natural course of many significant medical discoveries. The natural history of most such discoveries follows a sine curve. A technique when first introduced is embraced glowingly and uncritically by many as "the greatest thing that ever happened." Then, as the rate of complications—these are septic and metabolic in the case of parenteral nutrition— becomes increasingly apparent, the curve moves rapidly on the downswing. Most of us have gone through this biphasic curve and are now trying to discern just where the technique will finally come to rest in the armamentarium of the physician attempting to care for the nutritional needs of his patients.

The real problem of intravenous hyperalimentation lies in its deceptive simplicity. Many are led to think that all you have to do is insert a central venous line into a patient, run in the "nutritional goodies," and sit back and watch the patient thrive and grow. If one does this, he will almost certainly encounter an unacceptably high incidence of major complications. It was for this reason, coupled with the realization that the incidence of sepsis in our group of patients is only about 6%, whereas in some series it is as high as 67%,[19] that we were led to draw up guidelines. As I indicated earlier, these were discussed and approved by the participants of an interdisciplinary meeting on intravenous nutrition in the high-risk infant.[1]

The consensus of the participants was that a team approach is needed to implement properly the technique of parenteral nutrition using the central venous catheter in infants. Only with such a group can the rate and severity of complications be minimized. A diagram of the components of our team at the Babies Hospital in New York is shown in Figure 15. Details of the duties of each member of this group are outlined below. Institutions unable to bring together such a team should not attempt to use this technique in infants and probably not in any high-risk patient.

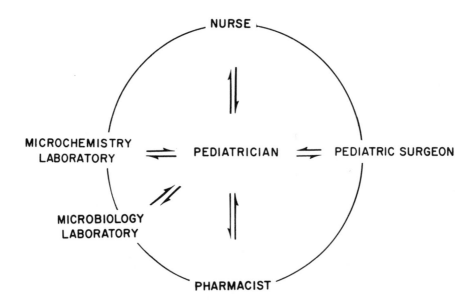

Fig 15. Parenteral alimentation team at Babies Hospital, New York.

Patient Housing

High-risk patients receiving intravenous alimentation should not be admitted to general medical or surgical wards but to intensive care units (neonatal, medical, or surgical) or to specified areas where intensive care is possible. Such special units should be equipped with the necessary facilities for care of the underlying disease process and should be staffed by competent personnel (see below).

Personnel

Around-the-clock coverage by *competent nursing* and *paramedical personnel* is an absolute necessity. Such personnel should be well trained in care of the seriously ill in the intensive observation of very sick patients, in the problems and techniques of frequent blood sampling, in care and maintenance of central venous or umbilical catheters, in the problems of infection, and in use and maintenance of monitoring equipment and constant infusion pumps. A patient-to-nurse ratio of 2:1 will insure careful observation of each patient.

Experience with intravenous alimentation has demonstrated the need for close observation of each patient by *physicians*. Specifically, there should be 24-hour coverage by competent pediatric, medical, or surgical house officers as well as by a full-time attending pediatric medical staff and/or surgical staff with experience in supervising the entire therapeutic program and, especially, in recognizing and dealing with any complications that may arise.

An experienced *surgeon* is necessary for the insertion of the catheter and subsequent care of the site. The catheter should be inserted using strict aseptic technique, and triweekly dressing changes should be carried out under similarly rigid precautions.

Percutaneous subclavian catheterization is preferred in adults and in older children. In infants the internal jugular vein is the most common site chosen, but the brachial, subclavian, and common facial veins are also used. In the newborn, umbilical catheterization (with usual precautions and full recognition of the hazards) may be used in the first few days of life, but the use of this route is a matter of individual professional judgment. Radiographic confirmation of the precise location of the catheter tip is mandatory.

Pharmacy

All infusates should be prepared in the hospital pharmacy, in close collaboration with the physician directing the therapy. Frequent adjustments in the composition of the fluid (eg, glucose, electrolyte concentrations), made in accordance with laboratory and clinical feedback information, are often necessary, and these require close communication with a pharmacist.

All mixing of fluids should be carried out under a laminar flow hood and passed through a Millipore filter.

At least one individual, preferably a pharmacist who is familiar with additive techniques and, specifically, with the rationale and complications of intravenous alimentation, should mix the infusates. Additional trained personnel to provide coverage for nights, weekends, and holidays is desirable, but the number of people preparing the infusates should be controlled in order to minimize human errors involving the procedure. Each bottle of infusate should be cultured and refrigerated in the dark for no longer than 48 to 72 hours. Random culturing rather than routine culturing may be used after sufficient experience has demonstrated that the technique of mixing and sterilization of fluids are satisfactory.

Microbiological Laboratory

The infusates used for intravenous alimentation are excellent growth media for some organisms, notably *Candida*. Continuous surveillance to detect bacterial or fungal contamination and the identification of any offending organism in episodes of sepsis or suspected sepsis requires a responsive microbiological laboratory. Cultures of the infusates before and after administration as well as culture of the Millipore filter and culture of the tip of the catheter—when it is removed—should be taken routinely. Random cultures of the filter and the infusate in the tubing after administration may be used after sufficient experience has been achieved to insure that all techniques are being satisfactorily carried out. With any evidence of sepsis, blood cultures through the catheter and through a peripheral vein should be drawn—as the catheter is removed—and appropriate sensitivity tests carried out. The catheter should be removed if sepsis is proved or strongly suspected.

Chemistry Laboratory

To assess the progress of intravenous alimentation, particularly in its initial stages, a number of chemical variables must be monitored. These are listed below. Because of the frequency of sampling, a responsive and competent chemistry laboratory is required, preferably on a 24-hour-a-day, seven-day-a-week basis. Micromethods are preferred in adults and are absolutely necessary in infants since the frequency of replacement transfusions and their attendant hazards might outweigh the potential advantages of the nutritional technique.

GUIDELINES FOR VARIABLES TO BE MONITORED

A number of variables, both clinical and chemical, should be systematically and serially monitored in patients receiving parenteral nutrition. Such monitoring is designed not only to judge the efficacy of the technique but also to minimize the rate and severity of complications.

Two general groups of complications may occur: those which are related to the catheter and those related to the patients' metabolic responses to the infusate. Complications relating to the catheter include dislodgment of the catheter, error in placement of the catheter, thrombosis of the superior vena cava, infection, especially with *Candida*, sterile inflammation of the vein, and venous perforation.

These catheter-related complications can be minimized by radiographic confirmation of the location of the catheter and meticulous aseptic technique in the mixing of fluids and in the care of the catheter site.

Metabolic complications may be numerous. A summary of those observed in infants is shown in Table 1 along with the probable cause(s). Monitoring of relevant chemical variables and appropriate adjustment of the composition of the infusate should minimize these complications. It may or may not be applicable to older patients, depending upon the degree of metabolic instability. This, obviously, is a matter of individual clinical judgment.

Table 1.—Physiological Complications

Complication	Probable Cause(s)
Hyperglycemia, glucosuria, osmotic diuresis, dehydration	Too rapid infusion of glucose, particularly in stressed or septic patients or in low-birth-weight infants prior to adaptation
Hyper- or hyponatremia	Inappropriate sodium intake in relation to water intake, particularly in the face of abnormal losses (eg, GI losses, osmotic diuresis, etc.)
Hypokalemia	Insufficient potassium intake associated with protein anabolism
Hyperkalemia	Excessive potassium intake, particularly with presence of acidosis
Hypocalcemia	Insufficient calcium intake
Hypercalcemia	Excessive calcium intake and/or insufficient inorganic phosphate intake
Hypophosphatemia	Insufficient inorganic phosphate intake
Hypoglycemia	Sudden cessation of infusion
Congestive failure and pulmonary edema	Excessively rapid infusion of hypertonic infusate
Hyperchloremic metabolic acidosis	Use of synthetic amino acid mixtures (FreAmine, Neo-Aminosol) containing excessive cationic amino acid; rarely seen with hydrolysates
Hyperammonemia	Excessive administration of free ammonia present in hydrolysates; ? hepatic damage; ? amino acid imbalance
Hypomagnesemia	Inadequate intake of magnesium, particularly with casein hydrolysates
Anemia	Failure to replace blood loss; iron deficiency, folic acid and B_{12} deficiency; copper deficiency
Rises in SGOT, SGPT and alkaline phosphate; hepatomegaly	? Hepatotoxicity due to amino acid imbalance; excessive glycogen and/or fat deposition in liver
Bleeding	Deficiency of vitamin K
Demineralization of bone; rickets	Inadequate calcium, inorganic phosphate and/or vitamin D intake
Hypervitaminoses A and D	Excessive administration of vitamin mixture due to error in mixing
Azotemia	Excessive administration of amino acids

Schedule of Monitoring

Table 2 shows the specific variables to be monitored and gives the suggested frequency of monitoring. The scheduled frequency of monitoring has been divided arbitrarily into two time periods, (Phase I and Phase II). Phase I is generally applicable to the initial period when the patient is adapting to the increasing parenteral loads of glucose, amino acids, and other nutrients. In infants, this period lasts approximately one week on the average. This phase, however, is also applicable to periods when the patient is ill or is showing evidence of a metabolically unstable state at any time during the course of intravenous alimentation. Phase II applies to the period when the patient is stable. The suggested sampling frequency should be modified if there is evidence of any specific complication.

Table 2.—Variables to be Monitored

Variable to be Monitored	Suggested Frequency	
	Phase I*	Phase II*
Growth variables		
Body weight	Daily	Daily
Body length (in infants)	Biweekly	Biweekly
Head circumference (in infants)	Weekly	Weekly
Metabolic variables		
Blood measurements		
Plasma electrolytes (Na$^+$, K$^+$, CL$^-$)	Daily	2-3 x weekly
Blood urea nitrogen	3 x weekly	2 x weekly
Plasma osmolarity†	Daily	2-3 x weekly
Plasma total calcium, inorganic phosphorus, magnesium	3 x weekly	2 x weekly
Blood glucose	Daily	2-3 x weekly
Plasma transaminases, alkaline phosphatase and bilirubin	3 x weekly	1-2 x weekly
Plasma total protein and fractions	2 x weekly	Weekly
Blood acid-base status	Daily	2-3 x weekly
Hemogram	Weekly	Weekly
Blood ammonia	1-2 x weekly	1-2 x weekly
Urine measurements		
Glucose	4-6 x daily	2 x daily
Specific gravity or osmolarity	2-4 x daily	Daily
General measurements		
Volume of infusate	Daily	Daily
Oral intake (if any)	Daily	Daily
Urinary output	Daily total and each voiding	Daily
Extrarenal losses (if any)	Daily	Daily
Prevention and detection of infection		
Clinical observation (activity, temperature, etc.)	Daily	Daily
WBC count and differential	As indicated	As indicated
Blood culture and culture of infusate and filter	As indicated	As indicated

*See text for definition of Phase I and Phase II.
†If the plasma concentration of Na$^+$ and glucose are known, osmolarity can be closely approximated by the relationship: plasma osmolarity (mOsm/kg H_2O) $= 2 \times$ plasma Na$^+$ (mEq/1) + plasma glucose concentration (mg/100 ml $\div$ 18).

References

1. Winters RW (ed): *Intravenous Nutrition of the High Risk Infant.* National Institute of Child Health and Human Development Conference, Oct 26-29, 1972, Government Printing Office. In press.

2. Winick M: Malnutrition and brain development. *J Pediatr* **74:**667-679, 1969.

3. Driscoll JM Jr, Heird WC, Schullinger JN, et al: Total intravenous alimentation in low-birth infants: A preliminary report. *J Pediatr* **81:**145-153, 1972.

4. Dudrick SJ, Wilmore DW, Vars HM: Long-term total parenteral nutrition with growth, development, and positive nitrogen balance. *Surgery* **64:**134-142, 1968.

5. Wilmore DW, Curreri PW, Spitzer KW, et al: Supranormal dietary intake in thermally injured hypermetabolic patients. *Surg Gynecol Obstet* **132:**881-886, 1971.

6. Heird WC, Driscoll JM Jr, Schullinger JN, et al: Intravenous alimentation in pediatric patients. *J Pediatr* **80:**351-372, 1972.

7. Curreri PW, Wilmore DW, Mason AD Jr, et al: Intercellular cation alterations following major trauma: Effect of supranormal caloric intake. *J Trauma* **11:**390-396, 1971.

8. Wilmore DW, Dudrick SJ, Daly JM, et al: The role of nutrition in the adaptation of the small intestine after massive resection. *Surg Gynecol Obstet* **132:**673-680, 1971.

9. Abel RM, Beck CH Jr, Abbott WM, et al: Improved survival from acute renal failure after treatment with intravenous essential L-amino acids and glucose. Results of a prospective double-blind study. *N Eng J Med* **288:** 695-699, 1973.

10. Walser M: Reduction of blood urea by feeding essential keto-acids, abstracted. *Am Soc Nephrology,* p 87, 1971.

11. Johnson JD, Albritton WL, Sunshine P: Hyperammonemia accompanying parenteral nutrition in newborn infants. *J Pediatr* **81:**154, 1972.

12. Webster LT Jr, Davidson CS: Cirrhosis of the liver: Impending hepatic coma and increased blood ammonium concentrations during protein hydrolysate infusion. *J Lab Clin Med* **50:**1-10, 1957.

13. Walker FA: Ammonia in fibrin hydrolysates. *N Eng J Med* **285:**1324-1325, 1971.

14. Heird WC, Nicholson JF, Driscoll JM Jr, et al: Hyperammonemia resulting from intravenous alimentation using a mixture of synthetic L-amino acids: A preliminary report. *J Pediatr* **81:**162-165, 1972.

15. Wallace WM: Nitrogen content of the body and its relation to retention and loss of nitrogen. *Fed Proc* **18:**1125-1130, 1959.

16. Kildeberg P: *Clinical Acid-Based Physiology: Studies in neonates, infants and young children.* Baltimore, Williams & Wilkins, 1968.

17. Travis SF, Sugarman HJ, Ruberg RL, et al: Alterations of red-cell glycolytic intermediates and oxygen transport as a consequence of hypophosphatemia in patients recovering from intravenous hyperalimentation. *N Eng J Med* **285:**763-768, 1971.

18. Rickham PP, Johnston JH (eds): *Neonatal Surgery.* New York, Appleton-Century-Crofts, 1969.

19. Curry CR, Quie PG: Fungal septicemia in patients receiving parenteral hyperalimentation. *N Eng J Med* **285:**1221-1225, 1971.

20. Duma RJ: First of all do no harm (editorial). *N Eng J Med* **285:** 1258-1259, 1971.

Digest of Colloquium

The multiple benefits and applicability of intravenous feedings to the critically ill patient became apparent several years ago when hypertonic nutrient solutions were administered by the central venous route. The deceptive simplicity of this technique and its dramatic results led to enthusiastic use of parenteral feedings in many quarters, especially on pediatric and surgical services. As a result, a wide variety of patients with complex nutritive problems was exposed to many variant forms of total parenteral nutrition administered by just as many enthusiastic and self-professed parenteral nutritionists.

Throughout 1969 and 1970, an abundance of reports describing clinical results with the technique of central venous feedings was found in the literature and in the nonliterature. A deluge of inquiries, constant visitations by experienced proponents of the methodology, and enthusiastic, well-attended meetings on parenteral therapy provided some feedback on the initial, highly individualized field trials which occurred. These inescapable conclusions followed:

> The technique of central venous feeding is being widely used, but in some cases indiscriminately;
>
> Research data generated lack proper design generally and proper controls; and
>
> Clinical experience and/or scientific data are, in many instances, being obtained at the expense of an unacceptably high rate of major complications.

Accordingly, we endeavored to recommend guidelines for the application of present-day techniques of parenteral nutrition. These guidelines are specific. They are subject to change and modification, depending on the hospital involved, the experience of the personnel, the underlying disease process of the patient, the type of nutrient solution infused, and the technique of administration.

INDICATIONS FOR USE OF TPN

Infants and Children

Among infants, parenteral therapy would be indicated in *surgical neonates* with gastrointestinal dysfunction which prevents enteral feedings for 10 to 14 days, eg, a patient with omphalocele, or short bowel syndrome, following massive intestinal resection.

Parenteral therapy would also be beneficial in infants or young children with nutritional depletion secondary to *chronic diarrhea or malabsorption syndrome* who prove refractory to most conventional management. These patients should, of course, have a complete diagnostic workup and trial of specialized oral diets before total parenteral therapy is initiated.

Selected *low-birth-weight infants,* in whom there is difficulty establishing a completely adequate enteral intake safely and promptly, constitute an *experimental* group in which the efficacy of total parenteral nutrition has not yet been determined. Intravenous feedings in these infants should be carried out in neonatal units with an adequately designed study which includes long-term neurological evaluations to determine the influence of total parenteral nutrition on mortality, morbidity, growth, and central nervous system development.

Adults

Among adults, parenteral therapy is indicated in *surgical patients with gastrointestinal dysfunction* which can be relieved by an operative procedure and which has resulted in a weight loss of about 10% or more of ideal body weight. An example would be a patient with chronic intestinal obstruction or pyloric stenosis. If, in the judgment of the surgeon, an immediate operation is required, prompt correction of fluid and electrolyte abnormalities, correction of blood volume deficiencies, and restoration of colloid osmotic pressure should be attempted before operation. Postoperatively, the patient should receive intravenous nutritional support if adequate enteral feedings cannot be established within seven to ten days of the procedure. In some patients, correction of nutritional deficits is necessary before operation is attempted, and, in these cases, two to four weeks of preoperative parenteral support may be necessary.

Patients with chronic gastrointestinal disease which precludes enteral intake (eg, regional enteritis, inflammatory disease of the colon, radiation enteritis, small bowel fistulas, and pancreatitis). Again if weight loss exceeds 10% of ideal body weight, and if the disease process appears to exceed 10 to 12 days of inadequate oral nutrition parenteral support should be initiated.

The 10% weight loss was agreed upon rather arbitrarily, for one of the discussants noted that he already was 7% below ideal body weight. Evidence was presented that there is an increased benefit from being slightly heavy if one undergoes long-term starvation, sepsis, or injury from burns.

In patients with burns or in individuals with multiple injuries or peritonitis, for example, there are increased metabolic demands which cannot be satisfied by enteral feedings. Again, if weight loss exceeds about 10% of ideal body weight, and resolution of the disease process does not appear self-limiting and early grafting is planned, then additional caloric support should be provided by the parenteral route.

Data on patients in whom *anabolism aids resolution or modification of the disease process* are more controversial; hence, further investigation is required. Among these patients are those who have undergone massive resection of the small intestine, in whom intravenous feedings may aid in villus hypertrophy and intestinal compensation. There is some evidence that modified intravenous feedings in acute renal failure may benefit patients with this disorder. At least, there is a decrease in acidosis, hyperkalemia, and hyperphosphatemia. But several participants of the Colloquium emphasized that the real benefits of parenteral feeding in patients with renal failure may be determined by a reutilization of renal failure toxin; at present there is no evidence for or against this possibility.

GUIDELINES FOR TPN

Physical Facilities

Guidelines for intravenous nutrition in critically ill patients are idealized. They are not applicable to all hospitals or to all patients. The critically ill patient should be cared for in an intensive care area, a specialized metabolic unit, or a neonatal area. These intensive care units are generally equipped with all necessary facilities for the care of the underlying disease process—monitors, infusion pumps, Millipore filters, and portable x-ray facilities—and are staffed with competent personnel. It is impractical to keep chronic patients who are not as ill in intensive care areas. Some participants recommended that they should be located together in one area of the hospital, simply from the standpoint of equipment and staffing.

Nursing Personnel

Around-the-clock coverage by highly competent nursing and paramedical personnel is absolutely necessary. Personnel in specialized units are generally trained in the care of high intensity illnesses, with emphasis on observation of these patients, care and maintenance of central venous catheters, and use of constant infusion pumps. In addition, in-house training on the care of the central venous catheter or umbilical catheter in infants, on the maintenance of the IV, and on monitoring of the infusion pumps should be carried out. For the critically ill patient, an ideal ratio would be two patients to one nurse.

Physicians

Twenty-four hour coverage should be provided by physicians. If a house staff member is present, a full-time attending staff member with experience in metabolic support and/or surgical skills should be in attendance. These individuals must supervise the entire program and deal with complications. The physicians are in charge of catheter care, which should be carried out at least three times a week. The external jugular, internal jugular, subclavian, or common facial veins are the routes of choice for hypertonic infusates.

Pharmacy

A hospital pharmacist in close collaboration with the physician directing the therapy should prepare all infusates. Frequent adjustments of the composition of the fluids should be made in accordance with feedback information. This requires close communication with the pharmacist. Mixing of all fluids should, if possible, be carried out under a laminar air-flow hood, using strict aseptic techniques and, if necessary, passed through a Millipore filter. At least one pharmacist familiar with additive techniques, and specifically with the rationale and complications of intravenous alimentation, should be available to mix the infusates. Each bottle of the infusate, or each mixing batch, should be cultured and refrigerated for no longer than 48 to 72 hours.

Additional trained personnel to provide coverage for nights, weekends, and holidays is desirable, but the number of individuals preparing the infusate should be limited to minimize human errors.

Laboratories

In the microbiological laboratory, continuous bacterial surveillance is essential since the infusates are excellent growth media, notably for *Candida*.

In addition to cultures of the infusate, or of batches of the infusate, there should also be a surveillance system for culturing the bottles once they have been infused, for culturing the Millipore filters, and for culturing catheter tips.

The catheter should be removed if catheter sepsis is strongly suspected; cultures can be drawn through the catheter or by peripheral vein—as the catheter is removed—and appropriate sensitivity tests performed.

In the chemistry laboratory a number of chemical variables need to be monitored to assess the progress of total parenteral nutrition, particularly in its initial stages. Because of the frequency of the sampling and the quantity of blood drawn, microtechniques may be used. In newborn or premature infants, ultramicro laboratory techniques are preferred. With the use of the multichannel analyzer, a small amount of blood can serve to survey patients frequently.

Monitoring

The frequency with which variables must be monitored has been divided into two general time periods: Phase I, corresponding to the period during which the patient is adapting to the high glucose loads, and Phase II, when adaptation is complete. In more general terms, Phase I represents a metabolically unsteady state, whereas in Phase II the patient is in a steady state (Table 1).

These recommendations, based on critically ill patients and infants, may be liberalized. As an example, analyses of the transaminases (SGOT and SGPT) three times a week in the first week and two times a week thereafter may be too frequent in the patient without signs of liver disease.

Only through careful patient monitoring can complications be prevented. Complications include a wide variety of electrolyte disturbances, hyperglycemia and hyperosmolality, glycosuria, hypoglycemia with the sudden cessation of infusion, hypercalcemia, hypophosphatemia, hyperchloremic metabolic acidosis, anemias, deficiencies in vitamins, vitamin toxicities, and liver dysfunction.

General measurements include intake by all routes, extrarenal estimates, and accurate measurement of urinary output. These data should be summarized every 24 hours. Vital signs should be monitored with white cell count and cultures as indicated.

The effect of parenteral nutrition is assessed best in the clinical situation by improvement in the condition of the patient, by overall weight gain, and by nitrogen balance studies.

Table 1.—Intravenous Alimentation Monitoring

Variable to be Monitored	Suggested Frequency	
	Phase I	Phase II
Growth variables		
Weight	Daily	Daily
Length	Weekly	Weekly
Head circumference	Weekly	Weekly
Metabolic variables		
Blood measurements		
Plasma electrolytes (Na^+, K^+, Cl^-)	Daily	3 x weekly
Blood urea nitrogen	3 x weekly	2 x weekly
Plasma osmolarity*	Daily	3 x weekly
Plasma total calcium, inorganic phosphorus,		
magnesium	3 x weekly	2 x weekly
Blood glucose	Daily	3 x weekly
Plasma transaminases	3 x weekly	2 x weekly
Plasma total protein and fractions	2 x weekly	Weekly
Blood acid-base status	Daily	3 x weekly
Hemoglobin	Weekly	Weekly
Ammonia	2 x weekly	Weekly
Urine measurements		
Glucose	4-6 x daily	2 x daily
Specific gravity or osmolarity	2-4 x daily	Daily
General measurements		
Volume of infusate	Daily	Daily
Oral intake (if any)	Daily	Daily
Urinary output	Daily	Daily
Prevention and detection of infection		
Clinical observations (activity, temperature, etc.)	Daily	Daily
WBC count and differential	As indicated	As indicated
Cultures	As indicated	As indicated

*Plasma osmolarity need not be determined directly; if the plasma concentration of sodium and glucose are known, osmolarity can be closely approximated by the relationship: Plasma osmolarity (mOsm/kg H_2O) = 2 times plasma sodium concentration (mEq/1) plus plasma glucose concentration (mg/100 ml ÷ 18).

ANALYSIS AND RETRIEVAL OF DATA

A mechanism of intrahospital data collection and exchange should be developed so that reports of results, complications, and techniques are available for study and analysis. Collection of such information may aid predictability of the success or failure of parenteral nutrition in treating certain high-risk patients. More data are required to determine the critical length of small intestine which will support normal growth and normal brain development in an infant, for example. These data can only be obtained through pooling of information from surgeons who have measured residual bowel length and subsequently evaluated the growth and mental development of the child.

More data are necessary to provide information on cost analysis. Data presented on the care of infants in a New York hospital demonstrated that the cost of using total parenteral feedings, with adequate supervision, laboratory support, and a hospital pharmacist mixing the solution, ran about 2.5 times the basic bed rate in that hospital.

In summary, we hope these guidelines minimize the hazards while they maximize the therapeutic benefits of parenteral nutrition.

PART TWO

Section One

**Protein Hydrolysates and Amino Acids
Calories: Nitrogen: Disease and Injury Relationships**

2 Protein Hydrolysates and Amino Acids
  Hamish N. Munro, M.B., D.Sc.
3 Calories: Nitrogen: Disease and Injury Relationships
  John M. Kinney, M.D.

  Colloquium: Protein Hydrolysates and Amino Acids
               Calories: Nitrogen: Disease and Injury Relationships
  Digest of Colloquium
  Stanley M. Levenson, M.D., and Hans Fisher, Ph.D.

NUTRITIONAL COMPOSITION

Chapter 2

Protein Hydrolysates and Amino Acids

Hamish N. Munro, M.B., D.Sc.

A digest of the available information and opinion about the requirements of healthy infants, children, and adults for total protein and for individual essential amino acids is given with the adaptation of these requirements to intravenous nutrition, emphasizing differences in metabolism that might be anticipated as a result of bypassing the alimentary tract and liver. Amino acid mixtures and protein hydrolysates used for parenteral administration are examined. Changes in amino acid requirements resulting from disease are discussed.

The protein and amino acid requirements of man have been revised by an expert committee of the World Health Organization and of the Food and Agricultural Organization.[1] In addition to this report, the following account provides a summary of the evidence available on the magnitude of human needs for nitrogen as protein and for essential amino acids. It is condensed from a more detailed survey published elsewhere.[2]

DETERMINING PROTEIN REQUIREMENTS

One approach to estimation of the requirement of adults for protein has been to measure all losses of nitrogenous compounds from the body when the diet is devoid of protein. If the requirement for protein in the diet is due to these losses, an amount of high-quality dietary protein containing the same quantity of nitrogen as these obligatory nitrogen losses should meet the protein requirements of the adult human subject. This procedure is termed the factorial method of determining protein requirements. It is based on adding up a series of factors that represent obligatory nitrogen losses from the body which must be replaced from dietary protein in order to achieve N equilibrium.

A second means of estimating protein requirements is to determine directly the minimum amount of dietary protein that will keep the subject in nitrogen equilibrium. This includes minor as well as major sources of nitrogen loss. Ideally, the two methods should provide similar estimates of dietary protein needs. It is also evident that, for infants and children, optimal growth and not nitrogen equilibrium is the criterion.

The Factorial Method

The factorial method of measuring dietary protein requirements of adults depends on adding the organic nitrogen losses of a subject receiving a nitrogen-free diet. When a protein-free diet is taken by a human subject, urinary N output decreases rapidly for a few days, followed after seven to ten days by a plateau or near plateau. Two extensive studies of young adults on protein-free diets give similar plateau levels of urinary N excretion on protein-free diets of about 37 mg of N/kg.[3, 4] Subjects on such protein-free diets continue to have a fecal excretion of nitrogenous end products representing unabsorbed secretions. Based on the two series of studies cited above and other published data, an average fecal N output of 12 mg N/kg would be representative of the best evidence available. In addition, nitrogenous compounds are lost through the skin to the extent of 3 mg/kg by subjects on a diet low in protein; at an ordinary level of protein intake, 5 mg/kg are lost.[5] A series of minor routes of N excretion include[6]: a small amount of ammonia excreted in the breath; menstruation by the female and seminal ejaculations in the male; nasal secretions, saliva, and sputum. For these minor routes, an estimate of 2 mg N/kg for men and 3 mg N/kg for women can be accepted.

Table 1 shows the sum of urinary, fecal, cutaneous, and minor routes of N loss to be 54 mg N/kg. The thesis of the factorial approach is that protein requirements are the amounts of protein needed in the diet to replace all those obligatory losses of nitrogen. Accordingly, these estimates of obligatory N loss have also been given in Table 1 as amounts of body protein that have to be replaced daily from dietary sources (conversion factor N x 6.25). This shows that the obligatory N losses represent a daily wastage of 0.34 gm body protein per kg. This wastage has to be replaced from the diet. Note that this estimate of protein requirement is an average figure for adults.

Table 1.—Obligatory Nitrogen and Protein Losses by Adult Men on Protein-Free Diets and the Equivalent Loss of Body Protein

Obligatory Losses (in adult men)	Daily Nitrogen Loss (mg/kg body weight)	Equivalent Amount of Protein (gm/kg body weight)
Urine	37	0.23
Feces	12	0.08
	49	0.31
Cutaneous	3	0.02
Minor routes	2	0.01
Total (average)	54	0.34
Total (upper limit for individual*)	70	0.45

*Additional 30% to cover upper level of individual requirements extending two standard deviations above the mean.

To make safe recommendations for the protein needs of individuals catabolizing body protein in excess of these mean figures, we must know the statistical distribution of obligatory N losses. In the two studies referred to earlier, the obligatory losses of nitrogen showed a coefficient of variation of ±15%.[3, 4] Consequently, almost all of this population would fall within the range ±30%. Increasing the final *average* estimate of protein needs by 30% will take care of almost all individuals with higher than normal needs. The upper limit of the amount of body protein to be replaced daily thus becomes 0.45

gm/kg of body weight. The factorial method predicts what amount of dietary protein should be provided in order to achieve N equilibrium; in this case 0.34 gm/kg for the average subject, with an *upper* limit of 0.45 gm/kg for individual subjects.

Determining Protein Requirements for Nitrogen Equilibrium

It should be possible to test these predictions of protein requirements for nitrogen equilibrium directly by feeding different amounts of protein and finding the minimum amount compatible with N equilibrium in healthy people. A diet of fixed composition except for the amount of protein is given, and the effect of stepwise increments of protein on N balance is recorded. By plotting N balance against protein intake, a line is obtained from which the intake corresponding to N equilibrium can be read off. Figure 1 shows such a line plotted from N balance data published for four elderly people, in whom equilibrium has been obtained at 0.6 gm protein per kg. A limited number of studies of this type have been published and will now be reviewed.

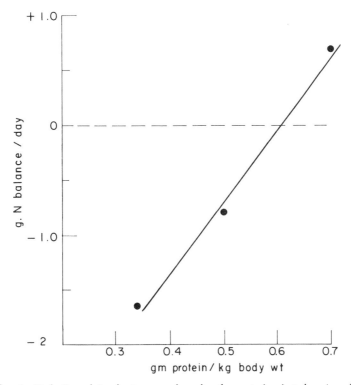

Fig 1. Relationship between level of protein intake (gm/kg body weight daily) and N balance in elderly men.

Since in these studies the dietary protein is replacing obligatory N losses, the amount of protein needed to achieve N equilibrium should vary inversely with the nutritive quality of the protein. Egg protein is generally accepted as being fully utilized for maximum growth of the young rat or for maintenance of the adult rat when fed at levels below requirements; accordingly, it has a utilization value close to 100% and has been assigned a chemical score of 100. This implies that whole egg protein contains optimal concentrations of the essential amino acids, although dilution studies suggest that some amino acids may be present in excess even for maximal growth of the rat.[7] The concentrations of essential amino acids in egg protein have been used to evaluate the amino acid pattern of other dietary proteins, which have been assigned chemical scores depending on the least abundant essential amino acid present. These scores provide a reasonable prediction of the biological utilization of food proteins in the growing rat.[8] The chemical scores of the food proteins shown in Table 2 range down to 53. It would be anticipated that a much larger amount of cow's milk or soy flour than of egg protein is required to achieve N equilibrium in man. Nevertheless, with the exception of wheat flour, essential amino acid content (chemical score) of these dietary proteins bears no relationship to the amount required in the diet to obtain N equilibrium as shown in Table 2. Even in the case of whole egg protein, the amount needed to achieve N equilibrium (0.47 gm/kg) is considerably higher than obligatory N losses in urine and feces would suggest (0.34 gm/kg, shown in Table 1).

Table 2.—Minimum Intakes of Protein Sustaining Nitrogen Equilibrium in Adults*

Protein	Chemical* Score	Minimum Intake* (gm protein/kg body weight)
Whole egg	100	0.47
Cow's milk	95	0.43
Casein	60	0.51
Soy flour	74	0.45
Rice	67	0.56
Wheat flour	53	0.73
Factorial estimate of requirements†		0.34

*Calculated from FAO/WHO Report on Energy and Protein Requirements (1973) for a 70-kg adult.
†See Table 1.

These findings have several implications: First, the minimum amount of protein needed in the diet for N equilibrium is greater than that calculated to replace obligatory N losses on a protein-free diet. Except for wheat flour protein, an average figure of 0.48 gm protein/kg is needed to achieve N equilibrium (Table 2) compared to an obligatory N loss in urine and feces equivalent to 0.34 gm body protein/kg (Table 1). Based on the N balance studies shown in Table 2, an intake of 0.48 gm protein/kg would thus be needed by the *average* subject and 0.6 gm protein/kg to cover the upper range of needs in a population with a coefficient of variation of 15%. (Note: The recent FAO/WHO Report[1] (1973) computes 0.57 gm/kg for males and 0.52 gm/kg for females.) This higher intake required to replace obligatory endogenous N output and achieve N equilibrium means that all dietary proteins are being used with some loss of efficiency. But proteins of rather different amino acid composition are probably used with similar efficiencies, indicating that the need of the adult for amino nitrogen is greater than for essential amino acids at levels of intake approximating requirement. Later, this last point will be seen to correlate well with the relatively small essential amino acid needs of adult men and women.

These estimates relate to dietary protein requirements for maintenance of young adults. In the case of the infant, requirement for human milk protein is taken as the minimum amount compatible with growth. Fomon and May observed in infants growing optimally on human milk that protein intake was 2.4 gm/kg during the first month and 1.5 gm/kg at four to six months.[9] The needs for optimal growth of older children are more difficult to estimate accurately.[10]

Finally, there has been some debate about whether protein requirements are different among the elderly. The few relevant studies of the protein needs of older subjects have been reviewed by Watkin[11] and Munro.[12] No single study provides definitive evidence, but calculations (Fig 1) of N balances obtained by Kountz et al,[13] on four elderly people suggest that their requirements for N equilibrium *averaged* 0.6 gm protein/kg, which is 25% greater than the *average* needs of young adults, namely, 0.48 gm/kg (Table 2).

ESSENTIAL AMINO ACID REQUIREMENTS

For adult man the eight essential amino acids are isoleucine, leucine, lysine, methionine, phenylalanine, threonine, tryptophan, and valine. Infants also require histidine. The amino acid needs of adults are based on N balance studies, whereas requirements for infants and children are defined as the least amount compatible with maximal growth. Human studies of amino acid needs —except for the report of Fisher et al[14]—were reviewed by Irwin and Hegsted.[15] These data are used to arrive at estimates of requirements for individual amino acids. The methodological limitations of such values are discussed in detail elsewhere[2] and are summarized here.

In the case of adults, subjects on diets containing adequate amounts of all other nutrients are given graded amounts of one essential amino acid until they pass from negative balance to equilibrium. The limitations of N balance techniques have been described frequently. The most serious problem is that N intake tends to be overestimated and N output underestimated, so that there is a tendency to an erroneously positive balance. A second problem is the criterion used to determine when the amino acid need has been met. As their end-point, Leverton et al[16] designated an equilibrium zone within 5% of balance, whereas Rose et al accepted the lowest amino acid intake compatible with a positive N balance and recognized the minimum requirement as the *highest* need of any subject in a series.[17] Third, we have to consider the other components of the diet used in these balance experiments. In addition to an amino acid mixture, the diet usually contains carbohydrate and fat sources low in protein, regarded as contributing negligible amounts of amino acids. However, studies on amino acid requirements of pigs show that cornstarch can be a significant source of essential amino acids.[18] Finally, other nutrients in the diet will influence amino acid utilization. In particular, N balance is affected by caloric intake.[19, 20]

Table 3.—Estimated Amino Acid Requirements of Young Adults

Essential Amino Acid	Number of Studies	Sex	Estimated Requirement (mg/day)	Author
Isoleucine	4	M	650-700	Rose et al (1955a)
	7	F	250-450	Swendseid and Dunn (1956)
	11	M & F	>422	Linkswiler et al (1960)
Leucine	5	M	500-1,100	Rose et al (1955a)
	13	F	170-710	Leverton et al (1956a)
	19	F	150	Fisher et al (1971)
Lysine	6	M	400-800	Rose et al (1955b)
	14	F	400-500	Jones et al (1956)
	10	M & F	500-900	Clark et al (1957)
	5	M	400-1,200	Clark et al (1960b)
	5	F	300-700	Clark et al (1960b)
	5	F	50	Fisher et al (1969)
Methionine	6	M	800-1,100*	Rose et al (1955c)
	8	F	150-350†	Swendseid et al (1956)
	20	F	300-550‡	Reynolds et al (1958)
	4	F	150*	Fisher et al (1971)
Phenylalanine (no tyrosine)	6	M	800-1,100	Rose et al (1955d)
	6	F	834-1,184	Tolbert and Watts (1963)
	13	F	600-700	Burril and Schuek (1964)
	9	M	900-1,000	Burril and Schuek (1964)
Threonine	3	M	300-500	Rose et al (1955c)
	15	F	103-305	Leverton et al (1956d)
Tryptophan	7	M	240	Denko and Grundy (1949)
	33	M	150-250	Rose et al (1954)
	5	M	225	Baldwin and Berg (1949)
	8	F	82-157	Leverton et al (1956b)
	5	F	50	Fisher et al (1969)
	2	M	6-9 mg/kg	Holt et al (1944)
	5	M	2-2.6 mg/kg	Young et al (1971)
Valine	5	M	400-800	Rose et al (1955e)
	7	F	465-650	Leverton et al (1956c)
	7	F	230-480	Linkswiler et al (1958)
	9	F	250	Fisher et al (1971)

*No cystine
†200 mg cystine
‡Total S-amino acids

Published estimates of essential amino acid requirements obtained by N balance measurements on adults are summarized in Table 3. These subjects display a wide range of estimated needs, even within a single study. To extract useful information from this confused literature, it was decided initially to accept Rose's studies, since they provide data for all essential amino acids studied under identical conditions on one sex. His estimates of requirements are expressed as ranges (Table 3), and these have been translated into midrange values per kilogram of body weight (Table 4). Inoue et al have made a study (unpublished) of the requirements of Japanese men for essential amino acids. They used the regression of N balance on intake of each amino acid to identify the point of N equilibrium. Table 4 shows that their estimates are close to the midrange values calculated from Rose's data. Finally, Hegsted[21] has applied regression equations to data published before 1963 for the amino acid requirements of women. His estimates are also in agreement with Rose's midrange values. Since it will emerge later that the values for the essential amino acid needs of young adults are proportionately much lower than those of infants and children, it should be noted that none of the data summarized in Table 3 would significantly increase the estimates selected for Table 4; indeed, some values might lower them further.

Table 4.—Essential Amino Acid and Protein Requirements in Mg/Kg Body Weight

Requirement	Infants (Holt)	Child, 10-12 yrs (Nakagawa)	Adult Man (Rose)	(Inoue)	Adult Woman (Hegsted)
Histidine	(25)	—	—	—	—
Isoleucine	111	28	10	11	10
Leucine	153	49	11	14	13
Lysine	96	59	9	12	10
Methionine & cystine	50*	27	14	11	13
Phenylalanine & tyrosine	90*	27	14	14	13
Threonine	66	34	6	6	7
Tryptophan	19	4	3	3	3
Valine	95	33	14	14	11
Total EAA (excl histidine)	680	261	81	87	80
Total protein needs (average)	1,700	700	425	425	425
EAA as % total	40	36	19	20	19

*Adding 50% of the mean requirement for methionine (39 mg/kg) and for phenylalanine (68 mg/kg) to include cystine and tyrosine needs respectively.

Table 4 displays estimates by Holt and Snyderman of the essential amino acid requirements of infants under six months of age growing maximally.[22] As in Rose's estimates on adults, the data were expressed in the original publication as ranges; Table 4 shows the midpoint of the range of values as the *average* need. Values of the same order have been obtained by Fomon and Filer who calculated the amino acid intakes of infants growing optimally on milk formula diets.[23] The requirements of older children 10 to 12 years of age have been estimated by Nakagawa and are reported in Table 4 as milligrams per kilogram of body weight.[24, 25] Finally, two groups have reported on the amino acid requirements of the elderly. A series of studies by Tuttle et al showed that double the intakes of methionine and lysine—and perhaps of other amino acids—were required to maintain elderly men in nitrogen equilibrium as compared to young men.[26, 27] But Watts and his co-workers could not demonstrate any increase in the needs of the older men for essential amino acids.[28] These contradictory findings are yet to be reconciled.

The preceding sections provide the best available estimates of the protein and amino acid requirements of infants, children, and adults. The figures in Table 4 show that, with increasing age from infancy onwards, the needs for both protein and amino acids decline considerably, but *not* in parallel. The proportion of total protein needs represented by essential amino acids falls from 40% in the case of infants to 36% for older children and to 19% to 20% for young adults (Table 4 and Fig 2). The recent FAO/WHO Report[1]

Table 5.— Proportion of Essential Amino Acids for Human Protein Needs and in Typical Dietary Proteins

Group	Percentage of Essential Amino Acids
Requirements*	
Infants	40
Schoolchildren	36
Adults	19
Dietary proteins†	
Casein	52
Whole egg	51
Human milk	50
Rice	52
Soy flour	41
Wheat flour	33

*Taken from Table 4.
†Calculated from WHO/FAO Report (1965).

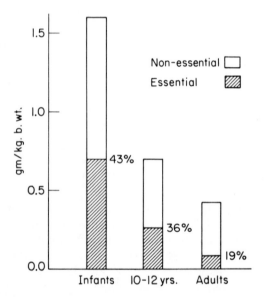

Fig 2. Requirements for total protein and essential amino acids by human subjects of various ages.

arrives at slightly lower percentages: 36%, 33%, and 15%. These figures can be compared with the percentages of essential amino acids in several representative dietary proteins. Table 5 shows that many proteins provide half their weight as essential amino acids (soy flour falls to 41%; wheat flour, to 33%). Wheat flour protein also suffers from a specially low content of lysine and threonine. For most of the proteins shown in Table 5, all of the essential amino acids are likely to be provided in excess when the amount of protein nitrogen needed to bring adults into N equilibrium is provided in the diet. The requirement is thus for amino-nitrogen (ie, for nonessential amino acids). This is not likely to be true for the rapidly growing infant, where essential amino acids are needed in greater abundance for increase in tissue mass. In the infant, unlike the adult, one would expect proteins of different amino acid composition to show different efficiencies of utilization when fed at the level of requirements.

UTILIZATION OF AMINO ACIDS ORALLY AND PARENTERALLY

Developments in the study of regulatory mechanisms in protein metabolism provide a better picture of the utilization of amino acids after meals.[29] These studies are relevant to parenteral administration of amino acids and may also suggest novel ways in which patients undergoing parenteral feeding may be evaluated for the adequacy of their amino acid intake.

Role of digestive tract Dietary protein is completely hydrolyzed to free amino acids in the course of digestion and absorption.[30] The digestive enzymes of the alimentary secretions are not entirely responsible for this; small peptides are a major end product of their action. These are finally resolved to free amino acids by peptidases in the mucosal lining of the small intestine. In addition, the intestinal mucosa carries out transamination of glutamic and aspartic acids. Hence, only a restricted part of these dietary constituents are absorbed as such into the portal blood of dogs receiving large amounts of protein;[31] and there is evidence that the liver provides a second defense against elevated levels of absorbed glutamate, especially in the newborn animal.[32] This implies that parenteral solutions containing large amounts of glutamic or aspartic acids do not mimic the natural digestive fate of proteins when their amino acids reach the systemic circulation. Some hazards are also suggested in reports that administration of glutamate or aspartate causes brain damage[33, 34] and retinal damage,[35] especially in young animals. It is comforting that Stegink and Baker found that two protein hydrolysates containing considerable amounts of free glutamic and aspartic acids—casein hydrolysate (Amigen) and beef fibrin hydrolysate (Aminosol)—do not raise the blood glutamate and aspartate levels of infants and do not cause overt neurological changes.

Role of the liver After a meal of protein, the liver is subjected to a much greater increase in free amino acid supply than other tissues because of the considerably greater increase in free amino acid levels in the portal blood than in the systemic circulation.[36] Using dogs, Elwyn has evaluated the role of the liver in determining the fate of an incoming load of amino acids.[31] Cannulas were used to sample blood amino acid fluxes in the portal vein and the hepatic artery going to the liver and the hepatic vein leaving the liver. The dogs were fed a large meat meal. During the 12-hour period following this feeding, Elwyn estimated that, during the absorptive period, 57% of the absorbed amino acid nitrogen passed out of the liver into the systemic blood as urea, 6% was secreted from the liver as plasma proteins, 14% was retained in the liver as protein, and only 23% passed into the systemic circulation as free amino acids. Confirmatory evidence indicates that meals containing protein cause extensive but temporary changes in liver protein and RNA metabolism.[37] Consequently, these meal-related changes give rise to diurnal rhythms in protein synthesis and in the activities of degradative enzymes such as tyrosine transaminase.[38]

As a result of these adaptive liver responses, the systemic circulation is protected against excessive changes in free amino acid concentration entering the body. Elwyn's results were obtained following a large protein meal. Other studies suggest that these proportions would be different if a diet lower in protein had been fed, and that a larger fraction of the incoming amino acids would pass into the general circulation, notably the essential amino acids. Thus, many of the enzymes of amino acid metabolism undergo adaptive changes related to alterations in amino acid supply (see Kaplan and Pitot for review[39]).

Harper examined the behavior of enzymes degrading essential amino acids when there is a subadequate intake of a given amino acid or when the diet provides an excess of the amino acid over requirements.[40] Young rats were given different levels of dietary casein from insufficient to excessive quantities. Threonine-serine dehydratase activity in the liver remained low until the casein content of the diet reached 20% which is optimal for growth of the rat. At casein intakes above 20%, enzyme activity rose sharply (Fig 3). But a transaminase handling the nonessential glutamic acid increased linearly in proportion to the intake of casein over the whole range of casein intakes.

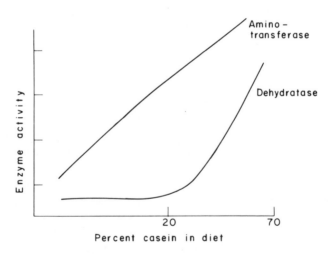

Fig 3. Activity in the liver of glutamic acid-oxaloacetate aminotransferase and threonine-serine dehydratase at different levels of protein intake (drawn from results of Harper, 1968).[40]

While these observations satisfy the prediction that dietary essential amino acids will not be extensively degraded in the liver until they are eaten in excessive quantities, the picture is probably more complex than these data suggest. Some of the liver enzymes involved in amino acid catabolism show changes in activity related to intake of tryptophan and not to intake of their substrate.[39] Also, the degradation of essential amino acids is not exclusively confined to the liver. Seven of the essential amino acids are degraded in that organ, but the branched-chain amino acids are destroyed mainly in the carcass,[41] where a low intake of protein does not reduce their activity.[42] The picture is finally complicated by the presence of multiple transaminases in the cell sap and in mitochondria.[43] These respond differently to protein deficiency.[44]

Peripheral blood amino acid levels The liver reduces impact of a protein meal on the levels of amino acids in the peripheral blood. In addition, the change is selective, since only seven of the ten essential amino acids are extensively degraded in the liver. A greater proportion of the branched-chain amino acids pass into the systemic circulation.[31] Consequently, increments in systemic blood amino acid levels are often not impressive. Some authors have been unable to correlate the pattern of change in individual amino acid levels with the pattern in the protein fed.[29] A more striking change occurs when a single essential amino acid is varied. Several investigators have added increasing amounts of the limiting essential amino acid to a deficient diet and observed the changes occurring in the free amino levels in the blood as the intake of the limiting amino acid progressed from insufficient to excess.[45-49]

As an example of this approach, Young and Munro[50] have examined the response of the plasma tryptophan level in the rat to different dietary levels of tryptophan. Both weanling and mature rats were fed for two weeks

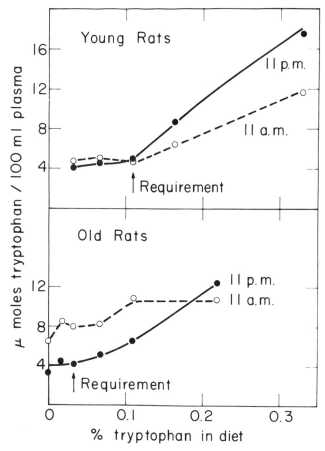

Fig 4. Plasma tryptophan levels of young and mature rats fed amino acid diets containing variable amounts of tryptophan.

on diets providing several levels of tryptophan—from insufficient to more than adequate—and animals were killed either in the absorptive or the post-absorptive stage. Figure 4 shows that the plasma tryptophan level rose sharply when intake exceeded requirements, especially in animals killed in the absorptive phase. Note that simultaneous increases in intake of all essential amino acids do not produce this sharp increase in amino acid level;[51] presumably the simultaneous availability of all amino acids stimulates temporary deposition of protein and thus prevents accumulation of one essential amino acid. These observations suggest an approach that could prove useful in measuring the amino acid requirements of human subjects, including those in various phases of injury or disease. Young et al[52] studied the effect on the free tryptophan content of plasma and on N balance in young adults given increasing levels of tryptophan (Fig 5). Their investigation confirms the usefulness of blood levels of amino acids in judging the adequacy of amino acid intake. The sharp increment at intake of 3 mg was taken to mean that the requirements of the subjects had been met at this point, in agreement with requirements based on N balance. These studies consequently support the use of blood amino acid measurement as an alternative means of determining the amino acid needs of man and other mammals.

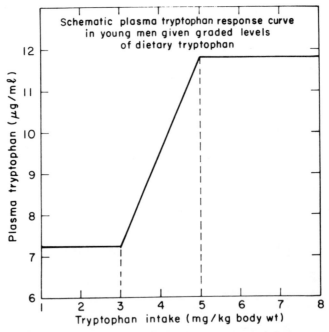

Fig 5. Relationship between plasma tryptophan concentration and tryptophan intake in man. Diagram is schematic representation of the data of Young et al for five young adults.[52]

Impact of oral and parenteral amino acid supply on body protein metabolism From what has just been said about the response of the body to a meal containing protein, it might be assumed that amino acids administered parenterally would be utilized rather differently because of the role of the gut and the liver in modifying the impact of amino acids derived from the meal. Evidence on such differences comes from comparisons of nitrogen balance and of amino acid utilization when similar levels of amino acids are fed by each route. In addition, these rather scanty observations can be supplemented by examining the daily flux of amino acids within the body. Each source of evidence will now be considered.

A comparison of the data on oral amino acid needs for nitrogen equilibrium (discussed earlier) is given in Table 6 with some conclusions about the amounts of amino acid required parenterally for N equilibrium. Josephson and his colleagues examined the N balances of healthy women. The subjects received daily 5 gm of amino acid nitrogen intravenously (770 mg total amino acids per kg of body weight) providing different proportions of essential amino acids.[53] Nitrogen balance was similar and in approximate equilibrium down to the lowest proportion (25%) of essential amino acids used. Since the authors did not attempt to find the minimum levels for total and essential N intakes, their studies show that not more than 770 mg total amino acids and 140 mg essential amino acids per kg are adequate to maintain N balance in healthy subjects fed parenterally. These figures are not greatly in excess of the corresponding estimates of requirements for adults fed orally (Table 6) and suggest that total and essential amino acid needs are probably similar by both routes. The table also shows figures for parenteral requirements of adults and infants with various illnesses. These are calculated from recommendations on parenteral nutrition tentatively suggested by Bassler et al (to be published). The suggested levels for normal subjects are greater than those found experimentally.

Table 6.—Comparison of Oral and Parenteral Requirements for Total and Essential Amino Acids

Route	Requirement Category	Group	Requirement (mg/kg)		
			Total Amino Acid	Essential Amino Acid	Essential as Percent
Oral	Observed average*	Infants	1,700	680	40
		10-12 yrs	700	260	36
		Adults	425	80	19
Parenteral	Observed average†	Adults (normal)	770	140	25
Parenteral	Recommended range‡	Infants (post-op)	2,000-3,000	500-1,500	25-50
		Adults (post-op)	1,600-2,000	400-1,000	25-50
		Adults (normal)	800-1,600	200-800	25-50
		Adults (uremic)	400	100-200	25-50

*From Table 4.

†Calculated from the data of Furst et al (1970) on healthy women receiving amino acids intravenously.[53]

‡Bassler et al (1971).

It will obviously be desirable to refine these estimates by further clinical observation. It is also probable that the proportions of essential amino acids required will vary according to the clinical condition of the patient; patients repleting their tissues after a serious illness may need the high proportions of essential amino acids required by the rapidly growing infant.

The considerable effect of the liver on incoming amino acids absorbed from the intestine suggests that parenterally administered amino acids may be treated rather differently. The data of Furst et al[53] show that requirements for total essential amino acids are not significantly higher when given parenterally (Table 6). In earlier studies from this group,[54] urea production was less in healthy subjects and uremic patients when a solution of essential amino acids was given intravenously than when introduced directly into the stomach by drip. In subsequent studies,[55] however, this difference disappeared when the gastric drip was given as slowly as the intravenous administration. It is thus evident that an excessive urea output is obtained on oral feeding only when absorption is too rapid. A real difference was observed for utilization of nonessential nitrogen, since intravenously infused ^{15}N-labeled ammonium acetate was found to pass more readily into muscle protein and less readily into liver-synthesized plasma protein than when given by mouth.[56] This type of metabolic comparison must be pursued further. The pattern of essential amino acids best utilized parenterally may differ from the oral pattern, since seven of the essential amino acids are exclusively catabolized in the liver,[41] and the amino acid spectrum emerging into the general circulation tends to be richer in the branched-chain amino acids and poorer in the other seven essential amino acids.[31]

Another view of the capacity of the body to accept amino acids parenterally can be obtained by calculating various components of amino acid utilization for a man weighing 70 kg. These are shown diagrammatically in Figure 6, which emphasizes the considerable daily turnover of body protein; some of its components (eg, plasma protein and gut protein turnover) can be individually quantitated. Against this large turnover, the intake of dietary amino acids, especially at the calculated average minimum of 32 gm for a man of 70 kg, represents only a fraction of the daily flux of amino acids in the body. This, of course, confirms much evidence from animal studies of the rapid turnover of plasma amino acids.[29]

The free amino acid pools of the body have to accept and provide the substrate for the daily turnover of 300 gm of body protein. Half of this daily body protein turnover represents uptake and release of essential amino acids; in consequence the minimum daily requirement of only 6 gm of essential amino acids from the diet (87 mg/kg for a 70 kg man, see Table 4) indicates the high degree of efficiency of reutilization of amino acids released by turnover; this remains true even if body protein turnover diminishes somewhat at minimum levels of protein intake. Under these circumstances, the recommended parenteral intakes of amino acids are well within the capacity of the system. This opinion is confirmed by the normal or even subnormal levels of plasma amino acids observed a few minutes after terminating infusions[58] or even during caval infusion.[32]

PRACTICAL APPLICATIONS TO TPN

In the preceding two sections of this review, the minimum amino acid needs of human subjects and the metabolic changes occurring within the body have been summarized. From this survey, it is possible to suggest some-

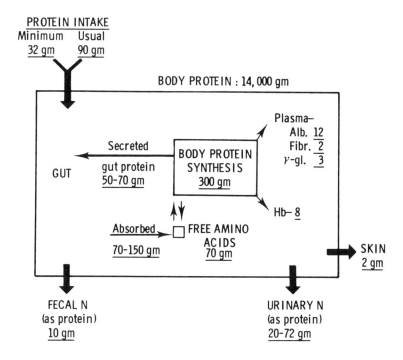

Fig 6. Protein and amino acid turnover for a 70-kg adult subject. The minimum protein intake is taken from the average needs of subjects for attaining N equilibrium: 0.45 gm/kg (Table 2). The usual intake on a Western diet of 90 gm, the endogenous secretion of protein into the gut, the fecal output, the amount absorbed, the total body daily synthesis of plasma proteins and hemoglobin are taken from Table V of Fanconneau and Michel.[30] The size of the free amino acid pool of the tissues is based on data obtained on rats.[29] These can be taken to be similar to those of man on the basis of comparison of various species.[57]

what tentatively the composition of a parenteral amino acid mixture that would most rationally provide the requirements of a *healthy* infant or adult:

• The requirement for total N is probably no greater parenterally than by mouth, so that the total amino acid levels for oral administration (shown in Table 4) are probably applicable to parenteral feeding.

• The higher percentage of essential amino acids for infants (40%) and children (35%) than for adults (19%) should be reflected in the composition of the mixture. In Table 7, requirements of each amino acid have been recalculated for infants and adults as percentages of total amino acid intake. The twofold reduction in the proportion of essential amino acids from infants to adults (from 40% to 19%) is not uniform, since there is only a small difference in the percentage of tryptophan needed in the amino acid intake of infants and adults and none in the percentage of methionine required by each group. The pattern of essential amino acids is thus different for infants and adults.

74

Table 7.—Essential Amino Acid Requirements as a Percentage of Total Protein Needs

Amino Acid	Requirements* Infant	Adult
Isoleucine	6.5%	2.4%
Leucine	9.0	3.0
Lysine	5.6	2.4
Methionine + cystine	3.0	3.0
Phenylalanine + tyrosine	5.3	3.3
Threonine	3.9	1.5
Tryptophan	1.1	0.7
Valine	5.6	3.0
Total Essential	40%	19%

*Calculated from data given in Table 4.

• Modification of the essential amino acid pattern after passage through the liver suggests that parenteral mixtures should have higher levels of the branched-chain amino acids (isoleucine, leucine, and valine) relative to the other essential amino acids. The proportions of these branched-chain amino acids should be given careful consideration, since excess of one can depress the utilization of the other two.[59]

• The phenylalanine requirement should be given partly as tyrosine. A significant proportion (2%) of the population (apparently healthy people) cannot tolerate large levels of phenylalanine since they are heterozygotes for phenylketonuria and have low levels of liver phenylalanine hydroxylase. Similarly, the premature infant is unable to form tyrosine and cysteine,[60] which at this stage become essential amino acids.

• The nonessential amino acids are also significant. No toxicity from parenteral use of glutamic acid has been reported,[32] but there is no advantage in including it. High levels of glycine should also be avoided. Tuttle et al[61] found N equilibrium more difficult to achieve in adults receiving amino acid mixtures containing large amounts of glycine. Tweedle reported N balance to be more favorable when postoperative cases were infused with amino acid solutions containing low levels of glycine (Aminosol and Vamin) than when given mixtures containing high levels of glycine (Aminofusin and Trophysan).[62] Since alanine is a main form of transport for amino nitrogen between tissues[29] it would be preferable as a major portion of the nonessential amino acids given parenterally.

In manipulating the mixture for parenteral use, consideration must be paid to imbalances, antagonisms, and toxicities of amino acids. Harper[59] finds imbalance created by changing the proportions of amino acids in the diet to produce a depression in growth and N balance which is alleviated by adding the essential amino acid in least abundance in relation to requirements. Thus histidine imbalance and consequent growth retardation can be produced in the growing rat by adding an amino acid mixture lacking histidine to a diet containing 6% fibrin as its protein source.[63] Under such conditions, utilization of the growth-limiting amino acid, histidine, becomes depressed. This phenomenon is probably of no significance for parenteral nutrition, since the mechanism of imbalance involves a reduction in *voluntary* food intake and occurs at suboptimal levels of protein intake only. But it is unacceptable to increase levels of amino acids indiscriminately, especially if one amino acid is increased without concomitant incremental increases in other amino acids.

Two major problems make it difficult to use the preceding criteria in appraising available parenteral sources of amino acids. First, discrepancies are apparent between analyses made on these solutions by different groups.[32] Second, the effects of various pathological conditions on amino acid requirements are virtually unknown. Accordingly, we shall assume that a major function of parenteral amino acid administration in most appropriate clinical cases is to promote regeneration of damaged or depleted tissue, and the amino acid requirements for tissue repletion resemble more closely those of the infant than those of the adult. Studies on the amino acid requirements of depleted adult rats provide support for this view.[64] Lower (maintenance) intakes of amino acids may be desirable under special circumstances, as in chronic renal failure.[55]

Administration of different amino acid sources causes predictable though not severe changes in plasma free amino acid patterns: Casein hydrolysate produces a high plasma ratio of phenylalanine to tyrosine, reflecting the composition of casein; fibrin hydrolysate induces a much lower ratio.[32] More studies of this kind should be assembled and analyzed to evaluate the effect of different infusions on the normal free amino acid pattern of plasma. Finally, it should be noted that the carbohydrate content of the infusion promotes removal of plasma amino acids into muscle. This action differs in extent for different amino acids.[29] Any study of the effects of infusions on amino acid metabolism must take these concomitant carbohydrate-dependent changes into account. A committee convened by the National Institutes of Health is reporting on the optimal amino acid pattern for infusion of infants.

References

1. *Energy and Protein Requirements,* FAO/WHO Export Report, World Health Organization Technical Report Series No. 522. Geneva, WHO, 1973.

2. Munro HN: Amino acid requirements and metabolism and their relevance to parenteral nutrition, in Wilkinson AW (ed): *Parenteral Nutrition.* Baltimore, The Williams & Wilkins Company, 1972, pp 34–67.

3. Young VR, Scrimshaw NS: Endogenous nitrogen metabolism and plasma free amino acids in young adults given a "protein-free" diet. *Brit J Nutr* **22:**9-20, 1968.

4. Calloway DH, Margen S: Variation in endogenous nitrogen excretion and dietary nitrogen utilization as determinants of human protein requirement. *J Nutr.* **101:**205-216, 1971.

5. Sirbu ER, Margen S, Calloway DH: Effect of reduced protein intake on nitrogen loss from the human integument. *Am J Clin Nutr* **20:**1158-1165, 1967.

6. Calloway DH, Odell AC, Margen S: Sweat and miscellaneous nitrogen losses in human balance studies. *J Nutr* **101**:775-786, 1971.

7. Bender AE: Determination of the nutritive value of proteins by chemical analysis, in *Meeting the Protein Needs in Infants and Children*, publication 843. Washington, National Academy of Sciences, 1961, pp 407-421.

8. Block RJ, Mitchell HH: Correlation of amino-acid composition of proteins with their nutritive value. *Nutr Abstr Rev* **16**:249-278, 1946.

9. Fomon SJ, May CD: Metabolic studies of normal full-term infants fed a prepared formula providing intermediate amounts of protein. *Pediatrics* **22**:1134-1147, 1958.

10. Demaeyer EM, Vanderbroght HL: Determination of the nutritive value of protein foods in the feeding of African children, in *Meeting the Protein Needs of Infants and Children*. Washington, National Academy of Sciences, publication 843, pp 143-145.

11. Watkin DM: Protein metabolism and requirements in the elderly, in Munro HN, Allison JB (eds): *Mammalian Protein Metabolism*, vol 2. New York, Academic Press, 1964, pp 247-263.

12. Munro HN: Protein requirements and metabolism in aging, in Carlson LA (ed): *Nutrition in Old Age*. Uppsala, Uppsala Swedish Nutrition Foundation, 1972, pp 32-52.

13. Kountz WB, Hofstatter L, Ackermann PG: Nitrogen balance studies in four elderly men. *J Gerontol* **6**:20-33, 1951.

14. Fisher H, Brush MK, Griminger P: Reassessment of amino acid requirements of young women on low nitrogen diets. II. Leucine, methionine, and valine. *Am J Clin Nutr* **24**:1216-1223, 1971.

15. Irwin MI, Hegsted DM: A conspectus of research on amino acid requirements of man. *J Nutr* **101**:539-566, 1971.

16. Leverton RM, Ellison J, Johnson N, et al: Quantitative amino acid requirements of young women. V. Leucine. *J Nutr* **58**:355-365, 1956.

17. Rose WC, Lambert GF, Coon MJ: The amino acid requirements of man. VII. General procedures; the tryptophan requirement. *J Biol Chem* **211**:815-827, 1954.

18. Baker DH, Allee GL: Effect of dietary carbohydrate on assessment of the leucine need for maintenance of adult swine. *J Nutr* **100**:277-280, 1970.

19. Munro HN: General aspects of the regulation of protein metabolism by diet and hormones, in Munro HN, Allison JB (eds): *Mammalian Protein Metabolism*, vol 1. New York, Academic Press, 1964, p 384.

20. Clark HE, Yang SP, Reitz LL, Mertz ET: Amino acid requirements of men and women. II. Relation of lysine requirement to sex, body size, basal caloric expenditure and creatinine excretion. *J Nutr* **71**:229-234, 1960.

21. Hegsted DM: Agriculture versus human nutrition. *Fed Proc* **22**:148-151, 1963.

22. Holt LE Jr, Snyderman SE: The amino acid requirements of children, in Nyhan WL (ed): *Amino Acid Metabolism and Genetic Variation*. New York, McGraw-Hill Book Co., 1967, pp 381-390.

23. Fomon SJ, Filer LJ: Amino acid requirements for normal growth, in Nyhan WL (ed): *Amino Acid Metabolism and Genetic Variation*. New York, McGraw-Hill Book Co., 1967, p 391.

24. Nakagawa I, Takahashi T, Suzuki T: Amino acid requirements of children. *J Nutr* **71:**176-181, 1960; *idem,* Amino acid requirements of children: Isoleucine and leucine, *J Nutr* **73:**186-190, 1961; *idem,* Amino acid requirements of children: Minimal needs of lysine and methionine based on nitrogen balance method, *J Nutr* **74:**401-407, 1961.

25. Nakagawa I, Takahashi T, Suzuki T, Kobayashi I: Amino acid requirements of children: Minimal needs of threonine, valine and phenylalanine based on nitrogen balance method. *J Nutr* **77:**61-68, 1962; *idem,* Amino acid requirements of children: Minimal needs of tryptophan, arginine and histidine based on nitrogen balance method, *J Nutr* **80:**305-310, 1964.

26. Tuttle SG, Swendseid ME, Mulcare D, et al: Study of the essential amino acid requirements of men over fifty. *Metabolism* **6:**564-573, 1957; *idem,* Essential amino acid requirements of older men in relation to total nitrogen intake, *Metabolism* **8:**61-72, 1959.

27. Tuttle SG, Bassett SH, Griffith WH, et al: Further observations on the amino acid requirements of older men. II. Methionine and lysine. *Am J Clin Nutr* **16:**229-231, 1965.

28. Watts JH, Mann AN, Bradley L, Thompson DJ: Nitrogen balances of men over 65 fed the FAO and milk patterns of essential amino acids. *J Gerontol* **19:**370-374, 1964.

29. Munro HN: A general survey of mechanisms regulating protein metabolism in mammals, in Munro HN (ed): *Mammalian Protein Metabolism,* vol 4. New York, Academic Press, 1970, pp 229-386.

30. Fauconneau G, Michel MC: The role of the gastrointestinal tract in the regulation of protein metabolism, in Munro HN (ed): *Mammalian Protein Metabolism,* vol 4. New York, Academic Press, 1970, pp 481-522.

31. Elwyn D: The role of the liver in regulation of amino acid and protein metabolism, in Munro HN (ed): *Mammalian Protein Metabolism,* vol 4. New York, Academic Press, 1970, pp 523-557.

32. Stegink LD, Baker GL: Infusion of protein hydrolysates in the newborn infant: Plasma amino acids concentrations. *J Pediatr* **78:**595-602, 1971.

33. Olney JW, Sharpe LG: Brain lesions in an infant rhesus monkey treated with monosodium glutamate. *Science* **166:**386-388, 1969.

34. Olney JW, Ho OL: Brain damage in infant mice following oral intake of glutamate, aspartate or cysteine. *Nature* **227:**609-611, 1970.

35. Olney JW: Glutamate-induced retinal degeneration in neonatal mice. Electron microscopy of the acutely evolving lesion. *J Neuropath Exp Neurol* **28:**455-474, 1969.

36. Denton AE, Elvehjem CA: Availability of amino acids in vivo. *J Biol Chem* **206:**449-454, 1954.

37. Munro HN: Role of amino acid supply in regulating ribosome function. *Fed Proc* **27:**1231-1237, 1968.

38. Fishman B, Wurtman RJ, Munro HN: Daily rhythms in hepatic polysome profiles and tyrosine transaminase activity: Role of dietary protein. *Proc Nat Acad Sci* **64:**677-682, 1969.

39. Kaplan JH, Pitot HC: The regulation of intermediary amino acid metabolism in animal tissues, in Munro HN (ed): *Mammalian Protein Metabolism,* vol 4. New York, Academic Press, 1970, pp 387-443.

40. Harper AE: Diet and plasma amino acids. *Am J Clin Nutr* **21:**358-366, 1968.

41. Miller LL: The role of the liver and non-hepatic tissues in the regulation of free amino acid levels in the blood, in Holden JT (ed): *Amino Acid Pools,* Amsterdam, Elsevier, 1962, pp 708-721.

42. Mimura T, Yamada C, Swendseid ME: Influence of dietary protein levels and hydrocortisone administration on the branched-chain amino acid transaminase activity in rat tissues. *J Nutr* **95:**493-497, 1968.

43. Munro HN: A general survey of mechanisms regulating protein metabolism, in Munro HN (ed): *Mammalian Protein Metabolism,* vol. 4. New York, Academic Press, 1970, p 3.

44. McFarlane IG, von Holt C: Metabolism of amino acids in protein-calorie-deficient rats. *Biochem J* **111:**557-563, 1969.

45. Zimmerman RA, Scott HM: Interrelationship of plasma amino acid levels and weight gain in the chick as influenced by suboptimal and superoptimal dietary concentrations of single amino acids. *J Nutr* **87:**13-18, 1965.

46. Mitchell JR, Becker DE, Jensen AH, et al: Determination of the amino acid needs of the young pig by nitrogen balance and plasma free amino acids. *J Animal Sci* **27:**1327-1331, 1968.

47. Pawlak M, Pion R: Influence de la supplémentation des protéines de blé par des doses croissantes de lysine sur la teneur en acides aminés libres du sang et du muscle du rat en croissance. *Ann Biol anim Biochim Biophys* **8:**517-530, 1968.

48. Stockland WL, Meade RJ, Melliere AL: Lysine requirement of the growing rat: Plasma-free lysine as a response criterion. *J Nutr* **100:**925-933, 1970.

49. Stockland WL, Lai YF, Meade RJ, et al: L-phenylalanine and L-tyrosine requirements of the growing rat. *J Nutr* **101:**177-184, 1971.

50. Young VR, Munro HN: Plasma and tissue tryptophan levels in relation to tryptophan requirements of weanling and adult rats. *J Nutr,* to be published.

51. Anderson HL, Benevenga JJ, Harper AE: Associations among food and protein intake, serine dehydratase, and plasma amino acids. *Am J Physiol* **214:**1008-1013, 1968.

52. Young VR, Hussein MA, Murray E, Scrimshaw NS: Plasma Tryptophan response curve and its relation to tryptophan requirements in young adult men. *J Nutr* **101:**45-49, 1971.

53. Furst P, Josephson B, Vinnars E: The effect on the nitrogen balance of the ratio essential-non-essential amino acids in intravenously infused solutions. *Scand J Clin Lab Invest* **26:**319-326, 1970.

54. Josephson B, Bergstrom J, Bucht H, et al: Amino acid treatment in uremia. *Proceedings 4th International Congress on Nephrology* **2:**203-211, 1969.

55. Bergstrom J, Furst P, Josephson B, Noree LO: Factors influencing the utilisation of amino acids in the uraemic patient, in Wilkinson AW (ed): *Parenteral Nutrition.* Baltimore, The Williams & Wilkins Company, 1972, pp 198-207.

56. Furst P, Jonsson A, Josephson B, Vinnars E: Distribution in muscle and liver vein protein of ^{15}N administered as ammonium acetate to man. *J Appl Physiol* **29:**307-312, 1970.

57. Munro HN: Evolution of protein metabolism in mammals, in Munro HN (ed): *Mammalian Protein Metabolism*, vol 3. New York, Academic Press, 1969, p 133.

58. Knauff HG, Hamelmann H, Seybold D, Kanters A: Die Auswirkung einer portocavalen Anastomose bei Lebercirrhose auf frei Plasmaaminosaüren und Blutammioniak nach oraler Proteinzufuhr. *Klin Wochschr* **44:**147-154, 1966.

59. Harper AE: Amino acid toxicities and imbalances, in Munro HN, Allison JB (eds): *Mammalian Protein Metabolism*, vol 2. New York, Academic Press, 1964, pp 87-134.

60. Sturman JA, Gaull G, Raiha NC: Absence of cystathionase in human fetal liver: Is cystine essential? *Science* **169:**74-76, 1970.

61. Tuttle SG, Swendseid ME, Mulcare D, et al: Essential amino acid requirements of older men in relation to total nitrogen intake. *Metabolism* **8:**61-72, 1959.

62. Johnston IDA, Tweedle D, Spivey J: Intravenous feeding after surgical operation, in Wilkinson AW (ed): *Parenteral Nutrition*. Baltimore, The Williams & Wilkins Company, 1972, pp 189-197.

63. Kumta US, Harper AE: Amino acid balance and imbalance. III, Quantitative studies of imbalances in diets containing fibrin. *J Nutr* **70:**141-146, 1960.

64. Cannon PR, Frazier LE, Hughes RH: Fat emulsions as caloric supplements in parenteral nutrition, with particular reference to amino acid utilization. *J Lab Clin Med* **44:**250-260, 1954.

Chapter 3

Calories:Nitrogen: Disease and Injury Relationships

John M. Kinney, M.D.

The effects of acute injury and infection on nitrogen loss and calorie expenditure are delineated for consideration in determining appropriate calorie-nitrogen ratios for use in total parenteral nutrition.

Requirements for calories and nitrogen in normal nutrition are not precisely known but have been reasonably well established within a range of values for each. During periods of acute illness and injury, the situation is much less clear, yet these are the cases in which proper use of parenteral nutrition is of greatest importance. Although my information in this area has been gleaned from experience with adult surgical patients, I hope that some of it will be equally applicable to nonsurgical conditions and all age groups.

BODY WEIGHT

Do you remember the familiar picture of Sanctorius sitting on a large scale and adjusting the amount he ate and drank in order to keep his body weight exactly in balance from day to day? In contrast to this picture, the critically ill or acutely injured patient will be lying in bed receiving most or all of his nutritional intake by the intravenous route. In addition to the altered nutritional requirements arising from the disease or injury, this patient has lost control of nutritional intake normally exerted by his appetite. He experiences changes in tissue fuel associated with physical inactivity. The normal middle-aged adult is able to maintain his body weight within $\pm 1\%$ of its total over many days and often for many months. Yet when this individual undergoes acute illness or injury, he will sustain loss of weight, the extent of which will roughly correspond to the severity of the metabolic insult to his body. Thus the clinician is often guided in his nutritional efforts by observations of body weight. I suspect the same is often true with the decisions about when and how much parenteral hyperalimentation or central venous feeding is utilized.

Temporary medical illnesses or elective surgical operations are commonly associated with weight losses of 4% to 8%. Patients with more serious forms of injury (eg, major fractures) will often lose 10% to 25% of their body weight during convalescence. Similar degrees of weight loss occur with major sepsis, although the rate of weight loss is usually more rapid.

A perspective for thinking about these losses should come from an analysis of average body composition of a middle-aged 70-kg adult male. Data in Figure 1 show that between 55% to 60% of the body weight is total body water, and around 40% of the total body weight is organic material.[1]

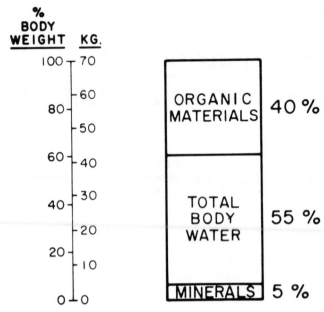

Fig 1. The relative proportions of aqueous and organic materials are shown for the body composition of an average adult male.[1]

Figure 2 also illustrates representative values for the adult male, an average composition of the organic portion of an adult male body in which the protein (estimated to be from 14% to 18% of body weight) is shown as approximately 11,000 gm. In addition to a few hundred grams of carbohydrate, mostly as glycogen, the remainder of the organic material is predominantly body fat. This, of course, varies significantly among individuals, but an average figure would appear to be in the range of 25% to 30% of body weight with an average value shown here of 18,000 gm. Intake of foodstuffs is compared with the output each day in a middle-aged adult male with only mild physical activity. Note that the food proportions in the average American diet —with approximately half the calories coming from carbohydrate—is in sharp contrast to the amounts of fat, carbohydrate, and protein in the normal body composition.

With greater activity, the intake might be over 3,000 kcal/day, although this might not be associated with an increase in the nitrogen intake. Increased physical activity during the adult years does not require increased nitrogen intake for nitrogen balance as long as the caloric needs are met satisfactorily. Therefore, the conventional calorie-nitrogen ratio in the normal adult diet is variable but is customarily between 200 to 300 kcal/gm N.

FACTORS GOVERNING NITROGEN EXCRETION

Factors governing nitrogen excretion in the adult include age, sex, body size, and body composition. The largest resting nitrogen excretion is customarily associated with the young muscular male. Above the basal level

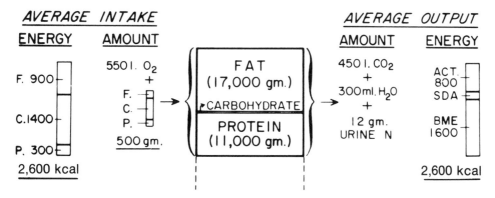

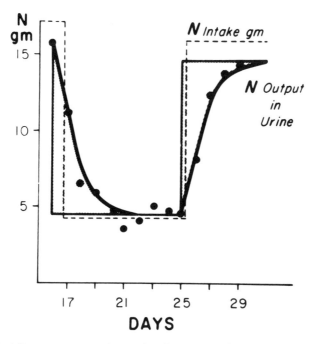

Fig 2. Average values for fat, carbohydrate, and protein in the adult male body are shown in relation to the daily energy balance.[1]

of nitrogen intake referred to by Munro (p 60), the nitrogen excretion will adapt over a few days to sharp changes in nitrogen intake. This is emphasized in Figure 3, where the nitrogen excretion is shown to reach equilibration within approximately five days after a sharp change in intake.[2] This factor is important. Nitrogen excretion following disease and injury may not seem significantly increased from that in normal life, but the effect of the disease or injury on increasing nitrogen excretion may have been just enough to offset the decrease which would normally have occurred with little or no nitrogen intake at that time.

Fig 3. Nitrogen excretion of a human subject is shown for three levels of intake.[2]

84

The observations of DuBois and associates during the early part of this century established some of the increased nutritional needs of patients during various medical conditions, particularly those associated with fever.[3] They recognized that severe infection was associated with great difficulty in establishing nitrogen equilibrium. They observed that to prevent loss of body protein extreme conditions might require far more calories than the calculated heat production, although "it is doubtful if this is necessary or advisable." They also commented on the fact that with extensive loss of body protein and fat the resulting depletion might become a special hazard from decreased resistance to infection. Metabolic studies to establish nitrogen loss as well as increased excretion of other urinary constituents were performed by Cuthbertson following long-bone fracture.[4] In this condition there appeared to be a parallel increase in urinary nitrogen excretion and in basal oxygen consumption (Fig 4). Since these pioneering observations, many laboratories have confirmed that nitrogen excretion is increased following injury and infection, with the increase roughly proportional to the degree of clinical severity. Many textbooks refer to this negative nitrogen balance without separating the part due to decreased intake from that due to an increased output. Mild to moderate clinical conditions are associated with a negative nitrogen balance, largely because of decreased intake. In contrast, moderate to extreme conditions are associated with a decreased intake in combination with an increase in output, largely as urea.

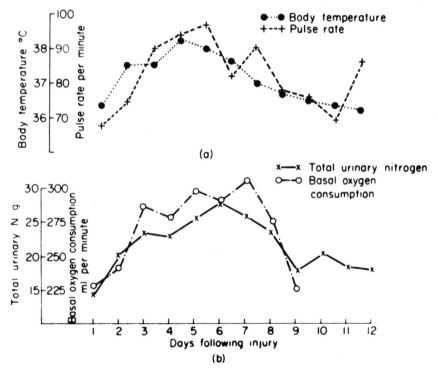

Fig 4. Correlation of vital signs and metabolic data on a 34-year-old man following long-bone fracture.[4]

An abrupt gain or loss of body weight in excess of 400 to 500 gm/day must include selective changes in body water beyond any changes in fat or lean tissue. But the slower, steady loss or gain of body weight bears a rough parallel to changes in nitrogen balance. Cumulative nitrogen losses in male adult surgical patients (not receiving parenteral nutrition beyond the conventional intravenous intake of 5% dextrose in water) will amount to 30 to 70 gm for uncomplicated major operations and reach a 200- to 300-gm loss during the prolonged, stressful convalescence of a major burn. These nitrogen losses are correspondingly less for the female, the elderly, and the poorly nourished, who also have less dramatic loss of body weight.

Repletion vs depletion Early animal studies by Munro and Cuthbertson revealed that the increase in nitrogen excretion following injury could largely be abolished in animals if they were fasted prior to the injury.[5] Johnston has shown similar findings in the nitrogen excretion following two forms of surgery (Fig 5).[6] Gastric operations on patients who had satisfactory nutrition prior to the operation were associated with a significant increase in nitrogen loss in contrast to patients undergoing colon resection for chronic inflammatory disease whose nutrition was poor and whose nitrogen excretion following surgery was not increased. Thus, the level of previous nutrition will strongly influence the nitrogen excretion following injury or infection. The patients who are depleted and have the least increase would appear to get the greatest clinical benefit from parenteral nutrition.

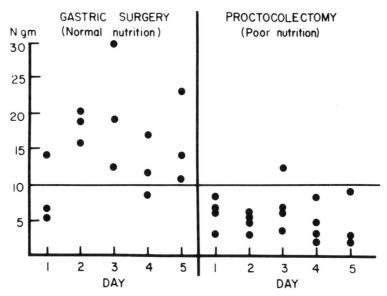

Fig 5. The influence of normal versus poor preoperative nutrition on postoperative nitrogen excretion.[6]

CAUSE AND PHYSIOLOGIC SIGNIFICANCE OF NITROGEN LOSS

The literature has offered many speculations as to the cause and physiologic significance of increased nitrogen loss (negative nitrogen balance).

It has been suggested that increased nitrogen loss is primarily a function of starvation. This does not seem reasonable since the starving patient without disease or injury will slowly decrease his nitrogen loss and caloric expenditure to a new lower level over two to three weeks as depletion develops.

Another possibility is the excretion of certain toxic breakdown products from body protein. But this seems unlikely since the great majority of the increased nitrogen loss is as urea, notably nontoxic in the concentrations which occur in such patients.

Still another suggestion: Perhaps the body is breaking down protein to obtain amino acids as building blocks for healing a wound. However, the degree of extra amino acid mobilization would appear to greatly exceed the amount needed to heal most wounds. In addition, the elderly or depleted patient who does not demonstrate an increased nitrogen loss in the presence of major injury customarily will heal his wounds to a satisfactory tensile strength. Every surgeon is aware of occasional exceptions to this experience, in which certain elderly patients develop a wound dehiscence after abdominal surgery. A fascinating unanswered question is whether such patients would have been able to heal their wounds had they been subjected to a period of intensive parenteral nutrition.

Another reason suggested for the nitrogen loss after acute disease and injury is that protein in the body is being torn down to supply extra fuel since the disease or injury is increasing the resting metabolic expenditure. This suggestion seems unlikely since the nitrogen loss is associated with deamination of amino acids which will provide relatively few calories upon ultimate combustion to CO_2 and water. In addition, there is no direct evidence that the oxidation of fat is inhibited during conditions of acute disease and injury. In fact, Carlson has suggested the possibility of a threat from over-mobilization of fat with the resultant deposition of excess fat in the liver.[7]

RELATIONSHIP BETWEEN CALORIC EXPENDITURE AND NITROGEN EXCRETION

An understanding of the nitrogen balance following acute disease and injury requires an understanding of the caloric expenditure of the body. The surgical literature has suggested that acute disease and injury may increase the resting metabolic expenditure (RME) by amounts up to 3 to 3½ times normal in extreme conditions. Such speculation seemed consistent with the impression that protein must be torn down in an effort to provide body fuel for these greatly increased calorie needs.

A special system for prolonged measurement of oxygen consumption and CO_2 production under clinical situations has been designed and applied to a variety of surgical conditions.[8]

From this type of measurement it is clear that an ordinary elective abdominal operation is followed by no significant change from the pre-operative level. Multiple fractures are followed by two to three weeks of increased caloric expenditure, as much as 20%. Major sepsis causes sustained increases of 10% to 40%. The only form of injury which is associated with sustained increases above 40% is major burns, in which calorie expenditure may be doubled for prolonged periods (Fig 6). As mentioned before, the increase in nitrogen excretion tends in an approximate way to parallel the increases in resting metabolic expenditure. The patient showing the largest increases in the resting metabolic expenditure and in nitrogen excretion is the young, previously well-nourished, muscular male. In contrast, there will be less response from females, from older patients, and from the poorly nourished.

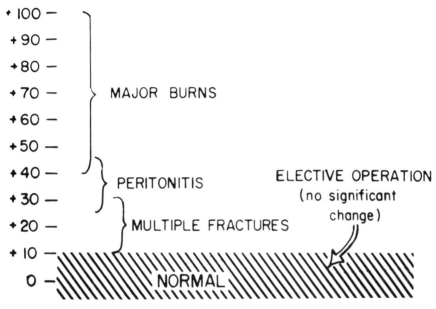

Fig 6. The ranges of increase in resting metabolic expenditure to be seen in well-nourished adult males following various forms of injury and sepsis.[8]

Duke and others reviewed the relationship between nitrogen and calorie balance in pre- and postoperative patients, patients with septicemia, patients with abdominal infection, patients suffering multiple trauma, and patients with major burns.[9] These patients were studied by plotting the urinary nitrogen against the resting metabolic expenditure, using an arbitrary relationship of 100 kcal/gm N (Fig 7). This relationship provided a surprisingly close correlation during periods of both positive and negative balance, representing the response to conventional treatment, most of which was 5% dextrose and water prior to the time when oral intake was possible. These studies emphasized that nitrogen excretion and calorie expenditure tended to move in parallel. They also suggested that, on a percentage basis, nitrogen excretion decreased more than calorie expenditure during periods of negative balance without acute disease or injury; and it increased more during the peak reactions to major infection.

This parallel behavior of RME and nitrogen excretion appears to be evident with increases of RME to approximately 40% above normal. Patients with major burns present special problems in measuring total nitrogen loss because of surface losses. Yet when reasonable estimates for this are added

88

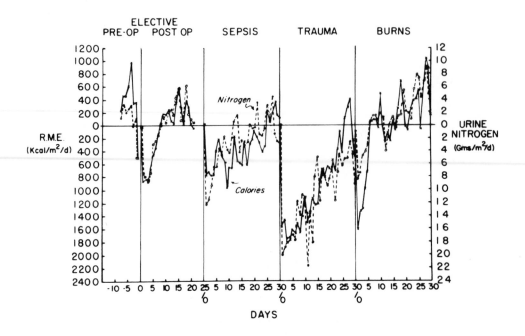

Fig 7. The correlation between daily balances of nitrogen and calories in four types of injury and/or sepsis.[9]

to other routes of loss, the total nitrogen loss is in the range often seen with other conditions such as peritonitis, where increases in RME may be up to approximately 40%. Elevations of RME from 40% to 100% above normal in patients with major burns seem to exist without a corresponding increase in nitrogen excretion. One may speculate that the high level of caloric expenditure in such patients is related to problems unique to the burn injury such as accelerated evaporative water and heat loss. This may resemble the extra calorie requirements for exercise which do not place extra demands on nitrogen metabolism if the calorie requirements are met.

RELATION OF NITROGEN LOSS TO SYNTHESIS REQUIREMENTS

The question remains: Is nitrogen excretion increased because body protein is being used as a primary source of extra calories? The main pathways relating the three organic portions of the average 70-kg male adult are shown in Figure 8. It now seems apparent that nitrogen excretion after injury has

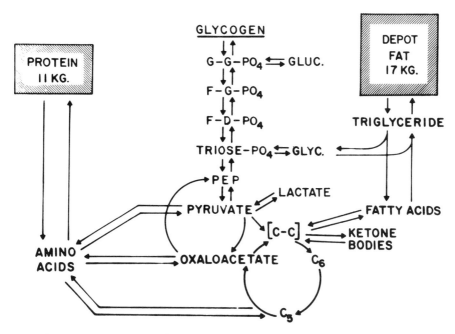

Fig 8. An abbreviated diagram of the major pathways of intermediary metabolism which interconnects the three foodstuffs.

been thought of entirely in terms of providing two-carbon fuel for the Krebs citric acid cycle. If fatty acids can provide two-carbon fragments readily when extra fuel is needed in most tissues, it becomes necessary to look for other needs for amino acid deamination beyond simply providing fuel. Certain synthetic needs for carbohydrate intermediates cannot be met by a supply of fatty acids.[10] Considerable biochemical evidence exists to indicate that a net gain of glucose or glycogen is not possible from the direct utilization of fatty acids or ketone bodies. The incorporation of tracer carbon from fatty acids into glucose or glycogen is thought to represent essentially an exchange of carbon atoms and not a true synthesis of new material. This may be important in consideration of the extra nitrogen loss following injury and sepsis. Since relatively few calories are made available by the increased deamination of amino acids and urea synthesis following injury and sepsis, it seems important to consider the synthetic needs for carbohydrate intermediates that the body is potentially faced with after injury and infection at a time when two-carbon fragments to fuel most tissues should be available from fatty acids. These synthetic needs include:

A continuing supply of new glucose as fuel for the central nervous system;
Intermediates such as oxaloacetate to supply the machinery for the Krebs citric acid cycle;
A continuing supply of new glycerol for the synthesis and deposition of triglycerides in adipose tissue; and

Carbon chains for the nonessential amino acids which the
body can synthesize.

This circumstantial evidence would suggest that an increased nitrogen loss largely represents a response of the body to provide carbohydrate intermediates to meet requirements for synthesis—which the breakdown of fatty acids cannot provide—rather than simply supplying additional two-carbon fragments for general fuel.

Calorie-nitrogen ratio The calorie-nitrogen ratio, which is normally somewhere between 200 and 300 kcal/gm N in the average diet, includes calories for physical activity and for the other activities of the body. When one considers the resting metabolic expenditures (the basal metabolism plus whatever additional amount is associated with food intake), the caloric requirements per gram of nitrogen normally fall in the range of 150 to 220 kilocalories. Preliminary evidence indicates that acute injury and infection are associated with a greater increase in nitrogen loss than calorie expenditure, with the resultant tendency to lower the calorie-nitrogen ratio in the tissue fuel to the range of 120 to 200 kcal/gm N. Current studies on the tissue composition of weight loss in surgical patients indicate that protein accounts for 8% to 12% and fat for 15% to 30% following acute injury and infection. Therefore, pending further study, it appears that appropriate parenteral nutrition for acute conditions where physical activity is minimal should provide a calorie-nitrogen ratio of 150 or lower, rather than the higher ratios indicated for the total diet needs of the active individual.

References

1. Kinney JM, Moore FD: Surgical metabolism and metabolism of body fluids, in Zimmerman LM, Levine R (eds): *Physiological Principles of Surgery.* Philadelphia, WB Saunders, 1964, chap 7.

2. Munro HN: General aspects of the regulation of protein metabolism by diet and hormones, in Munro HN, Allison JB (eds): *Mammalian Protein Metabolism,* vol 1. New York, Academic Press, 1964, chap 10.

3. Du Bois EF: *Basal Metabolism in Health and Disease.* Philadelphia, Lea and Febiger, 1924, p 338.

4. Cuthbertson DP: Observations on the disturbance of metabolism produced by injury of the limbs. *Q J Med* **25**:233–246, 1932.

5. Munro HN, Cuthbertson DP: The response of protein metabolism in injury. *Biochem J* **37**:xii, 1943.

6. Johnston IDA: The endocrine response to trauma. *Sci Basis Med Ann Rev,* pp 224–241, 1968.

7. Carlson LA: Mobilization and utilization of lipids after trauma: Relation to caloric homeostasis, in Porter R, Knight J (eds): *Energy Metabolism in Trauma,* A Ciba Foundation Symposium.

8. Kinney JM, Duke JN Jr, Long CL, Gump FE: Tissue fuel and weight loss after injury. *J Clin Path* **23** (suppl):65, 1970.

9. Duke JH Jr, Jørgensen SB, Broell JR, et al: Contribution of protein to caloric expenditure following surgery. *Surgery* **68:**168-174, 1970.

10. Coleman JE: Metabolic interrelationships between carbohydrates, lipids and proteins, in Bondy PK (ed): *Diseases of Metabolism.* Philadelphia, WB Saunders, 1969, chap 5, p 89.

Amino Acids and Protein Hydrolysates; Calories: Nitrogen: Disease and Injury Relationships

Colloquium

Stanley M. Levenson, M.D., chairman and editor
Hans Fisher, Ph.D., rapporteur

Dr. Levenson: Our group is charged with the task of defining the optimal calorie:amino acid:protein hydrolysate:protein requirements of patients in various states of nutrition, both pre- and postinjury or illness, and with varying degrees and types of injury and illness when the patients are fed parenterally. Clearly, this is a monumental task; we cannot hope to discuss all these matters in the depth required. To help limit the scope of our task, we will talk chiefly about patients who were in good health prior to injury or illness and their requirements from the points of view of (1) maintenance of the patients in good nutritional state and (2) correcting any malnutrition which may have developed.

We all recognize that information to enable firm recommendations is inadequate in some areas, but we should attempt to arrive at what we consider the most appropriate guidelines for current parenteral therapy and to point out where the important informational gaps exist and where additional investigation is required. Let us begin with an area which fits into the latter category.

    I. Nutritional role of peptides
   II. Amino acid requirements
      A. Essential and nonessential amino acids
  III. Effect of parenteral amino acid and protein hydrolysate alimentation on acid-base balance
  IV. Problems of patients with liver disease
   V. Hyperammoniemia
  VI. Amino acid mixtures
 VII. Calorie-nitrogen ratio
      A. Wound healing
      B. Resistance to infection
VIII. Intermittent vs continuous infusions
  IX. Quality control and labeling of commercial solutions
   X. Infusion of plasma protein
  XI. Infusion of red blood cells
 XII. Transition from TPN to oral diets; elemental diets

NUTRITIONAL ROLE OF PEPTIDES

Dr. Levenson: Will you comment on the nutritional role of peptides, Dr. Munro?

Dr. Munro: A significant proportion of the enzymic hydrolysates currently in use for parenteral administration is in peptide form. The question is, "Are these peptides utilized, and are they utilized efficiently?"

Some peptides are used. Apparently two major mechanisms are involved for the utilization of certain injected peptides:

> If denatured plasma proteins are injected into man or into animals, the denatured proteins are taken out of the circulation by the reticuloendothelial system (RES) and are efficiently turned into free amino acids.

> The kidney glomeruli filter smaller proteins and peptides such as the Bence Jones immunoglobulins. These are partly reabsorbed and returned to the blood by the renal tubules as free amino acids.

Both of these mechanisms are operational, except in severe renal dysfunction or severe dysfunction of the RES. I presume that utilization of injected peptides is moderately efficient although some appear in the urine.

Dr. Levenson: It is an open question whether there may be specific roles for specific peptides. At the moment this is a theoretical rather than a practical consideration. Is there a place for hydrolysates in parenteral use? Is there a disadvantage to using free L-amino acids as opposed to protein hydrolysates or some special mixture of hydrolysates and L-amino acids? Enzyme induction is an important consideration, particularly for the infant, perhaps also for the adult. We know relatively little about the efficiency—to use the term loosely—of infused peptides versus free amino acids in enzyme induction.

AMINO ACID REQUIREMENTS

Dr. Levenson: Dr. Munro pointed out that, in addition to the ingested protein in the gut, very large amounts of endogenous protein—perhaps as much as 180 gm/day—may be secreted into the lumen of the gut in adults. When digested, this large quantity of endogenous protein can modulate the composition of amino acids and peptides that result from the digestion of ingested proteins. The data of Nasset[1] on changes in amino acid composition as the ingested proteins pass down the gut indicate the gut's function in control of the amino acid composition of its contents and, consequently, of what is presented for absorption and utilization.

Another point Dr. Munro made is that all amino acids absorbed from the gut go through the portal system, the liver, the lung, then into the systemic circulation. In parenteral alimentation the infused amino acids go directly into the systemic plasma amino acid pool; subsequently a portion passes through the liver.

Dr. Stegink: One concept holds that once inside the cell all amino acids are essential in terms of their metabolic effects. In 1970 Sturman et al published data indicating that the liver in the human fetus and in the premature infant has little cystothionase.[2] This handicaps the ability of that organ and, therefore, of the total organism to carry out the conversion of methionine to cystine or cyst(e)ine.

Essential and Nonessential Amino Acids

Dr. Stegink: Studies of Holt and Snyderman on growth and development of orally-fed premature infants indicate that approximately one-third required cyst(e)ine or cystine.[3] They also pointed out that tyrosine was an essential amino acid for a certain group of premature infants. This is not an extraordinary finding, since we know about maturational differences in induction of the various enzymes involved in amino acid metabolism. Certainly we know about transient tyrosinosis of the premature infant. We're aware that certain cases of hyperphenylalanemia may be the result of a delayed maturation of the phenylalanine hydroxylase system. According to the data of Sturman et al,[2] the enzyme cystothionase also is relatively late in its induction; thus cyst(e)ine and tyrosine also may be essential amino acids for the premature infant.

Industry tells us that these two amino acids are "bad actors" when one tries to make solutions of them. Cystine is notorious for its insolubility, as is tyrosine, and both present formulation problems. Cyst(e)ine tends to severely discolor a product by its release of sulfur.

The adult may have a cyst(e)ine requirement. Normal adult volunteers were fed eucalorically a cyst(e)ine-free protein-hydrolysate-dextrose solution.[4] One group of four patients was fed first for two weeks intravenously through the superior vena cava and then for two weeks by the nasogastric route. In each case, the mixture was given by constant drip over a 24-hour period. During the parenteral nutrition period, the plasma cyst(e)ine levels dropped promptly within six hours, then continued to drop to approximately one-third to one-fifth of normal levels and stayed there during the two-week period. Plasma taurine dropped also.

When the subjects were switched to the nasogastric route, plasma cyst(e)ine levels rose to approximately two-thirds of the normal level. Normal levels were regained only when the subjects went back on a general diet and ingested some cyst(e)ine. A rebound phenomenon may evolve during the interim period of switch-over to the normal diet. This sort of response is helpful when looking for possible imbalances in amino acid mixtures. The converse of these changes in plasma cyst(e)ine levels occurred in the groups receiving the hydrolysate-glucose mixture by the nasogastric route first, then by the intravenous route. In contrast to man, monkeys infused with similar solutions have no problems maintaining plasma cyst(e)ine and taurine levels. In human subjects receiving cyst(e)ine-free parenteral solutions, the taurocholic acid concentration in bile decreased.

I have suggested an "ideal" synthetic amino acid mixture of both essential and nonessential amino acids for the parenteral feeding of infants, in which I used an additional criterion to apply to the data of Harper and of Holt and Snyderman. I took the position that the fetus has the placenta to help control blood levels, but the premature infant who is being infused does not have a placenta to help it.

Maintenance of the plasma amino acid levels close to normal values found in orally fed, well-nourished infants is one attribute of appropriate amino acid mixtures for infusion. I have made my calculations based on (1) the composition of fetal blood as it leaves the placenta as reported by several

N-Bilanz: + 6,28 g N/13 Tage = ~ 235 g Gewebe

Körpergewicht: + 275 g/13 Tage

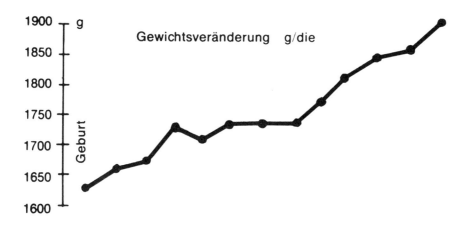

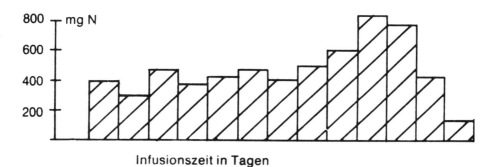

Infusionszeit in Tagen

Fig 1. Positive nitrogen balance and increase in weight of a premature infant nourished parenterally with an amino acid solution containing methionine as the sole source of sulfurous amino acids.

96

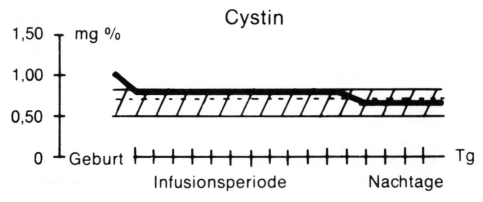

Fig 2. Plasma level of cystine during infusion of an amino acid mixture containing methionine as the sole source of sulfurous amino acids.

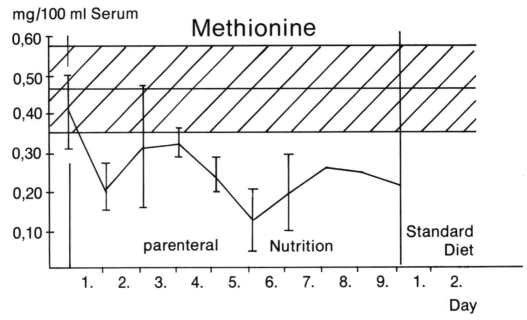

Fig 3. Plasma level of methionine after infusion of an amino acid mixture with low methionine content demonstrating the usefulness of the plasma pattern for measuring adequacy of an amino acid mixture.

groups, (2) studies of several synthetic amino acid mixtures on their effect on the plasma aminograms when infused into infants, and (3) the data of Holt and Snyderman[3] regarding amino acid requirements of orally fed infants.

Dr. Fekl: We nourished about 20 premature infants intravenously (the smallest weighing about 1,000 grams) with an amino acid mixture containing methionine but no cystine. The infants grew well, and the plasma cyst(e)ine levels remained in the normal range (Figures 1, 2, 3). If these infants had a need for "preformed" exogenous cyst(e)ine, the plasma level of cyst(e)ine would not have remained normal.[5]

Table 1.—Amino Acid Pattern of the Infusion Solution Used
     (Aminofusin RL 600)

	gm/liter
L-isoleucine	1.55
L-leucine	2.2
L-lysine (calc as base)	2.0
L-methionine	2.1
L-phenylalanine	2.2
L-threonine	1.0
L-tryptophan	0.45
L-valine	1.5
L-arginine (calc as base)	4.0
L-histidine (calc as base)	1.0
L-alanine	6.0
glycine	10.0
L-glutamic acid	9.0
L-proline	7.0
total N	7.6

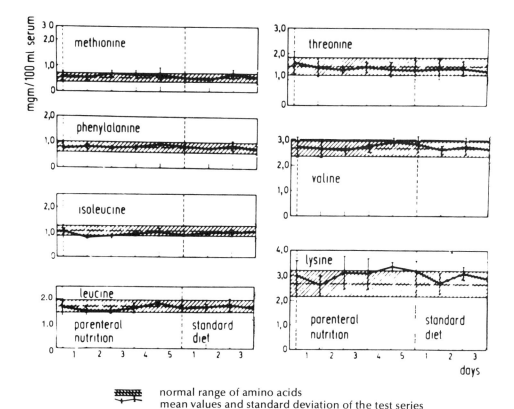

normal range of amino acids
mean values and standard deviation of the test series

Fig 4. Homeostasis of the essential plasma amino acids after infusion of Aminofusin[R] L 600.

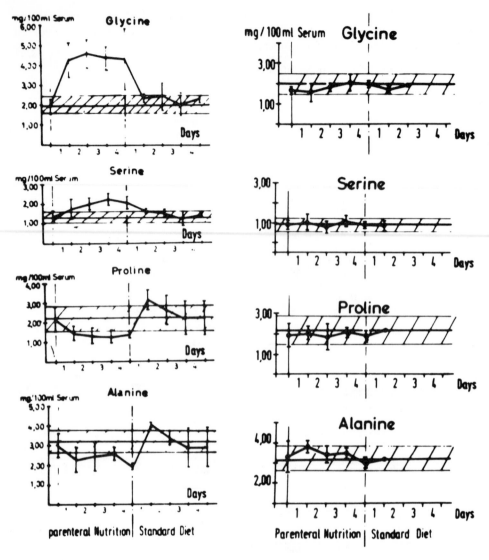

Fig 5. Disturbances in homeostasis of nonessential plasma amino acids after infusion of a mixture of essential amino acids supplemented with glycine as the sole source of nonspecific nitrogen.

Homeostasis of nonessential plasma amino acids after infusion of the same essential amino acid mixture supplemented with a proper mixture of glycine, proline, alanine, and glutamic acid as source of nonspecific nitrogen (Aminofusin[R] L 600).

If we give essential amino acids to infants or adults with a pattern adapted to their presumed requirements, along with an appropriate mixture of nonessential amino acids and an adequacy of calories, all of the essential amino acids remain in the normal range in the plasma (see Fig 4).

When we used glycine as the sole source of nonspecific nitrogen, we found an increase in plasma glycine and plasma serine; serine comes from

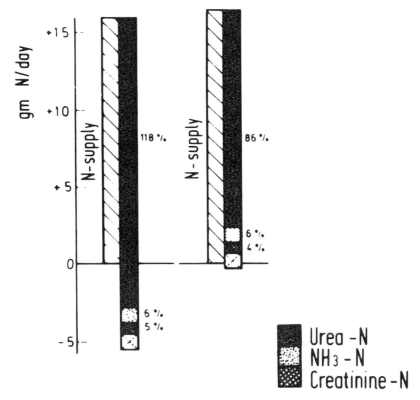

Fig 6. Left columns: Strongly negative nitrogen balance after infusion of an essential amino acid mixture supplemented with glycine as the sole source of nonspecific nitrogen.

Right columns: Equilibrated nitrogen balance by replacing glycine by a mixture of glycine, proline, alanine, and glutamic acid.

glycine metabolically (see Fig 5, Fig 6). It was interesting that there were enormous decreases in plasma proline and alanine. This may mean that proline and alanine are necessary for parenteral nutrition. We decreased the amount of administered glycine and added proline and alanine. Plasma glycine, serine, proline, and alanine remained in the normal range concomitant with a striking improvement in nitrogen balance. Additional improvement was obtained by adding glutamic acid to the infusion mixture. Glutamic acid must be limited in amount to ensure against abnormally high plasma levels of the acid, otherwise vomiting and nausea result.

The patients were in steady states in our studies, and we observed them for periods as long as four weeks. The plasma amino acid levels remained constant. We feel that more information is given by estimating the plasma amino acids in the steady state than by measurement of nitrogen balance. In Germany such studies were carried out by Dolif and Juergens,[6] also by Heller and coworkers.[7]

Dr. Levenson: Dr. Munro, the point has been made during this and other conferences that glutamic acid is a useful part of the nonessential amino acid mixture for parenteral nutrition. Nitrogen balance and maintenance of plasma amino acid levels are the criteria for judgment. You have suggested that glutamic acid and aspartic acid might be avoided for parenteral infusions. I assume you did not mean not to use glutamic acid or aspartic acid at all, but rather to limit the amounts used. As I recall, Greenstein, Winitz, and their colleagues, in studies with oral liquid amino acid diets (so-called chemically defined diets) for rats, found that proline and glutamic acid, among the nonessentials, were among the most efficacious in promoting growth of young rats.[8-18]

Dr. Munro: The gut participates extensively in the metabolism of glutamic acid and aspartic acid. In parenteral nutrition, the gut is bypassed to a large extent. Glutamic acid has been accused in a number of publications of causing mental damage, notably to young animals. On the other hand, Dr. Stegink has published, and I hope will discuss, data which indicate: (1) no evidence of mental impairment following the administration of high versus low glutamic-acid-containing protein hydrolysates to infants, and (2) relatively little effect on plasma amino acid concentrations.[19]

Nevertheless, if one is making up a mixture de novo of amino acids for infusion, I suggest that alanine would be better than glutamic acid for large quantity usage. Alanine is a major amino-nitrogen-transport mechanism for normal metabolic purposes.

Dr. Stegink: Glutamic acid has been accused of causing nausea and vomiting. I suspect that its bad reputation in parenteral administration is not well deserved and is related to high increases in the level of circulating glutamic acid, rather than to its metabolic properties. The concentration of glutamic acid in plasma is normally low, about $5\mu mol/100$ ml. Glutamine carries most of that particular carbon structure and is present normally in 60 to 80 $\mu mol/100$ ml of plasma.

When glutamic acid is ingested, some is converted to alanine. How much alanine depends on how much carbohydrate is available. One striking fact in our study of infant pigs was that the glutamic acid level in the portal blood is about 50 to 60 $\mu mol/100$ ml of plasma; upon passage through the liver, much is immediately converted to glucose and lactate as the major products and to small amounts of alpha-ketoglutarate and aspartate, with a marked drop in plasma glutamic acid levels in hepatic vein blood.

Evidence that monosodiumglutamate causes a specific neural toxicity in newborn mice is cited by Olney. This lesion can result in approximately three days. We are working on the neural toxicity but have been unable to demonstrate such a lesion in the newborn pig or in the newborn monkey. We have infused monkey fetuses in utero with high levels of glutamate and have been unable to obtain any evidence for the type of neural damage that Olney has described. [20, 21]

Dr. Law: We talked about bypassing the gut when amino acid solutions are infused and mentioned that 50% of the nitrogen in the gut is endogenous.

What are the data on parenterally administered amino acids and intraluminal makeup of amino acids? Do we have any information on how much of the amino acids infused actually bypasses the gut? The gut is certainly perfused by the infused amino acids.

Dr. Levenson: It is only the first pass-through that bypasses the gut. I don't know of any work in which anyone has attempted to determine the fate of the infused amino acids based on their appearance in the lumen of the gut.

One of the problems of getting cystine or cyst(e)ine in solution is their relatively low solubilities. In Greenstein and Winitz's original animal studies dealing with chemically defined liquid diets for oral use, cyst(e)ine ethyl ester and tyrosine ethyl ester were used for solubility reasons. The idea was that the tissue esterases would promptly hydrolyze the cyst(e)ine ethyl ester and the tyrosine ethyl ester. Hence, feeding the esters was considered to be equivalent roughly to feeding the free amino acids.

Evidence in our laboratory indicates that feeding cyst(e)ine ethyl ester as equivalent to cyst(e)ine is incorrect. The fed ester has substantially different properties from the free amino acid.[22-24]

We have reported that conventional rats develop progressive pancreatic acinar atrophy and fibrosis, azotemia and hemolytic anemia when fed certain formulations of chemically defined liquid amino acid diets. Germfree (GF) rats either do not develop the syndrome at all, or do so to a lesser extent. Our current experiments demonstrate:

> Cyst(e)ine ethyl ester (CEE) is critically involved. When it is absent, the syndrome does not develop. When it is present, the severity of the abnormalities is proportional to the amount of dietary CEE.
> Action of CEE is modified by other dietary components.
> CEE is more toxic in liquid diets than the same formulations fed in solid form.
> When cyst(e)ine hydrochloride is substituted for CEE, the syndrome does not develop.
> Monocontamination of GF rats with *Proteus spp* (saprophytes) makes them susceptible to CEE while GF rats monocontaminated with *E. coli* or bacteroides are not susceptible.
> CEE (but not cyst(e)ine hydrochloride in comparable doses) is toxic for rats, but its toxicity is conditioned by the physical state of the diet, the presence of other nutrients, and by specific intestinal bacteria.

Dr. Mohammed: To return to the use of cyst(e)ine ethyl ester, Johnson and Johnson have made formulations using both cyst(e)ine and cyst(e)ine ethyl esters. We had a problem similar to that mentioned by Dr. Levenson. When we fed cyst(e)ine ethyl ester to rats, pancreatic disorders developed resulting in fatty metamorphosis. At that point we got an increased prothrombin time, so we added menadione. We found that the menadione was inactivated by cyst(e)ine ethyl ester. Then we added menadione sodium bisulfide. The menadione sodium bisulfide was not inactivated, and we were able to bring the prothrombin times to normal. We found that technologically it was probably undesirable to include cyst(e)ine ethyl ester in the formulation. We dropped it, included methionine, and found that the methionine plus the cystine met the nutritional requirements.

Dr. Levenson: While cystine and cyst(e)ine may be similar for long-term feeding, particularly from the point of view of toxicity, cyst(e)ine has been used in few studies. In an extensive review by Harper and his colleagues,[25] the only reference to studies with cyst(e)ine is to some of their unpublished data. Studies on the use of cyst(e)ine in patients with schizophrenia are relatively short-term.[26]

EFFECT OF PROTEIN ALIMENTATION ON ACID-BASE BALANCE

Dr. Heird: I have information on the design of a pattern of amino acids for use in intravenous alimentation. This stems from observations made during the use of a synthetic formulation of amino acids (Neoaminosol). The essential amino acid pattern of this mixture is the same as that of a fibrin hydrolysate (Aminosol). The main difference between Neoaminosol and Aminosol is that peptides are missing in the former.

An acidosis was observed in five infants who were receiving Neo-aminosol.[27] Their blood pH, bicarbonate, and base excess were considerably lower than those of the infants receiving the hydrolysate. The pCO_2 of the patients receiving Neoaminosol was also somewhat lower, probably reflecting respiratory compensation. Plasma sodium and potassium concentrations were relatively normal, whereas plasma chloride concentration was universally higher in the infants receiving the synthetic amino acids. In some of the infants receiving Aminosol, serum chloride was also high, but it was matched by a simultaneous increase in concentration of plasma sodium.

The type of acidosis seen in infants receiving Neoaminosol was a hyper-chloremic metabolic acidosis. Among the possible reasons were excessive stool loss of base, excessive renal loss of base, infusion of an exogenous load of preformed acid, or an infusion of an exogenous load of potential acid.

We ruled out the first two possibilities by showing that the fecal unde-termined anion content was normal. The undetermined anion content is defined as the difference between the inorganic cations and inorganic anions, specifically the difference between sodium plus potassium plus calcium plus magnesium minus chloride plus phosphorus. Also the renal net acid excre-tion—a measure of the total renal acidification mechanism—was supernormal in most of the infants receiving Neoaminosol. Thus, neither excessive stool loss of base nor excessive renal loss of base was involved in causing the acidosis.

We then determined the titratable acidity (the amount of base required to titrate the infusion solutions) from their initial pH to pH 7.4, which occurs presumably when they are infused into the body. We also determined the cation and anion pattern of the infusates.

Examination of the inorganic cations and anionic composition of the two infusion fluids showed a greater cation gap in the synthetic amino acid mixture, whereas there is little difference in the anion gaps in the two solutions. The anion gap is caused by bicarbonate, by material metabolized to bicarbonate, or by material utilizing hydrogen ion on metabolism.

The greater cation gap in the synthetic amino acid mixture can be accounted for almost precisely by the lysine, arginine, and the small amount of histidine which are present as hydrochlorides in the synthetic amino acid mixture. Although the pH of both infusion solutions is low, the amount of preformed acid is only about one-fifth as much in the synthetic amino acid mixture as in the fibrin hydrolysate mixture. The latter when infused, does not cause acidosis, while the former does.

Dr. Stegink: The two solutions were infused in different concentrations, though: 2.5% for the Neoaminosol, and 5% for the Aminosol.

Dr. Heird: That is right, but if the Neoaminosol had been a 5% solution, the cation gap would have been that much greater than in the infused Aminosol.

We postulate that the reason for the acidosis in infants receiving Neoaminosol is related to the metabolism of the cationic amino acids. They can be catabolized to urea, carbon dioxide, and water, in which case there is a net release of hydrogen ions.

If these cationic amino acids, when incorporated into a peptide chain, retain a positive charge, the positively charged chains must be matched by negatively charged side chains. If the latter are present in the infusate (they are not in the synthetic amino acid mixture), then, of course, there would be no net acid-base effect; but if the body has to produce the negatively charged amino acids, hydrogen ion is released in the process of producing them before the organic acid anions are transaminated to the anionic amino acid.

If one reduces the amount of Neoaminosol infused from about 4 ml/kg to about 2 ml/kg, the acidosis is avoided. The acidosis can be avoided by the simultaneous administration of base, either sodium bicarbonate or sodium lactate.

This, then, is what we view as the mechanism of the acidosis following the infusion of Neoaminosol. We believe this has importance in the design of the amino acid mixture to be used in intravenous alimentation. If the cationic amino acids are used without either anionic amino acids to consume the hydrogen ion that is released on metabolism of the cationic amino acids or without some other agent (eg, an organic acid anion, such as acetate, citrate, or lactate), acidosis will result.

What I have said applies to Neoaminosol. It also is true for FreAmine but to a lesser extent, because FreAmine is titrated with acetic acid rather than hydrochloric acid. Two factors play a role: FreAmine contains fewer cationic amino acids, and part of the anion is acetate, which will consume the hydrogen ion on metabolism, presenting much less of a load of hydrogen ion. Despite this, we have observed five infants who became acidotic while receiving FreAmine.

Dr. Munro: Lysine accumulates in muscle in proportion to the dietary level. As you increase lysine intake the blood level rises, but muscle lysine rises quite out of proportion. Something like 80% of body lysine is present in muscle as compared with 40% to 50% of most other amino acids, probably because lysine replaces potassium as the cation in muscle.

One wonders, therefore, whether there is a corresponding urinary excretion of potassium after infusion with lysine.

Since the infant is deficient in muscle mass—he has only 25% as against 45% in the adult human subject—does this account to some extent for the inability of the infant to deal with loads of cationic amino acids which may be stored in muscular tissue?

Dr. Heird: The increase of potassium in the urine of infants receiving Neoaminosol is not large. I understand that adults also develop acidosis when receiving this amino acid mixture.

PROBLEMS OF PATIENTS WITH LIVER DISEASE

Dr. Law: I come seeking light, not shedding it. Our group at the University of New Mexico is interested in patients with liver disease because we see so many of them. In searching the literature, the patterns of plasma amino acid abnormalities that are found in patients with liver disease have been confusing to us and not consistent as reported. Plasma amino acid abnormalities are not clearly correlated with the clinical state of the patient, the type of liver disease, and the severity of the disease.

These patients are generally protein-starved, muscle-wasted, yet protein-intolerant. Prescription of utilizable nitrogen in the forms currently given is contraindicated. We would like to find an amino acid pattern of an infusate solution that would be acceptable and useful to people with severe liver disease.

We have compared the plasma amino acid levels—determined by ion exchange column chromatography—of a group of 11 male patients with severe alcoholic liver disease and jaundice with the plasma amino acid levels of a control group of faculty and house staff of similar age range, somewhat less alcoholic, and better nourished. Three of the 11 patients have died, three have been hospitalized for six months, and the other five are outpatients.

We have found significant diminution in plasma levels of alanine, valine, isoleucine, leucine, tryptophan, and lysine. The branched-chain amino acid levels seem to be lowest in the patients who are sickest. A clinical correlation exists among serum bilirubin levels, serum albumin levels, prothrombin times, and other measures of liver function. We plan to test the tolerance of such patients to infusions of various amino acids, measuring urinary amino acid losses and the ability of the infusion to bring the plasma amino acids to more normal levels. The effects of the infusions on the clinical courses of the patients will be observed. We recognize that development of a utilizable nitrogen source with minimal adverse side effects for people with severe liver disease will be a long and difficult task.

Dr. Munro: Iber has published information relevant to formulation of amino acid solutions for cirrhotic subjects.[28] He found, as I recollect, that the tolerance for the branched-chain amino acids was increased so that when one injected a test dose, the rate of removal by muscle was accelerated.

This means, in teleological terms, that the liver is no longer doing its job of guarding the body against intake of various nutrients. The enzymes in skeletal muscle concerned with the metabolism of those amino acids (ie, the branched-chain amino acids), which are catabolized largely in muscle, have adapted to the bigger load being imposed on them because of the metabolic failure of the liver. Other data in the literature also enable one to predict what sort of utilization of infused amino acids one can expect under these conditions.[29]

HYPERAMMONIEMIA

Dr. Stegink: Hyperammoniemia has been reported in the pediatric literature in patients receiving protein hydrolysates parenterally. The hyperammoniemia is an inevitability in view of the lability of glutamine and asparagine.

Dr. Dudrick: We have not seen hyperammoniemia in children, although we measured blood ammonia a few times during the course of infusions of protein hydrolysates. We did not make a point of measuring blood ammonia regularly, such as every other day, nor did we note any clinical syndrome or abnormal liver function test to indicate that the blood ammonia level might be awry. We knew that a significant proportion of the nitrogen in the hydrolysates might be in the form of ammonia. By spot checks of hydrolysates of different lots, we found a great variability in ammonia levels. This was confirmed by people who are knowledgeable about hydrolysate manufacture. The variability of ammonia levels in the lots was within a range that has not given problems when infused into adults.

We have not had hyperammoniemia problems in adults and we have reported using up to 3 liters/day of fibrin hydrolysate in a patient who had a serum ammonia concentration of 3.5 μg/ml at the start of the period of infusions. His serum ammonia level came down during the infusions. When we tried to feed him orally with about 40 gm/day of protein equivalent, his serum ammonia rose again, and he developed signs of encephalopathy.

We also watched the serum ammonia level come down in a patient who had rather severe hepatitis while on 3 liter/day of a protein hydrolysate infusion. But this will not always be the case. If one is caring for a chronic, poorly compensated, or virtually decompensated cirrhotic patient, I can guarantee that if hydrolysate is infused in substantial amounts, blood ammonia will rise.

Negligible amounts of ammonia were found in the crystalline amino acid solutions we tested. We are more worried about their chloride and hydrochloride content and have asked that acetates be used instead.

AMINO ACID MIXTURES

Dr. Levenson: Dr. Munro suggests that the requirements for amino acids of the adult who is sick, injured, or already malnourished are closer to those of the young growing child than to those of the healthy adult. It is implicit, then, that the proportion of nonessential amino acids to essential amino acids be reduced by a factor of two; Dr. Munro gave a figure for the infant of roughly 40% of essential amino acids as against 19% for the healthy adult (see p 65).

Is there agreement that this is a reasonable speculation, Dr. Munro?

Dr. Munro: It is a speculation supported by studies on adult rats which were depleted by dietary deprivation, then repleted by Cannon et al.[30-32] The requirements for repletion of such rats for essential amino acids were increased to be similar to those of young animals.

Dr. Fekl: The ratio of essential to nonessential amino acids is often misused. We need specific amounts of essential amino acids for specific metabolic purposes. Essential amino acids are not a good source of nonessential nitrogen, so we supplement the essential amino acids with nonessential amino acids. May we discuss what nonessential amino acids we should use and in what amounts? One view is that the ratio should be as high as in protein of high biological value, but that is not necessarily true. Snyderman has shown that for the infant nonessential nitrogen is a limiting factor in human milk.[33] Juergens and Dolif[34], also Scrimshaw and coworkers[35] have shown, that one can dilute proteins of high biological value to a low essential: nonessential amino acid ratio. Scrimshaw diluted egg protein approximately 1.5 times and found it satisfactory.

Dr. Munro: The dilution study was carried out by Scrimshaw on young adult students. The dilution by the New York University group, Holt and Snyderman, achieved something like 20% dilution for feeding infants. It was not a large dilution. The basic question is whether the surprisingly low proportion—19% of essential amino acids for the healthy adult—applies to people who must be repleted. Cannon and his colleagues studied this question in the late 1940s.[30-32] They found that the repleting rat—the adult rat which had been depleted by food deprivation and was making tissue again—required the type of amino acid pattern of the young animal. These findings suggest that the human subject who is recovering from injury or from illness requires a large proportion of essential amino acids.

Dr. Levenson: Do we have any concrete data on nonessential to essential amino acid ratio(s) desirable for the types of adult sick or injured patients we have been considering?

Dr. Stegink: Some hazards are encountered in applying the results of oral alimentation studies to parenteral alimentation. This represents an area of difficulty, especially as we gain greater knowledge of the role of the gut in amino acid and protein metabolism. We ought to look at the mixture of amino acids released from the liver of patients on oral feedings, since that is the mixture which is nourishing the rest of the body.

Fürst, Josephson, and Vinnars studied the effects of different ratios of essential to nonessential amino acids in normal adults.[36] No change in nitrogen balance was observed within a considerable range of such ratios. To me, this indicates no adverse effects from going to a higher level of essential amino acids for the adult who is ill compared with the healthy adult.

Dr. Fekl: We have worked in Europe for about 15 years with amino acid mixtures and can make better solutions with amino acids than with the hydrolysates. We do not believe we have the optimal mixtures yet but feel we can improve them, based on careful clinical investigation.

Dr. Levenson: Could you summarize what you think is a good mixture for injured, ill, or malnourished adult patients?

Dr. Fekl: *First,* we must have the eight essential amino acids. Dr. Munro's figures for essential amino acid requirements are good (see p 66). We support his proposal that they be increased by about 30% to meet the requirements of sick patients. The requirements were shown in different studies: Hegsted, Rose, and the FAO provisional patterns. [37, 38, 39] These are similar, and are superior to the pattern of fibrin or casein. We make amino acid solutions for adults and different ones for infants and children. For these, our figures for essential amino acids are those of my coworkers. We believe histidine and arginine must be added for both adults and children. Arginine has an important role, especially in parenteral nutrition, for the detoxification of ammonia. *Finally,* we must have enough of the nonessential amino acids. We know that glycine, for example, is not a good source of nonessential nitrogen. We must use alanine and proline. When these are used, better nitrogen balance is obtained. We also add glutamic acid and others. If we have adequate glycine in the infusate, we don't need to include serine.

The optimal relative amounts of these various amino acids are still in discussion, but we propose that the ratio of nonessential to essential amino acids be about 1 to 2 for adults. We are aware that this may not be optimal, but, if we make a solution in that range, we know it is better than available protein hydrolysates.

Use of amino acids offers the possibility of making specific formulations to meet specific requirements and the solution can be altered as our knowledge grows.

Other limiting factors to be considered are the caloric requirement and source, minerals, and vitamins. By supplying them all together, we can have a good parenteral solution which really works.

Dr. Levenson: Dr. Fekl, your statement that we can formulate an amino acid mixture which may be preferable to a mixture of amino acids that is preformed, say, in a casein or fibrin hydrolysate, seems to be based principally on nitrogen balance studies. That may not be a sufficient criterion. There may be others more subtle—and in the long run more important—than whether or not the efficiency of the infusate is 25%, 20%, or 30% from the point of view of nitrogen balance.

Dr. Wretlind: It is hard to tell what combination of amino acids is the optimal one for intravenous nutrition. The composition of some European commercial amino acid preparations for intravenous nutrition and the aminogram of egg protein are shown in Table 2. The relation between the essential amino acids in the amino acid mixtures seems to follow more or less the amino acid pattern found in egg protein. It is also about the same as the relation between the requirements of the essential amino acids found by Rose in nitrogen balance investigations of healthy men.[40]

We have investigated amino acid mixtures in dogs, studying the effect on nitrogen balance of various amino acid solutions. The dogs (Beagles) were given total, complete intravenous nutrition including fat (Intralipid) for periods of four to ten weeks. The intravenous solutions were administered during a period of five to seven hours daily, giving the infusions through a catheter in the superior vena cava. The dogs received complete intravenous nutrition during a two-week adaptation period prior to the commencement of the reported experimental periods. The amino acid solutions, included in Table 1, were administered to four dogs during separate experimental periods of seven days each.

The solutions were (1) a complete amino acid preparation containing the essential amino acids of egg protein, approximately, as well as the nonessential amino acids of egg protein and casein (Vamin); (2) a complete amino acid mixture with addition of asparagine and glutamine, but with a lower content of essential amino acids than egg protein (Aminonorm); (3) a mixture of essential amino acids in minimal amounts, plus arginine and histidine with a high glycine content (Intramin); (4) a mixture containing a higher concentration of essential amino acids than Intramin and a relatively large amount of glycine (Intramin Novum); (5) a preparation with a high content of essential amino acids and only small amounts of arginine, histidine, and glycine (Sohamin); and (6) a solution containing the essential amino acids and six nonessential amino acids (Aminofusin). Of the total supply of energy, 80% to 90% was derived from fats. The quantity of amino acids supplied corresponded on the average of 140 mg to 180 mg of nitrogen per kg per day.

The results from 2 to 34 weekly test periods are summarized in Figure 7. The nitrogen balance was positive and approximately the same with Vamin as with Aminonorm. These solutions contain both the essential and the nonessential amino acids present in proteins with high biological value. A positive nitrogen balance was also obtained with Sohamin, which consists mainly of essential amino acids (Table 2). Intramin and Intramin Novum gave negative nitrogen balances in this test system.

Investigation with the enzymatic casein hydrolysate, Aminosol-Vitrum (Table 2), proved in dogs that positive nitrogen balance could be obtained. Utilization seems to be somewhat less than with the complete intravenous crystalline amino acid preparations.

The explanation for the differences observed in utilization of the various types of amino acid solutions may be that certain of the nonessential amino acids are not present in some of the solutions. The degree of utilization may depend also on variations in the concentration of the essential amino acids in the solutions, which might be measured as the ratio of essential amino acids to total nitrogen in the mixture (E/T). During growth, the best results seem to be obtained when the E/T ratio is about the same as in body protein.

Table 2.—Amino Acid Contents in Egg Protein and Some Amino Acid Preparations

L-Amino Acids	Egg-protein g	Aminosol Vitrum* g	Amino-fusin† g	Amino-norm‡ g	Intramin§ g	Intramin novum§ g	Sohamin** g	Vamin* g
				Amount of Amino Acids in grams per 16 Grams of Nitrogen				
Isoleucine	6.6	7.3	2.5	2.6	2.5	4.0	8.1	6.6
Leucine	8.8	11.4	4.4	4.5	4.0	6.2	12.2	9.0
Lysine	6.4	7.4	3.6	7.2	2.9	4.5	18.7	6.6
Aromatic amino acids	10.0	6.9	4.0	4.7	4.0	6.2	11.7	10.2
Sulphur-containing amino acids	5.5	4.5	4.4	4.5	4.0	6.2	8.3	5.6
Threonine	5.1	4.4	1.8	4.1	1.8	2.8	8.6	5.1
Tryptophan	1.6	1.1	0.9	2.4	0.9	1.4	3.7	1.7
Valine	7.3	2.9	2.9	5.9	2.9	4.5	7.8	7.3
E = total amount of essential amino acids per 16 g total nitrogen (T)	51.3	48.2	24.5	35.8	23.0	35.8	79.1	52.1
Alanine	7.4	2.9	23.6	9.4				5.1
Arginine	6.1	2.9	11.8	5.0	4.0	6.2	11.0	5.6
Asparagine				2.6				
Aspartic acid	9.0	6.0		0.8				7.0
Glutamic acid	16.0	22.7		4.3				15.3
Glutamine				19.6				
Glycine	3.6	2.2	22.7	4.9	61.7	48.1	7.3	3.6
Histidine	2.4	2.6	2.7	4.4	2.0	3.1	4.2	4.1
Ornithine				2.4				
Proline	8.1	9.4	5.5	5.2				13.8
Serine	8.5	7.5		2.0				12.8
E/T ratio	3.2	3.0	1.5	2.24	1.44	2.2	4.9	3.2
E in per cent of total amino acids	46	46	27	38	25	38	78	44

Note: The amino acid values are given in grams per 16 g total nitrogen (T) of the protein or of the amino acid mixtures.

*Vitrum, Stockholm, Sweden
†J. Pfrimmer, Erlangen, Germany
‡B. Braun, Melsungen, Germany
§Astra, Södertälje, Sweden
**Tanabe, Seijaku Co., Osaka, Japan

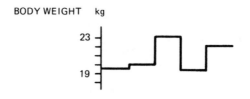

BODY WEIGHT kg

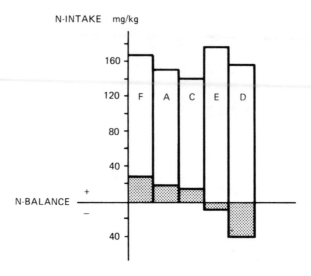

N-INTAKE mg/kg

N-BALANCE

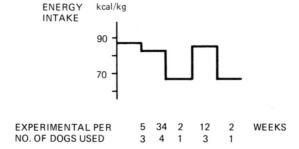

ENERGY kcal/kg
INTAKE

| EXPERIMENTAL PER | 5 | 34 | 2 | 12 | 2 | WEEKS |
| NO. OF DOGS USED | 3 | 4 | 1 | 3 | 1 | |

Fig 7. Effect on nitrogen balance of various amino acid preparations in beagles on complete intravenous nutrition. Each
test period covered one week. The figure shows the average
nitrogen intakes and nitrogen balances of all the tests performed with the five different amino acid preparations (Table 2).
A indicates Vamin; C, Aminonorm; D, Intramin; E, Intramin
novum; F, Sohamin. From the upper part of the columns down-
wards the nitrogen losses via urine and feces are marked. The
number of the test periods for each amino acid preparation is
given in the lower part of the diagram.

We investigated—in dogs on complete intravenous nutrition—the effects of amino acid mixtures with E/T ratios (grams of essential amino acid per one gram of total nitrogen) of 1, 2, 3, 4, and 5 (corresponding to 14%, 27%, 44%, 53%, and 66% essential amino acids of the amino acid total). The highest positive nitrogen balance observed was with amino acid mixtures having an E/T ratio of 3 to 5 containing 44% to 66% essential amino acids (Fig 8).

Seeking general background information, we took some of the amino acid mixtures shown in Table 2 and tested them in rats in the way oral proteins are tested to determine the protein efficiency ratio (PER, the weight gain of the growing animal divided by its protein intake) or nitrogen efficiency ratio (NER, the weight gained per gram nitrogen consumed). The content of nitrogen in the diets tested was 1.6%, corresponding to 10% protein.

During the 28-day test, growth of the rats receiving the complete amino acid mixture (Vamin) was the same as with an amino acid mixture having the amino acid pattern of egg protein. The NER value for Vamin was 22.7. The Sohamin preparation gave a NER value of 14.2. With Intramin Novum and Aminofusin, NER values of 9.1 and 0.3 were obtained respectively. Trophysan gave a reduction in body weight, because it lacks histidine, essential for rats.

When organs of the rats were weighed, we didn't observe the normal size of spleen with any of the amino acid mixtures tested. Probably the mixtures don't do the same job as the oral protein the rats normally get. The thymus practically disappeared when the rats were given an amino acid preparation without histidine. By this means, it might be possible to change the immunological reactivity of the animal. The thymus weight was normal only with a complete amino acid preparation. When the rat was given an amino acid preparation that did not promote good growth, an increase of the relative weight of the kidneys was noted.

The investigations in dogs and rats may not be directly transferable to man. But it is my opinion that an amino acid mixture intended for intravenous use in patients should—as a minimal requirement—produce the normal weight increases in rats that are anticipated from high quality protein or amino acid mixtures fed orally. One would not feed a protein to man unless it were possible to produce normal growth in rats with it. Thus, before a parenteral amino acid preparation is tested in man, it should be proved that the growth it produces in rats is about as good as that possible with oral feeding; also that it produces the positive nitrogen balance achieved in dogs through oral feedings.

Johnston of Newcastle on Tyne has made a similar investigation in man in postoperative periods.[41] During the first three postoperative days, he gave patients a complete intravenous feeding, including fat emulsion. He had five groups of six patients each. One group did not receive any amino acid preparation. Each of the other four groups received one of the following: Vamin, Aminosol, Aminofusin, or Trophysan. Nitrogen balances were performed. Johnston found that best utilization was obtained with Vamin and Aminosol. These observations accord with the results in dogs and rats.

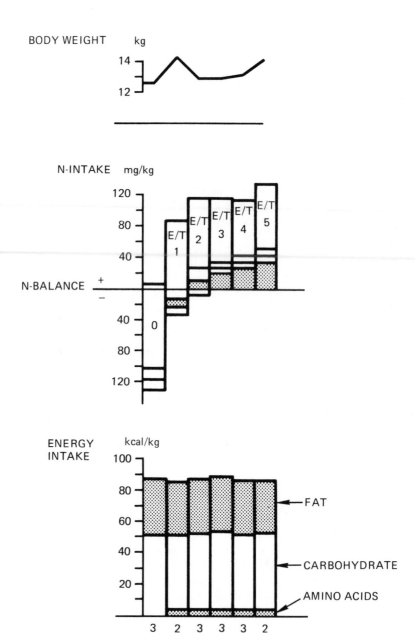

Fig 8. Nitrogen balance in beagles with amino acid mixtures of various E to T ratios. The dogs received complete intravenous feeding. Each period covered one week. During the first week the dogs received no amino acids, indicated in the column with "O." In the following periods amino acid solutions with an E/T ratio of 1, 2, 3, 4, or 5 were given. Solutions were prepared by mixing a solution of essential amino acids with a solution of nonessential amino acids.

SOLUTIONS

Essential amino acids		Nonessential amino acids	
Amount in mg/100 ml	Amino acid	Amount in mg/100 ml	Amino acid
240	L-histidine	300	L-alanine
390	L-isoleucine	330	L-arginine
525	L-leucine	405	L-aspartic acid
385	L-lysine	140	L-cysteine
545	L-phenylalanine	900	L-glutamic acid
300	L-threonine	210	glycine
100	L-tryptophan	810	L-proline
425	L-valine	750	L-serine
		50	L-tyrosine

From the upper part of the columns downward the nitrogen losses via urine and feces are marked. The horizontal heavy lines represent the average nitrogen balances, and the thinner horizontal lines indicate the daily variation of nitrogen balances during the period.

My opinion about intravenous amino acid preparations may be summarized as follows:

All studies concerning the utilization of amino acid mixtures indicate that an optimal amino acid preparation for intravenous nutrition should contain the essential as well as the nonessential amino acids in L-form and in the same proportions as found in the aminogram of egg protein or other proteins of high biological value.

The essential amino acids should provide about 45% to 50% of the total amino acids corresponding to an E/T ratio of 3 approximately.

A high content of glycine should be avoided.

Such a product should correspond to the nutritional quality requirements for a complete protein given orally.

An advantage of crystalline amino acid mixtures is that their composition can be altered readily, as results from new investigations indicate. Possibly we should reduce the contents of some amino acids as Dr. Munro and Dr. Fekl have suggested (eg, glutamic and aspartic acids) and exchange them for alanine. In this way, we might end up with better products than those we are now using; but all results indicate that the present formulations work.

The basal requirements for amino acids in mixtures of high biological value have been investigated with studies of total parenteral nutrition (TPN) in man. In one case (Vamin was used) the minimum daily quantity for positive nitrogen balance was found to be 80 mg N or 0.6 gm amino acids/kg of body weight per day. From results of various investigations, a daily amino acid allowance of more than 90 mg N or 0.7 gm amino acids/kg could be recommended for adults. This quantity exceeds the protein supply (calculated as protein with a net protein utilization [NPU] value of 100%) which one gets with a British or Swedish average national diet of 1,500 to 2,000 kcal/day.

Dr. Levenson: Dr. Wretlind, you said you did not demonstrate any significant advantage or disadvantage of protein hydrolysate versus a mixture of free amino acids.

Dr. Wretlind: Yes, that is correct. Johnston claims that the protein hydrolysates do exactly the same job as a complete crystalline amino acid mixture. Even though I was one of the first to use protein hydrolysates, I prefer to work with a crystalline amino acid mixture instead of a protein hydrolysate.

Dr. Levenson: Is your view a hunch, then, not really based on solid data?

Dr. Wretlind: That is right.

Dr. Munro: Were the dogs you used, Dr. Wretlind, growing or adult? Second, what was the E/T ratio? You had 1, 2, 3, 4, 5. What were the absolute values of these ratios? In other words, what were 1 and 2?

Dr. Wretlind: An E/T ratio (grams of essential amino acids per one gram of total nitrogen of the mixture) of 3 corresponds to about 50% essential amino acids and 50% nonessential amino acids. The ages of the dogs in most studies were 1 to 1.5 years of age. They were in good health. We have studied malnourished dogs several times, but the results are hard to deal with because it is easy to get a positive nitrogen balance in a depleted animal. You don't get such pronounced changes among different amino acid mixtures.

Dr. Levenson: Dr. Munro, you said that the biologic value of the protein made relatively little difference, at least in terms of nitrogen balance requirements for adults. In other words, it took about the same amount of casein, the same amount of egg protein to achieve nitrogen equilibrium in adults. Were you referring to healthy adults?

If we adopt one of our earlier premises—that nutritionally depleted adults, including those depleted consequent to severe injury or illness, have requirements close to those of the growing child or infant—the biologic value of the protein should make a difference.

How did others who have been working with mixtures of L-amino acids decide what mixtures to use?

Dr. Yoshimura: In our FreAmine solution, we adjusted the A/E ratio for each essential amino acid. We adjusted it such that the A/E ratio simulates that of whole egg.

In addition to that, we adjusted the E/T value to simulate egg, that is, 3 to 2.

Directions for use of protein hydrolysates included a recommendation to avoid fast infusion, thus eliminating certain untoward reactions, such as nausea and vomiting. Glutamic acid and aspartic acid were implicated in leading to nausea or vomiting, so we eliminated them.

Dr. Levenson: Therapy in the United States—using glucose as the major caloric source and not fat—precludes rapid infusion of amino acid-glucose solutions.

Dr. Fekl: In studies with man and with dogs, we found striking differences among different amino acid preparations (Fig 9, Fig 10). The worst formulation was a special amino acid solution adapted to the plasma amino acid pattern. We need recommendations and control. One preparation on the European market contains no tryptophan. We had a serious negative nitrogen

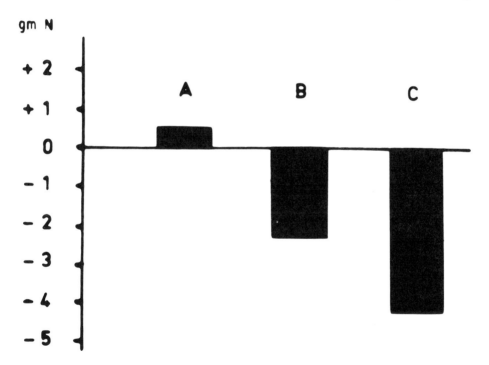

Fig 9. Average values of 4 healthy adults in each group:
   A—Amino acid composition according to the ROSE formula (Aminofusin L 600).
   B—Amino acid composition according to plasma pattern (Aminonorm).
   C—Casein hydrolysate (Aminosol).

Nitrogen balances with different amino acid solutions.

Pre-period: 3 days, 10 g N orally

Test period: 1 day, 10 g N parenterally

Total caloric supply daily: 2400 calories

116

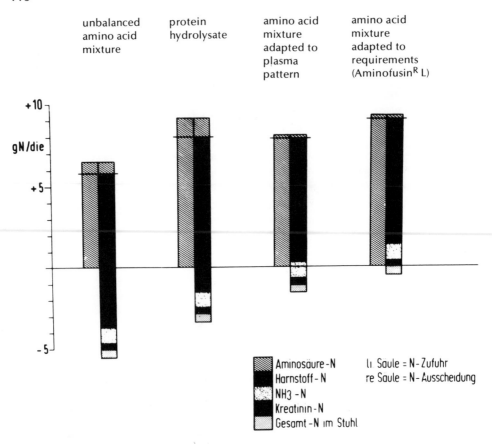

Fig 10. Nitrogen balances after various amino acid solutions.

balance with it. Aminoplasma was the preparation Dr. Wretlind mentioned as Aminonorm. It is a balanced amino acid preparation. Better nitrogen balance followed its use.

The data show that we can formulate amino acid mixtures which yield good clinical results. We are not satisfied. We want to improve. One goes step by step. If glycine is the only source of nonessential nitrogen, nitrogen balance is negative. We showed that alanine and proline are nearly essential— or let us say semiessential—in mixtures for parenteral nutrition.

Dr. Levenson: Our group holds this consensus on the composition of amino acid or hydrolysate preparations for the nutritionally depleted patient or for the patient who may be becoming depleted because of serious injury or illness: The proportion of essential amino acids to nonessential amino acids should be greater than that required to maintain the healthy adult in a steady state and nitrogen equilibrium. The danger of an excess of essential amino acids is related to the question of amino acid toxicity. Certain of the essential amino acids, particularly methionine, are the most toxic of the amino acids. It would seem that a reasonable proportion of essential amino acids would be fairly close to what Dr. Munro proposed, about 40% of the amino acid total. What did the group at the Belmont Conference recommend as the ratio of essential to nonessential amino acids for children?

Dr. Stegink: It was close to Dr. Munro's figure, which matches the amino acid concentration in the fluids available to the fetus. It also matches the figure we derived through clinical experience. We were measuring what may be an inadequate parameter, the response of plasma aminograms to different intravenous preparations of known amino acid composition.

Dr. Levenson: We have a general consensus on this point. This does not mean that it is right, but at least it reflects our present state of knowledge.

CALORIE-NITROGEN RATIO

Dr. Levenson: Dr. Kinney raised the question of the calorie-nitrogen ratio. What should the ratio of total calories to nitrogen intake be? Dr. Kinney reported that his studies suggested a ratio of about 100 kcal/gm N (see p 87). By calculation, this corresponds closely to data we obtained from studies of patients with extensive burns.[42] This relatively high nitrogen "requirement" may be a reflection, in part, of a general finding that, within a broad range, the greater the proportion of calories from protein, the better the growth of the animal and the better the deposition of body protein. Similarly, Cannon and his associates showed that, on a fixed protein intake, growth of rats was faster with higher caloric intake, within a fairly wide range.

I suspect that, at our present stage of knowledge of the metabolic reaction to injury, we are not feeding patients optimally, either by mouth or by vein. We may be feeding them satisfactorily, but not optimally.

Dr. Dudrick: The calorie-nitrogen ratio is a variable one. You may have a calorie-nitrogen ratio that is optimal for a growing baby. It can be standardized because most babies grow in a similar way. In the seriously ill and injured patient it is likely that a calorie-nitrogen ratio may be optimal for one patient but not for another. For some patients a calorie-nitrogen ratio of 100 to 1 may be desirable; but if the patient is severely burned and is fed with a parenteral mixture supplying a C/N ratio of 100 kcal/gm N, difficulties will ensue. This patient is burning up relatively much more than that. If he receives in a C/N ratio of 100 to 1 all of the calories he needs, he will be overwhelmed with nitrogen. He will have elevated blood urea nitrogens of 40, 50, 60 mg/100 ml of blood. Also, he won't look well; he is ill; he has GI symptoms. I would not advocate elevation of a metabolite which the patient has shown a lack of capacity to excrete.

Dr. Weston: In your study did you increase the nitrogen intake and leave the calories constant?

Dr. Dudrick: Yes. If a patient with burns receives 4,000 or 5,000 kilocalories daily through intravenous alimentation of a solution with a calorie-nitrogen ratio of about 120 to 150 kcal/gm N, his protein intake will be the equivalent perhaps of 150 to 200 gm of protein.

Dr. Weston: What if you kept the patient on a daily intake of 200 gm of protein and increased calories beyond 5,000 daily?

Dr. Dudrick: We have not been that fortunate. I don't know what would happen to the BUN or the patient. We studied patients who were fairly stable at an intake of 3,000 kilocalories intravenously. They had a disease process—regional enteritis—which had progressed beyond the acute phase. The inflammatory process cooled when their bowel was put at rest by feeding them parenterally. Two or three weeks later, when they no longer had fever and their diarrhea had subsided and they were fairly stable clinically, we maintained them at daily intakes of about 3,000 kilocalories and varied the nitrogen intake. The point after which there was no further increase in nitrogen balance positivity was a ratio of about 150 kcal/gm N.

Dr. Kinney has talked about ratios of 80 to 100 to 1. I believe his data are extracted from measurements of expenditures rather than replacement. Is that correct, Dr. Kinney?

Dr. Kinney: Yes.

Dr. Dudrick: There may be a subtle difference reflecting the techniques of arriving at the optimal calorie-nitrogen ratio. Dr. Kinney derives his data from showing what the organism is using as it is breaking down proteins and excreting nitrogen. I am talking about building proteins. There may be a subtle difference. We cannot say today that we are going to make all IV solutions at 80, 100, or 150 kcal/gm N. Different situations will require different ratios. It is simple to change the C/N ratio of the infusion fluid by varying the amount of concentrated sugar one adds to the amino acids. One will probably want to change the ratio during the clinical course of the patient. That is what we do. We watch the patient's course and the nitrogen balance and adapt the solutions we use accordingly.

Dr. Levenson: Dr. Dudrick used glucose as the main source of calories. The optimal C/N ratio may differ if fat is used. Dr. Dudrick's estimate is based on the intravenous route also. On an oral intake providing a C/N ratio of 100 to 1, patients with burns don't have the difficulties Dr. Dudrick described when such ratios are given intravenously. When fed orally, the patients were getting at least 50% of their calories from fat. The situations are not directly comparable.

Dr. Kinney: I agree with Dr. Dudrick about having a range of calorie-nitrogen ratios. How high did you go, Dr. Dudrick, and still find it effective by the intravenous route?

Dr. Dudrick: We have not gone higher than about 200 to 1 or 250 to 1 with positive nitrogen balance. When we went about 250 kcal/gm N, we did not find any effective positive nitrogen balance.

Dr. Curreri: The range of calorie-nitrogen intake for optimal utilization might vary, depending upon the patient and the patient's disease process. It is conceivable that we might recommend a lower calorie-nitrogen intake for the hypometabolic starved patient or the patient with chronic enterocutaneous fistula—who is efficiently using adipose tissue—than for the patient who has a high rate of metabolism, where prime defects are increased protein catabolism, negative nitrogen balance, and a negative caloric balance.

We have used C/N ratios of 250 to 1 for some patients. I don't know the best criteria for utilization; at least nitrogen balance is a useful criterion. We have found that with high caloric intakes to meet caloric expenditures as measured by following oxygen consumption continuously day after day, patients go into positive nitrogen balance.

Dr. Duke and Dr. Kinney reported that in patients with severe injury and/or sepsis and high metabolic expenditures, roughly 80% of the caloric expenditure was from fat or carbohydrate sources.[43]

Dr. Kinney: Turn it around and say that 15% to 20% of the caloric expenditure was from protein and the balance was from fat and carbohydrate, depending on what the patients were being given.

Dr. Curreri: But you would expect them to utilize the carbohydrate fairly quickly? We have given 10,000 kilocalories by combined enteral and parenteral means. The most I have given intravenously in a day (with glucose as the main caloric source) is 6,000 kilocalories. Most of the time we approximate 3,000 to 4,000 kilocalories by each route. The patients tolerate this well, but require attention. Dr. Kinney and Dr. Cahill both pointed out that the tolerance of such patients for carbohydrates is reduced, particularly if there is a septic problem in addition to the injury. Often our first sign of sepsis in the seriously injured patient is a greatly reduced tolerance for glucose. We have been able to maintain body weight over a period of eight to ten weeks in patients with extensive burns which averaged 60% of their body surface; during this time, a control paired population lost 25% of body weight. We offered this group of patients as much food as they could eat, and they received supplemental infusions of 5% glucose.

It is possible, then, to maintain weight in such patients who have a high mortality rate. I am not yet convinced of the benefits. We have demonstrated what we think are certain benefits in exchange of intracellular and extracellular ions, but we have not been able to accumulate enough data to demonstrate morbidity or mortality benefits.

Dr. Levenson: Dr. Kinney, may I ask you to clarify a point? When you spoke about increased oxygen consumption after injury, you indicated that the liver accounted for only 50% of the increase. I would put the emphasis differently, that the liver accounted for 50% of the increase, and the rest of the body for an equal amount.

Dr. Kinney: Years ago when nonshivering thermogenesis was discussed, it was thought that possibly the major contribution came from metabolic processes in the liver. Deamination and urea synthesis and gluconeogenesis all take place in the liver, supporting this suggestion. If this is heat associated with extra oxygen consumption of any major degree, one should be able to define it by measuring oxygen consumption across the splanchnic bed.

The experiments I reported reflected the metabolic processes of the entire splanchnic bed, not just the liver. Nonetheless, they indicate that probably about half of the extra oxygen consumption and heat production in patients with sepsis—at least in the 15 patients we studied—occurred in tissues other than the liver.

Dr. Carlo: Dr. Munro, concerning the variation in caloric requirements, we consider that 50 kilocalories are necessary normally to assimilate 1 gm N. If the individual takes in 10 gm N as protein, 500 kilocalories will be required. In some diseased states, patients may need 150 kilocalories/gm N. Why this difference? To synthesize the same amount of protein should require the same amount of energy in health or disease. Therefore, if there is a difference in caloric requirement, it is possibly because a lot of these calories go somewhere else and are utilized first before they are available for protein synthesis.

Dr. Munro: I am flattered that you have mistaken me for Dr. Kinney, who was speaking about calorie-nitrogen ratios. The relationship of calories to nitrogen is purely empirical, resulting from studies in animals and patients. The biosynthesis of protein requires three peptide bonds. ATP is required in the activation of amino acids with TRNA. GTP becomes GDP on attachment to the ribosome, and translocation to that position requires another breakdown of GTP to GDP. This amount of energy is nothing like the equivalent of energy required for growth where protein deposition occurs. Approximately 27 kilocalories are required for each gram of protein laid down in the growing animal. No one has satisfactorily explained the relationship of caloric requirements during growth. Various theoretical attempts have been made, none of which convinces me at the moment.

The second problem you raise is why the calorie-nitrogen ratio should differ under a variety of circumstances. As I understood Dr. Kinney, this depends upon the effect of the particular disease process on accelerating energy loss from the body, as in the form of evaporation in patients with burns. This demands a higher calorie intake. I think Dr. Kinney can elaborate better than I on this complex story.

Dr. Levenson: Dr. Munro, you said that 27 kilocalories were required per gram of protein synthesis for growth.

Dr. Munro: Yes.

Dr. Levenson: Multiplying 27 kilocalories by about 6.25 (to relate it to nitrogen) comes to about 170. This figure is close to the 150 to 1 calorie-nitrogen ratio that Dr. Dudrick was talking about in relation to positive nitrogen balance in adults who were being repleted. Dr. Kinney's data and our data suggest—at least for oral as opposed to parenteral feeding—that you do somewhat better at a lower calorie-nitrogen ratio, namely 100 to 1 in severely injured adults. Injured children don't present the same problem in excessive requirements. [44, 45]

Dr. Kinney: Dr. Munro, in the presence of widespread infection, where presumably certain steps in protein synthesis may be either inhibited or made more difficult, could there be a situation where a higher level of amino acids would tend to move in the direction of protein synthesis just by mass action?

Dr. Munro: It might facilitate the rate of protein synthesis. This is something in which I am considerably interested. I have no doubt that normally the supply of amino acids is the rate-limiting factor, but there are conditions under which energy supply can be limiting (eg, when you really reduce the energy available in the liver). It is conceivable that both factors operate.

The ATP level can be reduced in certain circumstances. An example is fructose administration, where you deplete ATP to make fructose-1,6-diphosphate, and the level falls.

Dr. Levenson: I would like to ask whether anyone has made measurements of heat production by the patient with severe sepsis who is hypothermic? That is the classical picture of severe gram negative sepsis, particularly in the patient with burns.

Dr. Kinney: That is in the terminal phase of sepsis.

Dr. Levenson: It depends on what you mean by terminal. It can go on for a week or more. Some patients recover. It is not necessarily irretrievably terminal. But as far as I know, the mechanism for the hypothermia has not been studied.

Dr. Kinney, is it possible (without heroic efforts) to minimize the period of negative nitrogen balance in the severely injured patient?

Wound Healing

Dr. Kinney: Surgeons have been taught that patients could not heal their wounds if they did not have adequate nutrition. This concept is a bit fallacious. We must emphasize that the patients in whom wounds literally fall apart—who don't have enough "vitality" in their wound healing processes to develop decent tensile strength—are not the patients in whom one sees the most severe negative nitrogen balance. Usually the most marked negative nitrogen balance after injury occurs in the previously well-nourished young, healthy, muscular male, the typical example being the young combat soldier in Vietnam with multiple visceral injuries. When he is operated on, despite having tremendous injury and perhaps many complications, he probably will heal his wounds to a good tensile strength. The patients in whom we have trouble with wound dehiscence usually are elderly and poorly nourished to begin with. These are the patients who do not tend to increase their urinary nitrogen excretion after injury. We have this peculiar paradox: The patient who heals his wound well is the patient who demonstrates the most derangement in terms of a negative nitrogen balance after injury. We don't really know what the negative nitrogen balance represents. I don't think we should assume that the negative nitrogen balance is bad and start out to treat it right away. But if one says it is all right to have some negative nitrogen balance, the question arises as to how much is acceptable and how much represents a threat to the patient? If one ignores increased urinary nitrogen excretion and weight loss until the patient has lost 5%, 10%, 15% of his body weight, at what point does one say, "Look, this is becoming a threat to convalescence"? I am not sure I know the answer. My philosophy is that I must try to avoid allowing my patient to lose more than 10% of body weight by ordinary or moderate means of therapy. We should attempt to prevent or, if present, treat a loss beyond 10% by hyperosmolar alimentation or supplemental nutrition.

Dr. Border: Could I agree with that and then disagree a little bit? Dr. Kinney has been presenting the problem of weight loss and its relationship to morbidity and mortality. This is an important relationship because weight loss can be measured easily.

I would disagree with equating the weight loss that follows severe sepsis and/or trauma with the weight loss that occurs with malnutrition. Animal studies indicate that organ distribution of the weight loss with starvation is different from organ distribution of weight loss following massive trauma and sepsis. I like the measurement of body weight because it can be made easily, but I am puzzled about how to interpret it. Dr. Kinney has worried about this, too, but he has not said it this way.

Dr. Dudrick: The wound healing question is a complex one. Peacock[46] says we should not be talking about wound healing, but about the phases of wound healing. Possibly the main reasons we have failure of wound healing or disruption of wounds are mechanical problems of dead space, surgical techniques that are poor, problems with muscular relaxation at closure, or postoperative distension, severe vomiting or coughing. Peacock thinks we should consider the components of wound contraction, collagen deposition, and epithelialization.

We should realize that various aspects of wound healing may be altered differently by nutritional factors in different patients. I agree with Dr. Kinney that in the average patient who is not drastically depleted wound healing is probably not affected very much. If the patients are seriously depleted nutritionally, wound healing is adversely affected.

We have been trying to study this problem in rats using colon anastomoses. We have been using the breaking strength of the anastomoses as a major index of the rate of healing.[47] In a study of rats with varying degrees of protein malnutrition induced by dietary restriction, decrease in breaking strength correlated closely with weight loss. As the percentage of weight loss increased, the strengths of the colon anastomoses at one week decreased. Serum albumin levels—not total plasma protein levels, just serum albumin levels—correlated in the same way (ie, the lower the serum albumin concentration, the lower the strength of the wounds). Measurement of only 2 of 10 or 12 parameters which correlated with diminution in breaking strength of the anastomoses suggested a range within which one can heal well. Beyond this range one finds some impairment of healing.

Dr. Levenson: When we talk about assessing wound healing in patients with our present modes of examination, we are using crude yardsticks (eg, the abdominal incision stays closed or it breaks open or a hernia develops). We may have situations in which wound healing is impaired substantially, but it would not be apparent since the wound might not break open or a hernia develop. Experimentally it is clear that very serious derangements of healing may be present without laparotomy wounds rupturing.

Wound healing is impaired in animals with severe injury (eg, burns or femoral fractures) or with infections at sites distant from the wound.[48-50] One can subject the wounds of experimental animals to biopsy, histologic and chemical observations, and measurements of breaking strength not used in our observations of healing in injured patients.

Do these experimental findings have clinical significance? We may not know until we begin using more precise criteria for assessing the rate of healing and convalescence of our patients. A much more detailed discussion of this appears in an article by Levenson.[51]

One ought not to speak of negative nitrogen balance in absolute terms only. The young, healthy, robust soldier whose leg is shot off with resultant muscular injury is going to show an enormous negative nitrogen balance, while the sick, nutritionally depleted, elderly individual with a carcinoma who has an extensive surgical procedure is going to show relatively less negative nitrogen balance. This may be large in relation to his body protein, however. We must think about the *proportionate* effects and responses.

Resistance to Infection

Dr. Kinney: Some of us have the clinical impression that the better-nourished patient resists infection better, that the therapy of hyperosmolar alimentation improves his chances of resisting infection. He survives the period of complications, but the patient without such nutritional support may go on to die from some intercurrent infection.

Dr. Levenson: Concrete data on the change in resistance of patients to infection imposed by injury is limited, particularly on the mechanism of this change. I don't know of any study in which the effect of "better" alimentation on resistance to bacterial and fungal infections has been determined objectively and unequivocally on previously well patients subjected to injury; the mechanism of this resistance especially needs further study.

Let us consider the diabetic. Surgeons and internists feel that the diabetic patient is remarkably prone to infection; yet the numbers of papers providing quantitative data on the mechanism of susceptibility to infection are few. We find data suggesting some defect in the ability of neutrophils of the diabetic patient to kill ingested bacteria. How the metabolic derangements associated with injury influence the response or the resistance of the individual to infection is an unplowed area.

Dr. Fekl: Some publications show that antibody formation is dependent upon the nutritional state of the individual.[52, 53]

Dr. Levenson: Agreed. Some studies have dealt with the induction of circulating antibodies. But in many infections the humoral antibodies are not the critical components. Alexander's studies provide evidence that in the severely burned patient the ability to ingest bacteria intracellularly is not impaired, but the ability to digest bacteria intracellularly is;[54] this seems to be analogous to the situation in the diabetic.[55] Balch found no change in the phagocytic properties of peripheral leukocytes of soldiers wounded recently.[56, 57] He also found no decrease in the rise of antibodies following injection of booster doses of tetanus toxoid into these soldiers. In a later study of a small number of patients with burns, Balch showed that the blood bactericidal capacity was greater than normal in the first few weeks following burning, but that the cellular response—especially of lymphocytes—to superficial skin trauma was decreased during this same period. Later there may be a decrease in blood bactericidal capacity in some patients. Phagocytic activity of the blood leukocytes was not impaired generally.

Dr. Weston: May I mention a serendipitous observation in support of Dr. Kinney's clinical impression? This evolved from studies of a small series of patients with acute renal tubular necrosis, particularly postoperative patients and patients with infections. The same observation has been made by others following studies of much larger series of patients.[58] When you treat such patients with a modified form of total parenteral nutrition, using a 70% dextrose solution to which about 250 cc or 2.5% of an essential amino acid solution are added, and maintain the patients with an adequacy of calories, they go into positive nitrogen balance. Their plasma potassium concentration drops, as do their plasma phosphorus and plasma magnesium levels. As their acute tubular necrosis approaches the diuretic phase, it is remarkable to see them not only healing their wounds—something they never did before, which we attribute to some peculiar uremic constituent—but their resistance to infection markedly increases. Their temperatures come down, and they respond to antibiotics, something we never saw before. Hence, we have been willing to hold off dialysis on some of them. We are seeing them heal better than they did before. We hope quantitative studies of these patients will be done on their resistance to infection under these circumstances.

Another interesting point is that these patients receive minimal amounts of essential amino acids but adequate amounts of calories. They synthesize their own nonessential amino acids, heal their wounds, and combat infection.

Dr. Border: One of our problems in trying to analyze the question of decreased susceptibility to infection is that we talk about it as though it were a general principle. Then we cite the humoral work and the white cell work to support this concept; but it is much more an organ effect than it is systemic resistance.

We studied a group of patients with fractured hips who were malnourished and would not eat. We questioned whether their pneumonias and other infectious complications were related to the protein catabolic state, even though it is relatively small in such patients. We provided hyperosmolar alimentation, but we could not show any improvement whatsoever in terms of cardiopulmonary measurements.

Since then, I have been doing the same thing with other aged malnourished patients. I shifted from studying patients with fractured hips to patients injured in automobile accidents. With active pulmonary physiotherapy—trying to do everything possible to keep the patients' lungs filled with air and to prevent atelectasis—pneumonia and pulmonary failure have been averted and the patients gained weight. Still, we keep such patients in nitrogen equilibrium, as their skeletal muscle protein mobilizes and skeletal muscle mass decreases.

A query on the relationship of the metabolic changes associated with injury and nutrition to sepsis is an organ-specific question. Ask it first about the factors involved in the lung, then ask about the factors involved in wounds.

Dr. Levenson: I am sure you meant also that one has to consider the nature of the specific infecting agent—whether it is a fungus, a bacteria, or a virus.

Dr. Border: The same thing (ie, organ specificity) can be said about catheter sepsis as a complication of intravenous hyperosmolar alimentation. If one waits until patients are severely malnourished, as is commonly done, catheter sepsis is more of a problem than if one starts early and keeps the patients from becoming malnourished.

Dr. Levenson: It would be good to have concrete data on this.

INTERMITTENT VS CONTINUOUS INFUSIONS

Dr. Levenson: Information is sparse or completely lacking, also, on the effect of continuous 24-hour infusions on various diurnal rhythms. How do such loads of nutrients infused continuously throughout the day, week after week, modify—if at all—adrenal function? Does it change the diurnal secretions of other hormones, such as growth hormone?

QUALITY CONTROL AND LABELING OF IV SOLUTIONS

Dr. Munro: Earlier I asked why the composition of certain protein hydrolysate solutions, stated on the labels of mixtures, was not replicated by investigators who submitted them to analysis. Is it possible to achieve some sort of agreement among the producers of these parenteral solutions and the users, who also are clinical investigators, regarding standard analytical procedures and some method of coordinating data?

Dr. Levenson: Perhaps you are asking what level of quality control is employed by commercial concerns manufacturing protein hydrolysates and amino acid solutions for parenteral use. I suspect that the question of the actual analysis of free amino acid composition is not a problem, particularly with the free amino acid solutions. If there is a problem with the amino acid solutions, it is probably a question of quality control. I don't mean to imply that quality control is inadequate. The problems with hydrolysates are more complex, since the degree of hydrolysis may vary among batches. Can the representatives of industry tell us something about the nature of the quality control? Also, are you aware of the sorts of differences in analyses mentioned by Dr. Munro, and have you been able to confirm them?

Dr. Yoshimura: I do not like to answer one question with another, but first let me ask the group if anyone has found the free amino acid content in FreAmine to be different from what is stated on the label? I ask this because the problem is different for the amino acid solutions than for the hydrolysates.

Dr. Levenson: You have not had any reports from investigators that their analyses of FreAmine don't check with yours?

Dr. Yoshimura: None. As far as I know, the amino acid values given on protein hydrolysate labels represent the total amino acid content: the free amino acids, also the amino acids present as peptides. In performing a free amino acid analysis on a protein hydrolysate solution without further hydrolysis, one would recover only part of what is listed on the label.

Dr. Levenson: I can't believe that it is as simple as that. I don't think an investigator would fall into that kind of trap.

Dr. Yoshimura: Let me ask the group how they analyze their hydrolysate solutions. Do you further hydrolyze the solutions before analysis? We know that the free amino acid content in the hydrolysate is lower than that indicated on the label.

Dr. Levenson: I am aware of that, but have you not had the problem of an investigator calling you and saying, "Look, I have analyzed Lot 368, and the figures I get are totally different from yours."

Dr. Yoshimura: No.

Dr. Levenson: How about other companies?

Dr. Carlo: In France we use a synthetic amino acid mixture, and the analyses are run systematically by autoanalyzer. Everyone knows the accuracy of an autoanalyzer. The composition does not vary within the theoretical range of the product, provided, of course, that all of the procedures have been accomplished adequately.

We are using an entirely computer-monitored system from the entrance of the product to the finished product. Solutions of extremely accurate and reproducible compositions result. I am sure that J. Pfrimmer & Co. in Germany is using the same method with the same accuracy.

Dr. Munro: I was raising the question primarily for protein hydrolysates. I know that Dr. Steginik has found the problem to be worth mentioning in his publications.

Dr. Stegink: We did not analyze for peptide nitrogen, as Dr. Yoshimura suggested. What the amino acid listing represented on the label was not clear. We found some amino acids present at higher levels than the labels indicated, if I recall correctly. We did this not so much to check the company's quality control, but for checking the response of patients to solutions of "known" amino acid composition.

Having analyzed a variety of batches, we can see that there is a variability of free amino acid and peptide compositions from batch to batch of protein hydrolysate. This is not surprising because of the kinetic principles of enzymic hydrolysis of such preparations. Batches of the casein hydrolysate are tested for their ability to support growth of rats.

Please correct me if I am wrong, but it is my impression that in some instances the amino acid analyses were carried out by microbiological methods. I am uncertain whether the microbiological methods used included analysis of both the free amino acids and the peptides, or whether this was a mixed response, depending on the particular amino acid studied.

Dr. Munro: Since we have already discussed the uncertainty of peptide utilization, the analytical difficulty provides another factor of variability, whether you are expressing free amino acids which are fully utilizable or peptides which are partially utilizable. Therefore, the use of protein hydrolysates adds further difficulty in trying to evaluate the results of what is being used. The free amino acid solutions, with quality control to check that they are correctly made up, provide a product with a reasonable degree of certainty and reproducibility. But in using hydrolysates, especially where the label does not indicate total or free amino acids, one is subject to some uncertainty about what the patient is getting and in interpreting metabolic data regarding utilization of the infusate.

Dr. Levenson: One specific recommendation would be for the manufacturers to indicate not only total amino nitrogen, which they do, but also the free amino acids. By difference, the rest presumably is bound amino nitrogen. Certainly there may be variation in free and bound amino acids from batch to batch of protein hydrolysate. Commercial acid hydrolysis preparations vary from 20% to 30% among those we have used for oral diets in rat studies. Does giving more detail on the label pose any special problems for the manufacturer?

Dr. Westman: No, not at all, except that sort of information is probably inadequate. To give the amino acid analysis of the free amino acids (eg, of casein hydrolysate), then the total amino nitrogen, is inadequate. If the peptide concentration is relatively significant, the pattern of what utilizable amino acids are being infused is not known, since one can't, at this point, assess the extent to which the peptides will be utilized. Therefore, I don't see what is gained. The best approach is to standardize by running an amino acid analysis of the total available amino acids, whether they are bound as peptides or whether they are free amino acids.

Dr. Levenson: How would you decide the available amount of each amino acid, including those in peptide form, since you have just indicated the inability to predict the extent to which the peptides are going to be utilized? At this stage, while we are all trying to learn more, wouldn't it be wise to have the maximum analytical information provided by the companies? The companies must analyze their preparations routinely for free and bound amino acids.

Dr. Shils, didn't you raise a question about the electrolyte content of some of these preparations?

Dr. Shils: I pointed out differences in sodium, calcium, and phosphorus content from the values on the labels as measured in my laboratory. It has varied significantly from batch to batch.

About a year or two ago, I wrote to companies that hydrolyze casein asking for information about which free amino acids were available and which were bound. I got a reply from only one of the four or five companies to which I had written. It was not particularly informative.

Dr. Levenson: We have representatives at this meeting from most of the companies in this country, and from some of the major European producers. Do you see any reasons why the information we have talked about can't be provided?

Dr. Carlo: We have analyzed some preparations of hydrolyzed casein on the autoanalyzer and have found some amino acids missing, histidine in some batches, cystine in others. In addition, Vinnars in Sweden found that the total nitrogen content of some protein hydrolysates (supposedly prepared the same way) will vary from 11 gm N to 14.8 gm N/100 gm casein hydrolyzed. With such wide variations, the manufacturer will refrain from giving data.

Dr. Levenson: Is the inference that the starting material has that range of "purity"?

Dr. Carlo: The problem is that when you start with casein, your hydrolysis cannot be totally controlled.

Dr. Levenson: Total nitrogen per gram of protein should not change that much if the protein has been relatively purified.

Dr. Carlo: These preparations are dialyzed to remove large peptides, and the amount of large peptides removed depends upon the amount of hydrolysis, which varies from batch to batch. Therefore, you may remove more nitrogen from one batch than from another.

Dr. Munro: Dr. Carlo, do the nondialyzable peptides have a random distribution of amino acids? Does the product reflect the original casein?

Dr. Carlo: No, it does not. Vinnars' analyses show that the variability among batches of protein hydrolysates is so great that some amino acids are totally lacking as free amino acids in certain preparations.

Dr. Levenson: Your information stresses the need for us, as users, to have as complete an analysis as possible of every batch, and that analysis should be listed on the label. Obviously it is much easier for the producer to make a reproducible solution starting with free amino acids than to make a reproducible protein hydrolysate solution.

Dr. Munro: We should regard the free amino acid mixture as the standard then, and the hydrolysates very much second best, unless they can be rigorously quality-controlled.

Dr. Levenson: Second best from the point of reproducibility and ease and precision of analysis, but not necessarily second best from the point of view of utilization by patients or clinical usefulness. Certainly, solutions of free amino acids are easier to control from the manufacturing point of view. Such solutions with various formulations, precisely controlled and easily reproducible, could be made and tested for usefulness, metabolically and clinically. Investigations to discern possible special metabolic and nutritional roles for peptides in parenteral alimentation might be carried out at the same time, first at the experimental animal level, later at the clinical level if the experimental evidence indicates this additional research. If and when such a peptide or complex of peptides is demonstrably useful, it could be synthesized and added to solutions in a controlled fashion.

Dr. Carlo: Vinnars also studied the utilization of peptides in a casein hydrolysate. He found that a large proportion—nearly all—of the peptides contained in that hydrolysate were utilized by healthy patients; but when patients underwent the stress of surgery, the average utilization of the peptides fell abruptly postoperatively. About 80% of the peptides were excreted. The healthy patient and the postoperative surgical patient differ in their abilities to utilize peptides. There was no differential in utilization of free amino acids.

INFUSION OF PLASMA PROTEIN

Dr. Levenson: It is unrealistic and inappropriate to neglect the use of whole protein for certain aspects of the parenteral feeding of patients. Would someone comment on the special role that infusion of whole protein may have in parenteral nutrition? The pioneering work of Elman[59] should not be forgotten.

Dr. Munro: In the late 1940s Whipple and his colleagues maintained their famous dogs in nitrogen equilibrium by infusing plasma proteins over long periods.[60] Allen and his colleagues demonstrated that puppies can grow "normally" when infused plasma is the only source of exogenous nitrogen.[61] This is undoubtedly due to the capacity of tissues to degrade these proteins, which they normally do. Also, certain tissues may depend on plasma protein degradation.[62] The kidney can degrade proteins on the way down the proximal tubule. This, presumably, is a source of amino acids for that organ.

Undoubtedly, infused plasma proteins can be used. Whether they are a practical source, I do not know. The difficulty of obtaining human plasma protein presents certain practical difficulties.

Dr. Border: We have been interested in patients with massive trauma, most of whom depend upon intravenous alimentation for some time after injury. Their serum albumin concentrations drop rapidly, even in the presence of an apparently adequate nitrogen intake. This occurs also in patients with severe sepsis. Many of our patients have serum albumins of 1.2 to 1.6 gm/100 ml of serum the day after they arrive. This continues for many weeks with ordinary intravenous alimentation (glucose and amino acids). Only by infusing serum albumin in the range of 40 gm to 70 gm/day could we maintain serum albumin concentrations of 2.5 gm to 3 gm/100 ml of serum. It is essential to maintain the serum albumin concentration at about these degrees in these patients to help reduce morbidity and mortality.

Dr. Weston: We demonstrated the marked impairment of albumin synthesis in man in the course of any type of stress, including acute illness, infection, and administration of large doses of the corticosteroids.[62] But I believe the only indications for the replacement of albumin by the administration of albumin-containing solutions is acute volume depletion when there is sufficient liver damage to seriously impair or prevent the manufacture of albumin.

Much of what has been taught about the need to have normal serum albumin concentrations before the body "can heal wounds or fight infection" is based on observations of Whipple.[63] Many years ago he demonstrated that the body has an enormous capacity to convert all types of protein into albumin if limited protein sources are available. Albumin appeared to be a high priority protein. Actually a patient with hypoalbuminemia heals wounds and fights infections long before his serum albumin level rises (ie, the limited amount of amino acids available to him is utilized for the healing of wounds and to combat infection, not for albumin synthesis).

This is one reason amino acid-glucose infusions are so efficacious. If you can get the amino acids into the tissues by intravenous infusion, bypassing the liver, the tissues which need amino acids for repair of wounds and for fighting infections can do so, leaving some amino acids for the liver to use for the synthesis of albumin. Short of acute volume depletion, administration of albumin solutions for nutritional purposes does not have clinical support.

Dr. Kinney: We have used albumin infusions as Dr. Border has. Considering priorities for protein synthesis, we have always placed hemoglobin near the top with some of the plasma proteins and enzymes farther down. We have no quantitative data, however.

Dr. Weston: In Madden and Whipple's review on plasma proteins they demonstrated that the hemoglobin fell in plasmapheresed dogs, and the available amino acids were used for synthesis of albumin.[64]

Dr. Levenson: I have a simplistic view on infusion of plasma proteins for nutritional purposes: In a nutritional deficiency which is physiologically significant of a known protein which can be supplied without complications, do it and correct thereby the physiologic abnormalities secondary to the deficiency. Since serum hepatitis is not a problem in giving serum albumin or a modified plasma protein solution (Plasmanate) and since—even if the liver of the injured or sick patient can make albumin—it is going to take time and will divert available amino acids from other metabolic uses, it makes sense to me to give plasma albumin if the patient is hypoalbuminemic, particularly if there is edema. I believe the evidence is good for giving preformed plasma protein under this circumstance.

Dr. Weston: Dr. Levenson, do you consider it necessary to give albumin? What level of serum albumin concentration are you willing to accept in patients?

Dr. Levenson: Looking at these questions clinically, I find that a level of serum albumin acceptable for one patient might not be acceptable for another. It depends wholly on the specific clinical problem.

Dr. Curreri: When one infuses serum albumin, how much of it is retained as albumin? When we infuse serum albumin to hypoalbuminemic patients, it takes an inordinate amount to raise their plasma levels and to maintain them at a near normal level. Patients have different sets of priorities for various synthetic processes, and albumin happens to be fairly low on the list for many. For example, hepatic synthesis of fibrinogen is fantastically increased early after injury.

Some of your studies, Dr. Levenson, showed that hepatic regeneration after hepatectomies was faster in injured rats with low serum albumin concentrations than in uninjured rats.[65] I am not sure that it is helpful in the long run to give albumin to an injured patient where hepatic synthesis of albumin is decreased. Albumin gets recycled into other amino acid and protein moieties.

Dr. Border: I give serum albumin because the colloid osmotic pressure falls and because I am concerned about pulmonary edema and the effects of tissue edema interfering with cellular nutrition.

Dr. Levenson: In answer to your comment, Dr. Curreri: when one infuses albumin, one does not expect it all to stay in the plasma. Some of it leaves through the capillaries promptly. The mass of albumin in the extracellular fluid—other than the plasma—is at least equal to that in the plasma. What is the rate of degradation of albumin in the injured individual? Is it faster than normal? Is it normal? Available data suggest that albumin catabolism is increased in the early period after injury.[66]

Dr. Weston: We showed decrease of albumin synthesis in certain patients and demonstrated that an enormously increased rate of turnover of albumin occurred in patients with infection and in subjects following the administration of adrenal corticoids. The point Dr. Curreri makes is important. The rate at which the albumin is catabolized is related to the plasma level of albumin. As one infuses albumin and raises the serum albumin level, albumin turnover increases rapidly, albumin catabolism is rapid. Because of the ensuing hypoalbuminemia, enormous amounts of albumin must be infused to raise and maintain serum albumin levels. Also, the amount of albumin in the extracellular fluid outside the vascular tree is about 1.5 times that in the vascular tree.

Infusion of albumin is a singularly uneconomic way of raising the serum albumin level. One must provide the patient with protein precursors (amino acids) as well. If the level is low enough to seriously impair osmotic pressure with a potential for edema, one should infuse albumin. But I object to

132

the view that one infuses albumin because the serum albumin is low. We have all seen patients with serum albumin concentrations of 1 to 1.5 gm/100 ml of serum who do not suffer edema. We handle their fluid metabolism by restricting sodium intake.

Dr. Levenson: When one must feed a patient parenterally, one must make use of all the nutrients which it is reasonable to use, and I would put plasma protein in that category, depending on each patient's specific clinical problem and nutritional state. One does not proceed by rote.

Dr. Stegink: One point related to Dr. Munro's comments concerning infused peptides and the various comments made about the use of albumin is to recall that Christensen demonstrated the effects of interaction of carbohydrate on the utilization of peptides in parenteral protein hydrolysate mixtures.[67, 68] Briefly, he found reasonable utilization of infused peptides if glucose and the protein hydrolysates were mixed together just prior to administration; but if the glucose and protein hydrolysates were mixed and allowed to stand for some time before administration, a large urinary loss of the peptide nitrogen resulted. These data suggest a combination (a Schiff base type) of the aldehydic groups of the glucose with some of the amino acids in the peptides or with some of the free amino acids which inhibited peptide utilization.

In some institutions, the albumin is administered along with the parenteral alimentation mixture (glucose and amino acid or protein hydrolysate solutions). The utilization of amino acids, peptides, and possibly protein might be inhibited if the mixtures are prepared far in advance. This might be as long as 12 hours prior to their administration.

Dr. Munro: The peptide or free amino acid-carbohydrate problem relates mainly to sterilization procedures (such as autoclaving) or to solutions standing in contact for a fair length of time. A thought has occurred to me which might be worth investigating. Can peptides containing cystine and tyrosine be synthesized (as peptides now can be synthesized) to get over the solubility problem, and are such peptides utilized metabolically? One could label cystine and tyrosine, synthesize an octopeptide or a quadripeptide, and find out whether the labeled amino acids find their way into tissue proteins when given parenterally. This may be the solution to the worries about the horrors of cysteine and tyrosine solubility.

INFUSION OF RED BLOOD CELLS

Dr. Levenson: The question of infusing plasma proteins for nutritional purposes is different, however, from the question of giving red blood cells for nutritional purposes. Considering the various serious risks of whole blood transfusions and the relatively slow entry of normal red blood cells into the metabolic pool, most physicians would agree, I believe, that red blood cells are not given for nutritional purposes. One gives red blood cells for hypovolemia secondary to bleeding, for air hunger, but not for nutritional reasons as such.[69-71]

TRANSITION FROM TPN TO ORAL DIETS; ELEMENTAL DIETS

Dr. Border: May we discuss elemental diets (diets made of amino acids, sugar, mineral, vitamins, and a limited amount of unsaturated fatty acids or fat)?

Dr. Levenson: You mean in terms of oral diets.

Dr. Border: In the transition from IV to elemental oral diets, it is clear in principle that the gastrointestinal mucosa must obtain significant amounts of nutrients from the contents in the lumen of the gut.

Evidence indicates that feeding so-called elemental diets has some effect on decreasing the occurrence or severity of stress ulcers.[72] Apparently oral elemental diets have a minimal effect in stimulating digestive enzymes. Start with IV alimentation then switch gradually to administration of an "elemental" orally or by nasogastric tube—at least for the massively injured patient who often has return of gut function before he comes out of coma or is able to eat—with the intent of providing adequate nutrition and doing something about the prevention of stress ulcers.

This is what we are doing. We can begin with nasogastric tube feeding long before we could otherwise begin oral or nasogastric feeding were we to use a whole protein liquid diet.

Dr. Levenson: Is that correct, Dr. Border? My own thought is that if one starts oral or nasogastric feedings gradually—taking several days or a week to reach the desired levels of calories and proteins—the patient probably can handle (and perhaps handles better) the whole protein formula type of diet than the so-called elemental diet. The elemental diets may be less damaging to the lungs than whole protein formulas if aspiration occurs. Where aspiration is a significant risk, this may be an overriding factor for the use of elemental liquid diets for nasogastric intubation feedings.

May we discuss Dr. Border's thesis, that giving the elemental type of diet does not greatly stimulate the secretion of digestive enzymes. My review of the literature and the results of some experiments in our laboratory by Ragins, Signer, Stanford, Levenson, and Seifter[73] suggest that if the elemental diet does not stimulate digestive enzyme secretion, it is almost certainly not because the elemental diet does not have whole protein, but because of its huge quantities of glucose and other carbohydrates. It seems clear that hypertonic glucose may inhibit pancreatic secretion, particularly if instilled into the jejunum, whereas certain of the free amino acids in 2% to 6% solution stimulate pancreatic secretion remarkably, perhaps to the same extent as proteins or peptides.

Dr. Curreri: I agree with the view that it is as easy, or easier, to get a patient with a functioning gastrointestinal tract to digest and absorb a complete liquid diet, building up the level of intake gradually in the same manner one would build up the intake of an elemental diet. There is a place in patient care for elemental diets. It is in a situation where one is trying to keep the secretions of the gastrointestinal tract relatively depressed.

That is not the purpose for the patient with severe injury. If such patients have an active functioning GI tract and can digest and absorb food, I see no reason to give them an elemental diet. I find it much easier to get more calories in with a complete diet than with an elemental diet. This has to do with the relatively high amount of glucose (which Dr. Levenson mentioned) in the elemental diet leading to the hyperosmolarity of such solutions.

Dr. Ali: May I ask a question about protein quality? We have heard that the amino acid pattern of amino acids in egg protein is "ideal." Dr. Munro, would you comment on the nutritive value of the mixed protein in the work coming from Germany reported by the Kofranyi and Deckner group?

Dr. Munro: I know about Dr. Kofranyi's studies.[74] Kofranyi has mixed egg protein—which is supposed to be ideal—with potato protein and found better nitrogen retention with the mixture than with the protein from egg alone. Two points emerge: first, Kofranyi is dealing with young healthy adult German students who are dependent presumably upon total nitrogen intake, rather than upon intake of essential amino acids; second, Kofranyi has been using rather high levels of nitrogen intake for his minimal comparisons, about 0.5 gm protein per kg of body weight. I suggested 0.42 gm as all that was necessary to achieve equilibrium. Because of the conditions of his study, I am not convinced he has demonstrated that supplementation with plant protein in the form of potato nitrogen has any relevance to whether the pattern of amino acids in egg protein is a good or a bad pattern. These are details of patternology, an obsession of people who work in this field of nutrition. But does it really help to discuss the precise patterns used in these studies upon young healthy adults? I don't think they help us to devise amino acid patterns for patients who are suffering from metabolic disturbances resulting from injury or disease.

References

1. Nasset ES: Role of the digestive tract in the utilization of protein and amino acids. *JAMA* **164:**172-177, 1957.

2. Sturman JA, Gaull G, Raiha NCR: Absence of cystathionase in human fetal liver: Is cystine essential? *Science* **169:**74-76, 1970.

3. Holt LE Jr, Snyderman SE: The amino acid requirements of infants. *JAMA* **175:**100-103, 1961.

4. Stegink LD, Den Besten L: Synthesis of cysteine from methionine in normal adult subjects: Effect of route of alimentation. *Science* **178:**514-516, 1972.

5. Fekl W: Some principles of modern parenteral nutrition. *Scand J Gastroenterol* 4, Suppl 3, 7-34, 1969.

6. Dolif D, Juergens P: Utilisation von Aminosäuren bei parenteraler Applikation, in Lang K, Fekl W, Berg G (eds): *Balanced nutrition and therapy,*

International Symposium in Nuremberg, April 10-12, 1970. Stuttgart, George Thieme Verlag, 1971, pp 160-174.

7. Heller L: Bilanzierte Ernährung in der Gynäkologie und Geburtshilfe, in Lang K, Fekl W, Berg G (eds): *Balanced nutrition and therapy*, International Symposium in Nuremberg, April 10-12, 1970. Stuttgart, George Thieme Verlag, 1971, pp 233-243.

8. Greenstein JP, Birnbaum SM, Winitz M, Otey MC: Quantitative nutritional studies with water-soluble, chemically defined diets. I. Growth, reproduction and lactation in rats. *Arch Biochem* **72(2):**396-416, 1957.

9. Birnbaum SM, Greenstein JP, Winitz M: Quantitative nutritional studies with water-soluble, chemically defined diets. II. Nitrogen balance and metabolism. *Arch Biochem Biophys* **72:**417-427, 1957.

10. Birnbaum SM, Winitz M, Greenstein JP: Quantitative nutritional studies with water-soluble, chemically defined diets. III. Individual amino acids as sources of non-essential nitrogen. *Arch Biochem Biophys* **72:**428-436, 1957.

11. Birnbaum SM, Greenstein ME, Winitz M, Greenstein JP: Quantitative nutritional studies with water-soluble, chemically defined diets. VI. Growth studies on mice. *Arch Biochem Biophys* **78:**245-247, 1958.

12. Greenstein JP, Otey MC, Birnbaum SM, Winitz M: Quantitative nutritional studies with water-soluble, chemically defined diets. X. Formulation of a nutritionally complete liquid diet. *J Nat Cancer Inst* **24:**211-219, 1960.

13. Winitz M, Birnbaum SM, Greenstein JP: Quantitative nutritional studies with water-soluble, chemically defined diets. IV. Influence of various carbohydrates on growth, with special reference to D-glucosamine. *Arch Biochem Biophys* **72:**437-447, 1957.

14. Winitz M, Greenstein JP, Birnbaum SM: Quantitative nutritional studies with water-soluble, chemically defined diets. V. Role of isomeric arginines in growth. *Arch Biochem Biophys* **72:**448-456, 1957.

15. Winitz M, Birnbaum SM, Sugimura T, Otey MC: Quantitative nutritional and *in vivo* metabolic studies with water-soluble chemically defined diets. *Amino acids, proteins and cancer biochemistry*, in: Edsall JT (ed): Jesse P. Greenstein Memorial Symposium. New York, Academic Press, 1960, p 9.

16. Winitz M, Graff J, Seedman DA: Effect of dietary carbohydrate on serum cholesterol levels. *Arch Biochem* **108:**576-579, 1964.

17. Winitz M, Graff J, Gallagher N, et al: Evaluation of chemical diets as nutrition for man-in-space. *Nature* (London) **205:**741-743, 1965.

18. Winitz M, Seedman DA, Graff J: Studies in metabolic nutrition employing chemically defined diets. I. Extended feeding of normal human adult males. *Am J Clin Nutr* **23:**525-545, 1970.

19. Steglink LD, Baker GL: Infusion of protein hydrolysates in the newborn infant: plasma amino acid concentrations. *J Pediatr* **78:**595-602, 1971.

20. Olney JW, Sharpe LG: Brain lesions in an infant rhesus monkey treated with monosodium glutamate. *Science* **166:**386-388, 1969.

21. Olney JW: Brain lesions, obesity, and other disturbances in mice treated with monosodium glutamate. *Science* **164:**719-721, 1969.

22. Geever EF, Seifter E, Levenson SM: Pancreatic pathology, chemically defined liquid diets and bacterial flora in the rat. *Br J Exp Pathol* **51:**341-347, 1970.

136

23. Levenson SM, Kan D, Gruber C, et al: Strange hemolytic anemia and pancreatic acinar atrophy and fibrosis. *Fed Proc* **30:**1785-1802, 1971.

24. Levenson SM, Seifter E: Amino acids and whole protein utilization in germfree animals in Brown H (ed): *Symposium on Protein Nutrition, Boston City Hospital.* Springfield, CC Thomas, 1971, chap 3.

25. Harper AE, Benevenga NJ, Wohlhueter RM: Effects of ingestion of disproportionate amounts of amino acids. *Physiol Rev* **50:**428-558, 1970.

26. Sprince H: An appraisal of methionine-tryptophan interrelation-ships in mental illness: methylation reactions involved. *Biol Psychiatry* **2:**109-117, 1970.

27. Heird WC, Driscoll JM Jr, Schidlinger JN, et al: Intravenous alimentation in pediatric patients, *J Pediatr* **80:**351-372, 1972.

28. Iber FL, Rosen H, Levenson SM, Chalmers TC: The plasma amino acids in patients with liver failure. *J Lab Clin Med* **50(3):**417-425, 1957.

29. Long JM, Dudrick SJ, Steiger E, et al: Use of intravenous hyperalimentation in patients with renal or liver failure, in Cowan GSM Jr, Scheetz WL (eds): *Intravenous Hyperalimentation.* Philadelphia, Lea and Febiger, 1972, chap 12.

30. Benditt EP, Humphreys EM, Wissler RW, et al: The dynamics of protein metabolism. I. The interrelationship between protein and caloric intakes and their influence upon the utilization of ingested protein for tissue synthesis by adult protein-depleted rat. *J Lab Clin Med* **33:**257-268, 1948.

31. Frazier LE, Wissler RW, Steffee CH, et al: Studies in amino acid utilization. I. The dietary utilization of mixtures of purified amino acids in protein-depleted adult albino rats. *J Nutr* **33:**65-84, 1947.

32. Wissler RW, Steffee CH, Frazier LE, et al: Studies in amino acid utilization. III. The role of the indispensable amino acids in maintenance of the adult albino rat. *J Nutr* **36:**245-262, 1948.

33. Snyderman SE, Holt LE Jr, Norton PM, et al: The plasma aminogram. I. Influence of the level of protein intake and a comparison of whole protein and amino acid diets. *Pediatr Res* **2:**131-144, 1968.

34. Juergens P, Dolif D: Die Bedeutung nichtessentieller Amino-säuren fur den Stickstoffhaushalt des Menschen unter parenteraler Ernährung. *Klin Wochenschr* **46:**131-143, 1968.

35. Scrimshaw NS, Young VR, Schwartz R, et al: Minimum dietary essential amino acid-to-total nitrogen ratio for whole egg protein fed to young men. *J Nutr* **89:**9-18, 1966.

36. Fürst P, Josephson B, Vinnars E: The effect on the nitrogen balance of the ratio of essential to nonessential amino acids in intravenously infused solutions. *Scand J Clin Lab Invest* **26:**319-326, 1970.

37. Hegsted DM: Protein and amino acid requirements in man, in Lang K, Fekl W, Berg G (eds): *Balanced Nutrition and Therapy.* Stuttgart, George Thieme Verlag, pp 12-21, 1971.

38. Rose WC: Nutritive significance of amino acids. *Physiol Rev* **18:**109-136, 1938.

39. World Health Organization: Protein requirements. Report of a Joint FAO/WHO Expert Group. WHO Technical Report Series No. 301, Geneva, 1965.

40. Rose WC: The amino acid requirements of adult man. *Nutr Abstr Rev* **27:**631-647, 1957.

41. Johnston IDA: Parenteral Feeding: *Practitioner* **206:**103-110, 1971.

42. Levenson SM, Lounds Elizabeth A, Morris Rosalyn: Oral fat emulsion in the feeding of patients with severe burns. *Ann NY Acad Sci* **56:** 37-45, 1952.

43. Kinney JM, Long CL, Duke JH: Carbohydrate and nitrogen metabolism after injury, in Porter R, Knight J (eds): *Energy Metabolism in Trauma.* London, J&A Churchill, 1970, p 103.

44. Levenson SM: Nutritional care of burn patients. Symposium on Burns, National Research Council, National Acad Sci, pp 142-147, Washington, 1951.

45. Sutherland AB: The nutritional response of the burned child. *J Royal Coll Surgeons,* Edinburgh **4(2):**149-152, 1959.

46. Peacock EE Jr, van Winkle W Jr: Surgery and biology of wound repair. Philadelphia, W. B. Saunders Company, 1970.

47. Steiger E, Allen TR, Daly JM, et al: Beneficial effects of immediate postoperative total parenteral nutrition. *Surgical Forum* **22:**89-90, 1971.

48. Levenson SM, Crowley LV, Oates JF, Glinos AD: Injury, wound healing and liver regeneration. Proc Second Army Sci Conf, West Point, NY **2:** 109-122, 1959.

49. Crowley L, Kriss P, Seifter E, et al: Nitrogen metabolism and wound healing in rats: Effects of femoral fracture, testosterone and environmental temperature. Fed Proc 31 (Abstr #2897), 1972.

50. Carrel A: Effet d'un abscès à distance sur la cicatrisation d'une plaie aseptique. *C R Soc Biol* (Paris) **XC:**333-335, 1924.

51. Levenson SM: Some challenging wound healing problems for clinicians and basic scientists, in Dunphy JE, Van Winkle W Jr (eds): *Repair and Regeneration, The Scientific Basis for Surgical Practice.* New York, McGraw-Hill, Inc, 1969, pp 309-337.

52. Cannon PR, Bendett EP, et al: *Recent advances in nutrition, with particular reference to protein metabolism,* Univ of Kansas Press, 1950.

53. Scrimshaw NS, Taylor CE, Gordon JE: Interactions of nutrition and infection. World Health Organization Monograph Series, No. 57, Geneva, 1968.

54. Alexander JW, Hegg ME, McCoy HV, et al: Neutrophil function and infection during immunosuppression and transplantation. *Surg Forum* **19:** 198-200, Cit No 4013244, 1968.

55. Johnson JE: Infection and diabetes, in Ellenberg M, Rifkin H (eds): *Diabetes Mellitus: Theory and practice.* New York, McGraw-Hill, 1970, chap 34, pp 430-437.

56. Balch HH: The effect of severe battle injury, and of post-traumatic renal failure on resistance to infection, in Howard JM (ed): *Recent advances in medicine and surgery* (based on professional medical experiences in Japan and Korea, 1950-53), *Medical Science Publication no 4,* Army Medical Service Graduate School, Walter Reed Army Medical Center, Washington, DC, 1954, pp 165-192.

57. Balch HH: Resistance to infection in burned patients. *Ann Surg* **157:**1-19, 1963.

138

58. Levenson SM: *Wound healing in patients with battle wounds and severe renal dysfunction*. Battle casualties in Korea, Studies of the Surg Res Team, vol IV, Post Traumatic Renal Insufficiency, Army Med Serv Grad School, WRAMC, Washington, DC, Chap 8, pp 127-155, 1954.

59. Elman R, Kelly FJ, Simonsen DH: Pure serum albumin compared with citrated plasma in the therapy of chronic hypoalbuminemia. *Ann Surg* **128:**195-209, 1948.

60. Terry R, Sandrock WE, Nye RE Jr, Whipple GH: Parenteral plasma protein maintains nitrogen equilibrium over long periods. *J Exp Med* **87:** 547-559, 1948.

61. Allen JF, Stemmer E, Head LR: Similar growth rates of litter mate puppies maintained on oral protein with those on the same quantity of protein as daily intravenous plasma for 99 days as only protein source. *Ann Surg* **144(3):**349-355, 1956.

62. Cahill GF Jr, Owen OE: The role of the kidney in the regulation of protein metabolism, in HN Munro (ed): *Mammalian Protein Metabolism, vol 4.* New York, Academic Press, 1970, pp 559-584.

63. Whipple GH: *The dynamic equilibrium of body proteins, hemoglobin, plasma proteins, organ and tissue proteins.* Springfield, Charles C. Thomas, 1956.

64. Madden SC, Whipple GH: Plasma proteins: Their source, production and utilization. *Physiol Rev* **20:**194-217, 1940.

65. Levenson SM, Crowley LV, Oates JF, Glinos AD: *Injury, wound healing, and liver regeneration.* Proc of the Second Army Sci Conf, West Point, NY **2:**109-122, 1959.

66. Birke G, Liljedahl SO, Plantin LO, Wetterfors J, et al: Albumin catabolism in burns, and following surgical procedures. *Acta Chir Scand* **118:** 353-366, 1960.

67. Christensen HN, Lynch EL, Decker DG, Powers JH: Conjugated, non-protein amino acids of plasma: Difference in utilization of peptides of hydrolysates of fibrin and casein. *J Clin Invest* **26:**849-852, 1947.

68. Christensen HN, et al: Conjugated, non-protein amino acids of plasma: study of clinical significance of peptidemia. *J Clin Invest* **26:**853-859, 1947.

69. Levenson SM, Birkhill FR, Maloney MA, Bell JA: Metabolic fate of infused erythrocyte. *Ann Surg* **130:**723-746, 1949.

70. Birkhill FR, Maloney MA, Levenson SM: Effect of transfusion polycythemia upon bone marrow activity and erythrocyte survival in man. *Blood* **6:** 1021-1033, 1951.

71. Levenson SM: Current status of some aspects of parenteral nutrition. *Am J Surg* **103:**330-341, 1962.

72. Voitk AJ, Chiu CJ, Gurd FN: The prophylactic effect of an elemental diet on porcine stress ulcers. *Surg Forum* **22:**328-329, 1971.

73. Ragins H, Levenson SM, Signer R, Stanford W, Seifter E: Intrajejunal administration of an elemental diet at neutral pH avoids pancreatic stimulation: Studies in dog and man. *Am J Surg* **126:**606-614, 1973.

74. Kofranyi E, Jekat F: Zur Bestimmung der biologischen Wertigkeit von Nahrungsproteinen, XII. Die Mischung von Ei mit Reis, Mais, Soja, Algen. *Hoppe-Seylers Z physiol Chem* **348:**84-88, 1967.

Digest of Colloquium

AMINO ACIDS AND HYDROLYSATES

Colloquium participants reviewed the limited amount of concrete data on specific amino acid requirements of recuperating patients receiving total parenteral nutrition (TPN). From these data they attempted to set guidelines for the amino acid composition of solutions for long-term parenteral infusions of seriously ill or injured patients.

The view held by most participants was that the amino acid requirements of adult patients receiving TPN are more likely to approximate those of the growing child than those of the healthy adult. As a starting point, the following guidelines to composition of an amino acid infusion mixture appear reasonable:

> The essential amino acids should be patterned after the needs of the growing child;
> The essential to nonessential amino acid ratios of the mixtures should be about 1 to 1.5;
> The nonessential amino acid component should contain alanine, proline, arginine, glycine, glutamic acid, and histidine;
> Tyrosine and cysteine might also be added.

Some investigators hold that the absence of cysteine or very low levels of cysteine in infused solutions led to reduced plasma cystine levels. Others, studying infants receiving IV infusions free of cysteine, observed normal plasma cystine levels in these patients. The studies cited were not comparable since a protein hydrolysate was used in the study by Stegink, and a mixture of free amino acids was used in the study reported by Fekl. Also, cysteine may be a required amino acid for premature infants and possibly for the full-term newborn.

The participants advanced reservations about the use of ester forms of cysteine and tyrosine to increase their solubility. They based their reservations on lack of knowledge about the metabolism of such esters when infused; also experimental evidence implicates cystine ethyl ester as a major pathogenic factor in an often lethal hemolytic anemia and pancreatic acinar atrophy and fibrosis occurring in rats fed certain "chemically defined" liquid amino acid diets.

A suggestion by Munro that the synthesis of peptides containing tyrosine and cystine be considered as a possible means of introducing these two amino acids into a parenteral infusion mixture evoked these questions: What are specific or special roles for the specific peptides that should be supplied parenterally? Why should we use hydrolysates at all, now that free amino acids are available at reasonable cost?

Responses to these queries emphasized the limited data on the metabolic fate of (and possible need for) infused peptides; hence, we could not state precisely the need for their incorporation in solutions for parenteral feeding. The limited data suggest that some infused peptides are metabolized while others may not be, or at least not rapidly enough to escape excretion by the kidney.

Discussion of the advantages for certain peptides over free amino acids centered on induction of enzymes involved in the metabolism of proteins and their metabolites. The participants agreed that intravenous alimentations of peptides could be advantageous to the premature or full-term neonate in combating possible amino acid toxicity from amino acid infusions. Certain peptides will combat certain amino acid ester and amino acid anti-metabolite toxicities, whereas a mixture of free amino acids will not.

Because of the difficult control problems in preparing truly reproducible hydrolysates, standardizing parenteral solutions for study is easier with mixtures of crystalline amino acids than with protein hydrolysates. The proportion of bound to free amino nitrogen generally varies from batch to batch of protein hydrolysate. It is impractical to control precisely the size and composition of the various peptides in the hydrolysate. In some preparations large peptides are dialyzed out, in others they are not. When infusing hydrolysates, therefore, the investigator is using an unknown solution. He does not have precise analytic data on concentrations of individual amino acids and peptides. Use of mixtures of L-amino acids may be a desirable starting point for standardization of solutions for study, but investigations should determine whether or not there are special roles for specific peptides.

Heird and Winters found the level of cationic amino acids—particularly in the free amino acid mixtures used for the parenteral feeding of infants—to be associated with a hyperchloremic metabolic acidosis. This finding should be considered when formulating amino acid patterns for parenteral infusion, especially for children. Lysine, for example, is present in a free amino acid parenteral preparation as the hydrochloride.

Munro pointed out that:

When lysine is injected intravenously, it leaves the plasma rapidly, going into the skeletal muscle;
Skeletal muscles contain 30 times more lysine than is in the plasma;
Skeletal muscle is proportionately less in the infant than in the adult.

These facts may explain why Heird and Winters observed difficulties in children using the amino acid solution, whereas others have not noticed any in adults using the same mixture.

Stegink mentioned the occurrence of hyperammonia in infants, traceable perhaps to increased ammonia content of the mixtures being infused, particularly the hydrolysates. No one had observed this in adults.

Law questioned whether infused amino acids enter the gut. (The consensus is that they do.) If they do, is the difference between the metabolic fate of ingested and intravenously injected amino acids referable primarily to the first pass through the circulation, whereby the amino acids infused into a peripheral vein bypass the liver, while those ingested go to the liver initially after absorption? After this first pass-through, the amino acids, infused or ingested, presumably would follow the same pathway.

The differences in handling glutamic acid and aspartic acid in the gut were discussed. Differences in amino acid levels in plasma are observed in humans receiving a protein hydrolysate intravenously and the same material intragastrically (eg, in plasma cystine and taurine levels). This pointed to the general view of significant differences when amino acids or peptides are given intravenously, as opposed to their being given by mouth. Studies are needed to determine the extent of these differences.

RED BLOOD CELLS AND PLASMA PROTEINS

Red blood cells and plasma protein are available materials with certain uses. Levenson stated that red blood cells should not be infused for nutritional purposes but may be infused for the correction of significant anemia or blood volume deficit. Studies dealing with the survival time of red blood cells in injured patients in both the catabolic and anabolic phases indicate unequivocally that red blood survival is normal. The amounts of amino acids which would be made available to the patient from the natural destruction of the red blood cells or reduced red blood cell production if the patient is made polycythemic are small, the equivalent of about an egg a day. The risk of transfusion of red blood cells far outweighs this minimal quantitative supply of amino acids.

Plasma protein infusion using commercially prepared plasma protein and albumin solutions avoids the risks of transfusion of whole blood. Some argued in favor of using plasma protein preparations and/or albumin as preformed protein in the presence of hypoproteinemia, while others disagreed with this concept, unless there was a blood volume deficit. The former group of participants felt that one would not use plasma proteins clinically as the only parenteral source of amino acids, peptides, and whole protein; but using them in conjunction with the infusion of amino acids and protein hydrolysates when physiologically significant hypoproteinemia is present seems eminently sensible and judicious.

CALORIE TO NITROGEN RATIO

From calculations of metabolic studies based on oral feedings, Kinney demonstrated an approximate calorie-nitrogen ratio of about 100 to 1 in patients with injury and/or sepsis during the catabolic and, later, during the anabolic phase. He did not imply that they were optimal levels.

Dudrick had attempted to use a calorie to nitrogen ratio of this order of magnitude in patients who received their total nutrient intake intravenously and who required large quantities of calories. He found he was infusing an excess of amino acids or protein hydrolysate. The patients did not look good and had increased blood urea concentrations.

Others have not found difficulties when these levels were used by the oral route. This raises again the question of differences in nutritional response of individuals to nitrogenous foodstuffs given orally and parenterally.

The usual oral feedings differ from parenteral infusions in protein versus amino acid and hydrolysate content and in nonprotein-containing calorie sources. The nonprotein caloric source in the intravenous feedings used by some investigators in the United States has been glucose, essentially, whereas the nonprotein caloric sources in oral diets have been largely carbohydrate polymers and fat. The possibility was suggested that it is the difference in caloric mixture which is critical, not the calorie-nitrogen ratio per se.

The physiologic and clinical significance of the negative balance period after injury, its duration and intensity were discussed. Controversy followed the question of whether or not one ought to do something about it; and, if so, at what time and at what rate.

Clear evidence was sought, other than clinical impression, that such patients were more susceptible to infection. There are a few *in vivo* studies on circulating antibodies and humoral agents possibly involved in the defense reaction; some measurements of white blood cell function also have been made.

INFUSION SOLUTIONS

Information is sparse or completely lacking, also, on the effect of continuous 24-hour infusions on various diurnal rhythms. How do such loads of nutrients infused continuously throughout the day, week after week, modify—if at all—adrenal function? Does it change the diurnal secretions of other hormones, such as growth hormone?

The majority of studies dealing with changes in formula have been carried out in Europe, in part because of our FDA regulations. In the European studies, the major criteria have been related to nitrogen balance. This is a useful and necessary measurement but is, by itself, probably insufficient. Clearly one would prefer a parenteral preparation that maintained a healthy adult in nitrogen equilibrium over one that resulted in a negative nitrogen balance; but this is only a first step in evaluation.

Many of the experimental studies have been conducted in healthy animals. Studies should be extended to "sick" animals: animals undernourished by nutrient means, animals subjected to injury, animals subjected to infections.

Along with nitrogen balance, measurement of plasma amino acid levels is a guide to the efficacy of the materials being infused. If the levels drop, the preparation is deficient in something (eg, an amino acid); if they go up, too much of something (eg, an amino acid) is being infused.

Problems of quality control of solutions for parenteral alimentation and provision of analytic data by commercial manufacturing concerns appear to relate principally to protein hydrolysates. This makes it critical that the precise analysis of each lot of protein hydrolysate—if not on the label—be given to the investigator. An investigator using protein hydrolysates should insist on this information. He should carry out spot-check analyses also.

To summarize, we have inadequate information to judge and formulate what the optimal parenteral amino acid and protein hydrolysate solutions are. Solutions of different compositions are required for different clinical situations, including age, sex, injury, and illness.

A need exists for the same type of systematic metabolic and nutritional studies in animals with the nutrients given intravenously as have been carried out when the foodstuffs have been given orally. Amino acid imbalances and amino acid toxicities should be studied. Such tests, not readily feasible in man, should be carried out first in injured and sick animals, as well as in healthy animals. After appropriate animal studies, controlled clinical investigations will be needed.

PART TWO

Section Two

Carbohydrates and Fats

4 Carbohydrates
George F. Cahill, M.D.
5 Fats
H. C. Meng, M.D., Ph.D.

Colloquium: Carbohydrates and Fats
Digest of Colloquium
Arvid Wretlind, Ph.D., and William Schumer, M.D.

NUTRITIONAL COMPOSITION

Chapter 4

Carbohydrates

George F. Cahill, M.D.

*Glucose is the sole carbohydrate or carbohydrate-related sub-
strate not possessing a charge at physiologic pH and which is
readily metabolized by all tissues. Low insulin levels control
glucose production, and high insulin levels control its
utilization.*

Certain general biological facts need emphasis in discussing carbohydrates in relation to parenteral nutrition: First, only three sugars gain access
to the bloodstream via the gastrointestinal tract in sufficient mass to satisfy
caloric requirements. These are glucose, fructose, and galactose. Second,
specific enzymatic pathways (mainly in the liver) are available for rapid
metabolism of fructose and galactose. With these two sugars, however,
there are problems.

Galactose is a substrate which is transported by the glucose carrier
across many cell membranes and thus is available for the almost ubiquitous
aldose reductase reaction, resulting in accumulation of dulcitol and, subsequently, in possible metabolic disarrangement in tissues such as nerve or the
lens of the eye.

Fructose, due to its high phosphorylation rate in liver, results in decreased levels of hepatic phosphate and high energy phosphate which has not
been shown to result directly in severe liver damage but is, nevertheless, an
unappealing fact to the biochemist.[1]

This leaves glucose. It is interesting to note the waves of clinical
enthusiasm first for fructose, then for its polyol, sorbitol, and most recently for
the pentitol, xylitol, as glucose substitutes.[2] None has been clearly demonstrated as a satisfactory replacement for glucose. It appears unlikely that any
substitute for glucose will be found for which adequate metabolic pathways
are available within the human body and which can be given parenterally.

GLUCOSE

A healthy man can dispose of up to 5 gm of glucose per minute and
possibly more, since no published studies on the upper limit are available.
Even this is a relatively phenomenal rate, being 15 to 20 times in calories the
rate of his basal energy expenditure. He can do this without osmotically
damaging erythrocytes since the gastrointestinal tract adds small increments of
isosmotic glucose-containing fluid to the capillaries perfusing the mucosa,
thereby providing hexose equilibration within the red cells, unlike pouring
glucose into the blood at a single site from the end of a catheter placed in a
vein or artery.

Where does all this glucose go? As yet, a certain answer cannot be
given. Recent experiments by Hultman and Nilsson[3] have shown the relative

lability of man's glucose reserves as reflected by changes in hepatic glycogen content; but, obviously, the greatest proportion of ingested calories ends up as fat, should the influx per unit time surpass the expenditure. This is supported by the rise in respiratory quotient after carbohydrate ingestion as observed by the classical nutritionists at the turn of the century and by many studies showing a brisk glucose uptake across adipose beds in man and animals.

If, however, carbohydrate intake is at a rate approximating the rate of expenditure, the lesser rise in insulin concentration compared to the large glucose infusion rate could result in glucose displacing fat as fuel, but probably in little net lipid synthesis. As the rate of glucose infusion is reduced to one-fourth to one-fifth of the rate of caloric expenditure, the brain still has sufficient glucose, sparing thereby the need for gluconeogenesis by the organism. The carcass would then rely primarily on its fat as fuel and conserve nitrogen, thanks to adequate exogenous carbohydrate for the central nervous system. With no glucose available, gluconeogenesis and its concomitants, ketogenesis and proteolysis, would occur. Thus, there is a spectrum of events, as shown in Table 1, whereby the relative concentration of insulin serves as the body's integrative signal initiating or suppressing metabolic events in the various tissues (Fig 1).

Table 1.—Hormone-Fuel Interrelationships in Man*

	Very Large Meal	Small Meal	Central Venous Line	"D/W"†	Fasting	Diabetic Ketoacidosis
Glucose balance (mg/min)	+5,000	+1,000	+500	+100	0	−100
Insulin concentration	+++++	++++	+++	++	+	0
Glucagon concentration	±	±	±	±	+	++
Liver						
Glycolysis & lipogenesis	++++	+++	++	±	0	0
Gluconeogenesis & ketogenesis	0	0	0	0	+	++
Adipose tissue						
Lipogenesis	++++	+++	++	±	0	0
Lipolysis	0	0	0	+	++	+++
Muscle						
Proteolysis (normal)	±	±	±	±	+	++
Proteolysis (trauma)	±	+	++	++++	++++	++++
Energy substrate (muscle)						
Glucose	++	++	++	±	0	0
Fatty acid	±	±	±	++	++	++

*Approximately 300 mg/min glucose is the caloric equivalent for a normal man, meaning that amount of substrate needed to satisfy total basal energy needs of approximately 1,700 kcal/day.
†Standard intravenous dextrose and water infusion.

Table 1 is a gross oversimplification, since it does not account for intake of fuels other than glucose, nor does it involve changes in rates as a function of time. For example, adipose tissue becomes more and more sensitive to insulin with continuous exposure to high insulin levels, probably due to increased synthesis of glucose-metabolizing enzymes inside the cell. Conversely, with decreased exposure to insulin, these enzymes decrease (due to their usual metabolic degradation) without being replaced; and the adipose tissue becomes more resistant—metabolically speaking—to insulin, contributing partly to the so-called "diabetes" of starvation or of carbohydrate deprivation.

CATABOLIC   ANABOLIC

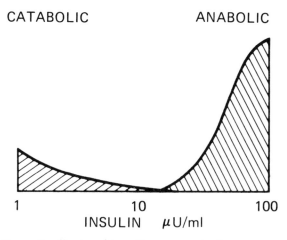

Fig 1. Overall effects of insulin concentrations on responsive cells such as adipose and muscle.

In trauma, the insulin suppression of muscle proteolysis becomes shifted to the left. This fact has been demonstrated by Hinton et al,[4] who found that large doses of insulin, up to 500 units/day, were capable of suppressing urea loss in patients with severe burns (Fig 2). Thus, insulin, which reacts with cell membrane to initiate some second messenger inside the cell (Fig 3) which, in turn, suppresses muscle proteolysis, needs to be in much higher concentration to oppose whatever the factor is that appears in trauma or sepsis and which provokes accelerated muscle catabolism. This fact makes one wonder whether all patients with acute trauma or sepsis should receive these very large doses of insulin to suppress this frequently lethal hypercatabolic state. This large dose of insulin, of course, necessitates continuous monitoring of glucose concentration, since fatal hypoglycemia could occur very rapidly were sufficient glucose not provided. Several laboratories are now working on either "on-line" glucose-analyzing systems or else implantable glucose-sensitive devices which can detect glucose concentration rapidly and accurately. Without this, these large insulin doses are fraught with danger.

150

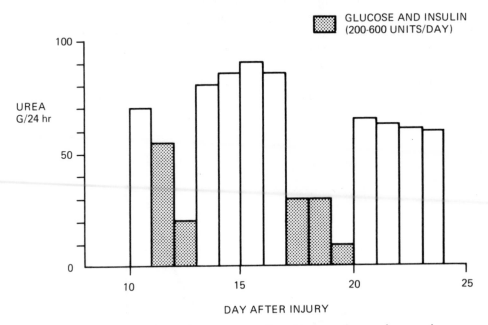

Fig 2. Suppression of urea excretion by very large doses of insulin.

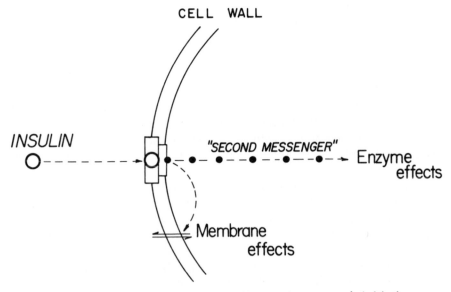

Fig 3. Insulin reacting on cell membrane and initiating a "second messenger," as yet unidentified, which then transmits insulin's metabolic effects.

The aforementioned can best be understood by assembling a simple scheme of a normal man's fuel depots and sites of fuel metabolism (Fig 4). These data are approximations of daily rates of substrate flux in a fasted man, showing central nervous system dependence on glucose and carcass metabolism of fatty acids and ketoacids.[5] Other glycolytic tissues, such as red cells, use glucose as does the brain, but only to the lactate stage which, is then recycled to the liver for glucose resynthesis. With trauma there is accelerated muscle protein catabolism and, as shown by Kinney (see p 84), accelerated gluconeogenesis to provide fuel for the reparative tissues (Fig 5). This accelerated protein catabolism can be suppressed by enormous quantities of insulin. Precisely how this works biochemically remains to be elucidated.

Cuatrecasas[6] has shown insulin to work solely on cell membrane, and, presumably, its effects on intracellular processes result from some form of second messenger (Fig 3). Thus, the concentration of insulin alters the metabolic response of a cell, presumably by the amount of this second messenger generated, and trauma initiates a need for a much higher concentration of insulin, moving the diagram (as shown in Fig 1) to the left. The factor produced in trauma that initiates this "insulin resistance" remains to be defined.

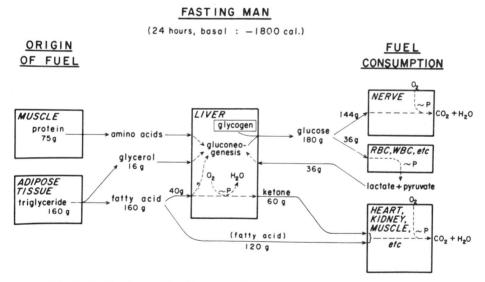

FASTING MAN

(24 hours, basal : −1800 cal.)

Fig 4. Daily flux of fuel in a totally starved man.

152

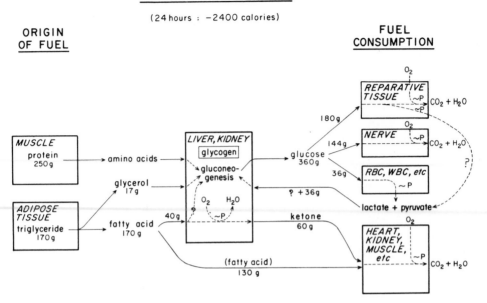

TRAUMATIZED MAN

(24 hours : −2400 calories)

Fig 5. Estimation of daily fuel flux with severe trauma.

References

1. Burch HB, Max P Jr, Chyce K, Lowry OH: Metabolic intermediates in liver of rats given large amounts of fructose or dihydroxy acetone. *Biochem Biophys Res Commun* **34:** 619-626, 1969.

2. Mehnert H, Förster H, Geser CA, et al: Clinical use of carbohydrates in parenteral nutrition, in Meng HC, Law DH (eds): *Parenteral Nutrition.* Springfield, C. C. Thomas, 1970, pp 112-138.

3. Hultman E and Nilsson LH: Liver glycogen in man. Effect of different diets and muscular exercise, in Pernow B, Saltin B (eds): *Muscle Metabolism in Exercise.* New York, Plenum Press, 1971, pp 143-151.

4. Hinton P, Allison SP, Littlejohn S, Lloyd J: Insulin and glucose to reduce catabolic response to injury in burned patients. *Lancet* **1:**767-769, 1971.

5. Cahill GF Jr: Physiology of Insulin in Man. *Diabetes* **20:**785-799, 1971.

6. Cuatrecasas P: Insulin-receptor interactions in adipose tissue cells: Direct measurement and properties. *Proc Nat Acad Sci USA* **68:**1264-1268, 1971.

Chapter 5

Fat Emulsions

H. C. Meng, M.D., Ph.D.

In both enteral and intravenous alimentation fat is a concentrated source of energy, yielding a greater number of calories per gram than carbohydrate or protein. Fat emulsions also provide essential fatty acids. Based on the evidence of serum fatty acid composition, the minimum and optimum daily dosages to meet the requirements are discussed. The intravenous requirement of triglycerides is not yet understood. In contrast to amino acid and concentrated carbohydrate solutions, fat emulsions may be administered into a peripheral vein. This may reduce the occurrence of phlebitis, thrombosis, and central venous catheter related sepsis. The undesirable long-term effects and contraindication of intravenous administration of fat emulsions are considered.

This review of information on the use of fat emulsions in parenteral nutrition is undertaken with the hope that it will stimulate further research toward solving problems that have been identified.

Reflecting on the calorie requirement in total parenteral nutrition evokes a response to the frequent query: Why is fat needed in parenteral nutrition? My answers are:

Fat is a concentrated source of energy, yielding 9 kcal/gm. Thus, the use of fat is advantageous in that a smaller volume furnishing a greater number of calories may be given as compared to carbohydrate.

There is no loss of the infused fat in the urine or feces.

Current research demonstrates the potential of triglycerides per se, even when adequate calories from carbohydrate and essential fatty acids are supplied.[1-3]

Fat supplies essential fatty acids, the fatty acids that we cannot make in the body.

Even a 30% fat emulsion is not hypertonic and it may be possible to administer a fat emulsion along with amino acids, carbohydrates, and other nutrients into the peripheral veins. Solutions for parenteral nutrition containing concentrated carbohydrate and amino acids or protein hydrolysate must be delivered into a central vein via an indwelling catheter. While central venous delivery is the best procedure available, problems such as sepsis and hyperosmolar syndrome, have been encountered. An advantage of infusing fat by way of a peripheral vein may be reduction in occurrence of phlebitis and/or thrombosis.

FAT EMULSION PREPARATIONS

Table 1 shows the composition of five oil-in-water emulsions:

A 10% or 20% soybean oil emulsion, emulsified by purified egg phosphatides (1.2%) in 2.5% glycerol (Intralipid);

A 15% cottonseed oil emulsion stabilized by soybean lecithin in 5% sorbitol (Lipiphysan). It also contains some α-tocopherol;

A 10% or 20% soybean oil emulsion (Lipofundin S). It is emulsified by soybean phosphatides in 5% xylitol;

A 15% cottonseed oil emulsion emulsified by purified soybean phosphatides and a nonionic detergent (pluronic F68), in 4% dextrose (Lipomul, IV).[4] Although this preparation has been withdrawn by the manufacturer, it has been included because of data obtained from studies using Lipomul.

A nonphosphatide emulsion (SR 695).

Nonphosphatide emulsions were included because phosphatides or phosphatide products were suspect as toxic agents in fat emulsions. Therefore, studies were designed to compare these two types of emulsions—phosphatide or nonphosphatide—to determine which is more acceptable. Of the five preparations, Intralipid, Lipiphysan, and Lipofundin S are commercially available (see Table 1).

Table 1.— Composition of Fat Emulsions

Component (gm/100 ml)	Intralipid	Lipiphysan	Lipofundin-S	Lipomul, IV	SR 695
Soybean oil	10 or 20	. . .	10 or 20	. . .	. . .
Cottonseed oil	. . .	15	. . .	15	15
Purified egg phosphatides	1.2	. . .	. . .	. . .	. . .
Purified soybean phosphatides	. . .	2.0	0.75 or 1.5	1.2	. . .
Pluronic F68	. . .	. . .	. . .	0.3	0.3
Polyethylene glycol monopalmitate	. . .	. . .	. . .	. . .	1.2
Drewmulse	. . .	. . .	. . .	. . .	0.3
Dextrose	. . .	. . .	. . .	4.0	5.0
Glycerol	2.5	. . .	. . .	. . .	. . .
Sorbitol	. . .	5.0	. . .	. . .	. . .
Xylitol	. . .	. . .	5.0	. . .	. . .
DL-α-tocopherol	. . .	0.5	. . .	. . .	. . .
Dist H_2O to	100 ml	100 ml	100 ml	100 ml	100 ml

Zilversmit et al prepared an anhydrous emulsion which could be stored more or less indefinitely.[5] For emergency use, one may add water or some other solution like dextrose, shaking and mixing to form an emulsion. Although not successful, it is deserving perhaps of further study.

Another emulsion is a preparation containing the medium-chain fatty acid triglycerides. Unfortunately, our preliminary study showed some toxic effects after intravenous injection in rats (H. C. Meng, unpublished data).

Wretlind reported short-chain fatty acids to be toxic in that they produce changes in blood pressure and in the brain.[6, 7] It may be worthwhile to take another look at the medium-chain fatty acid triglyceride emulsions.

Shafiroff and associates prepared an emulsion containing fat emulsified by gelatin, protein hydrolysate, and carbohydrate which was given intravenously to animals and patients.[8-11] The emulsion was prepared with sterile starting materials and homogenized in a homogenizer which had also been sterilized before use. Thus, the final preparation was expected to be sterile.

Although it is advantageous to have a preparation containing all of the essential nutrients, it may be difficult to maintain the stability of such a preparation. Geyer,[12] Edgren and Wretlind,[13] Wretlind,[14] and Meng[3] reviewed in detail the formulation and preparation of fat emulsions.

Available emulsions have two oil sources: soybean oil and cottonseed oil. Our experience and that of others indicate that the soybean oil emulsion has fewer adverse effects than cotton seed oil. I do not know why the soybean oil emulsion should be more acceptable. Differences in fatty acid composition between these two oils are not significant (Fig 1). The soybean oil contains more linoleic acid and less palmitic acid. In addition, there is some linolenic acid in the soybean oil, none in the cottonseed oil. The oleic acid and nonsaponifiable materials in both oils are about the same. I do not know if the presence of linolenic acid in the soybean oil could make this difference. Perhaps the soybean phosphatides versus egg phosphatides, or glycerol versus other carbohydrates, may make the difference.

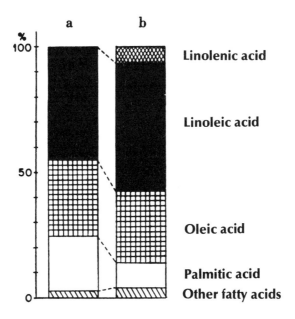

Fig 1. Fatty acid composition of the two oils, cottonseed oil (a) and soybean oil (b), used in the preparation of the commercially available fat emulsions for intravenous nutrition.[14]

158

Acute or immediate adverse effects of fat emulsions In the forties and fifties acute toxic effects were observed after intravenous infusion of fat emulsions.[12] These adverse effects were: changes in blood pressure, respiration and heart rate; histamine-like effect; back pain or "colloidal reactions"; and fever. With the currently available emulsions—including Intralipid—these types of reactions have not been encountered,[15, 16] (H. C. Meng, unpublished data).

Biological utilization of intravenously administered fat emulsion Reports have shown little or no accumulation in the body after infusion of large amounts of fat emulsion.[12] In addition, oxygen consumption increases, the respiratory quotient decreases, and blood ketones increase after fat infusion.

Geyer[17] has observed the increase in $^{14}CO_2$ after intravenous injection of an emulsion of triolein-1-^{14}C to the rat (Fig 2). Similar results were reported using ^{14}C-trilaurin and ^{14}C-tripalmitin.[12] In addition, increase in potassium retention and body weight were also observed during the period of intravenous administration of fat emulsion. [12, 15, 16, 18-25]

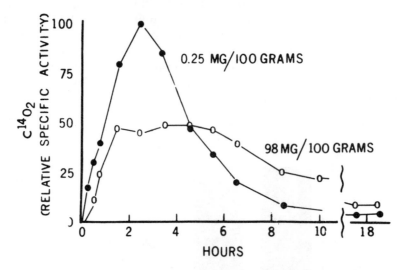

Fig 2. Oxidation of ^{14}C-1-triolein emulsion by the rat. ^{14}C-1-triolein, having a specific activity of 1 millicurie/millimol, was used; the same total radioactivity was supplied in both the high and low dose. Nonradioactive triolein was used as a carrier in the case of the 98-mg dose. Two percent soybean phosphatides (Upjohn) were used as the stabilizer. Injections were via the tail vein. Differences in actual specific activities were taken into account when calculating the relative specific activities.[17]

Figure 3 shows that dogs on a fat-free diet plus intravenous infusions of fat emulsions gained weight and exhibited a positive nitrogen balance. These results are comparable to those produced when the animals received a complete synthetic diet with all nutrients ingested orally. But the dogs lost weight and showed negative nitrogen balance when they were given a fat-free diet by mouth without infusions of fat emulsion.[3]

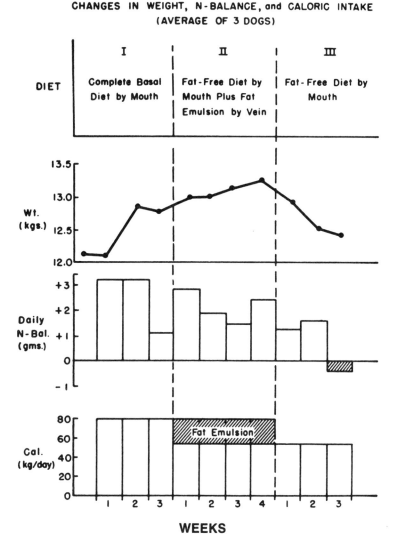

Fig 3. Changes in weight, nitrogen balance, and caloric intake (average of 3 dogs).[3]

Figure 4 illustrates that greater nitrogen and potassium retention and weight gain were observed in a patient during the period when additional calories in the form of fat emulsions were given.[3]

Findings of Abbott, Krieger, and associates are given in Figure 5.[26] Administration of dextrose alone resulted in a negative nitrogen balance. Dextrose plus amino acids or protein hydrolysate reduced the negative nitrogen balance. Dextrose, protein hydrolysate, and fat emulsion further reduced the negative nitrogen balance. In addition to the increased retention of nitrogen, marked weight loss was also checked when additional calories were given as fat.

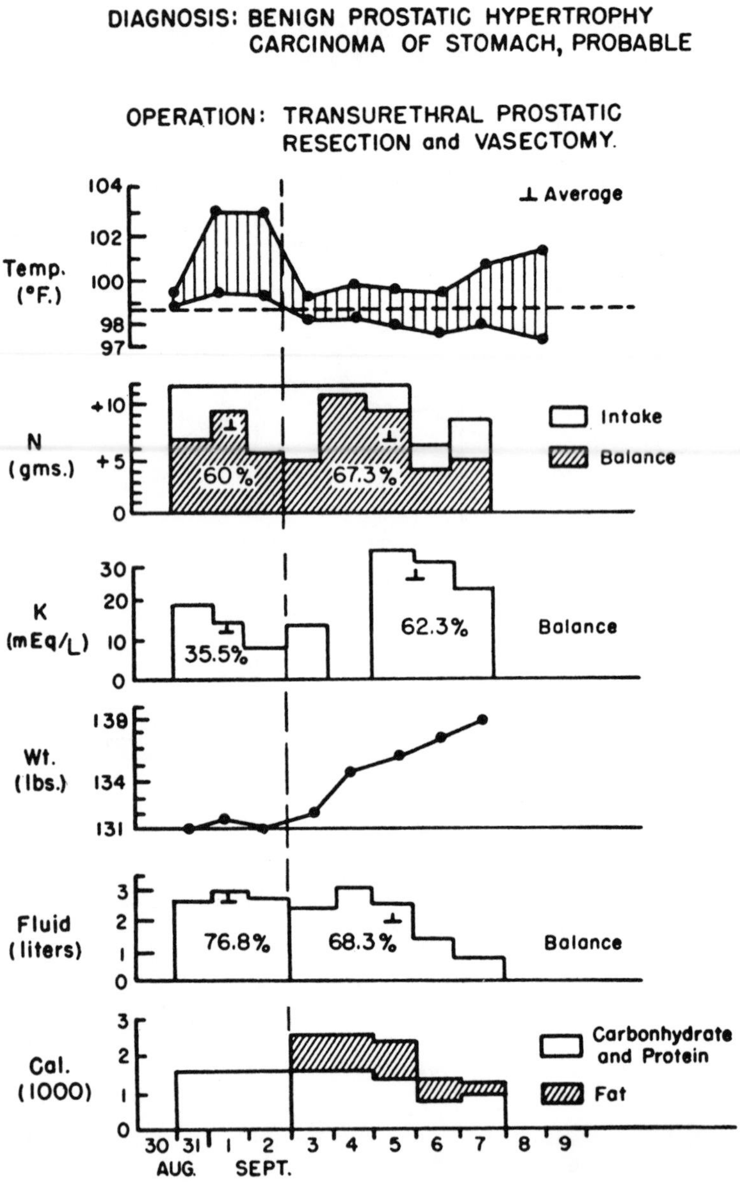

DIAGNOSIS: BENIGN PROSTATIC HYPERTROPHY
CARCINOMA OF STOMACH, PROBABLE

OPERATION: TRANSURETHRAL PROSTATIC
RESECTION and VASECTOMY.

Fig 4. Increase in nitrogen and potassium retention in a post-operative patient given a fat emulsion.[3]

Jacobson and Wretlind studied a patient who received parenteral nutrition with fat for a prolonged period (Fig 6). Weight gain and positive nitrogen balance were observed.[23] Obviously, the intravenously administered fat emulsion was being utilized for energy, a conclusion supported by the results of many investigators.[12, 15, 16, 18-25] Utilization of intravenously administered Intralipid in infants has also been reported.[27-29]

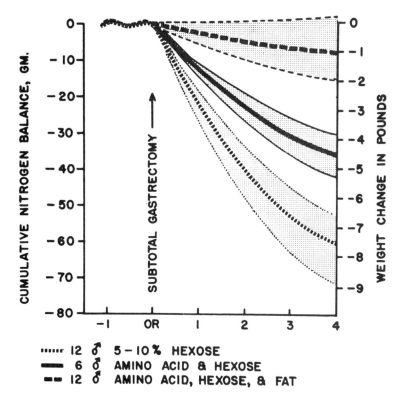

Fig 5. Cumulative nitrogen balances and changes in body weight for 30 male patients who were maintained on one of three different nutritional regimens following a subtotal gastrectomy.[26]

TRIGLYCERIDE IN IV NUTRITION

The importance of triglyceride other than its function as a source of essential fatty acids was first suggested by Deuel et al.[1] Some years ago, we undertook studies to determine the importance of triglyceride in long-term intravenous nutrition in dogs and obtained findings in support of this suggestion.[2,3,30] In the first part of our study, five young adult dogs were fed a complete synthetic diet furnishing 80 kcal/kg/day for three to four weeks as controls; 50% of the calorie total came from carbohydrate (sucrose, 10 gm/kg/day); 34% from fat (lard, 3 gm/kg/day); and 16% from protein (casein, 3 gm/kg/day). Immediately following the three or four weeks of oral feeding, four dogs were given a diet containing the same amount of carbohydrate, protein, and fat, but the diet was administered exclusively by vein. The carbohydrate was glucose; the protein, a casein hydrolysate (Amigen); and fat was given as a 10% olive oil emulsion. Minerals and vitamins were supplied in adequate amounts as during the period of oral feeding. Water was allowed ad libitum. The fifth dog received the same amount of carbohydrate, protein, minerals, and vitamins, but without the fat emulsion. The caloric intake of this dog during the period of parenteral nutrition was 53 kcal/kg/day.

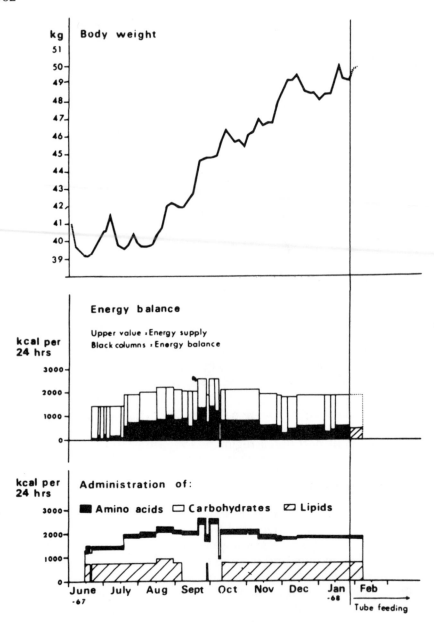

Fig 6. Changes in body weight and energy balance of a patient during complete intravenous nutrition for 7 months and 13 days.[23]

The nutrient solution and fat emulsion were administered into the superior vena cava through an indwelling catheter inserted percutaneously into the external jugular vein. All five dogs were maintained on parenteral nutrition for four weeks with nothing by mouth except water.

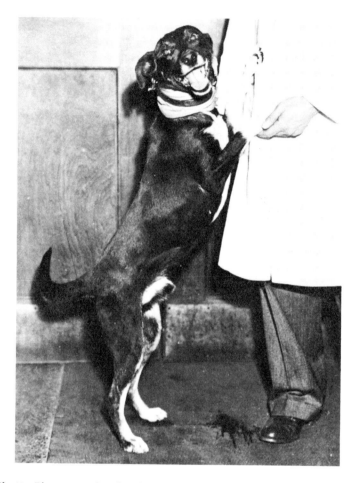

Fig 7. Photograph of a dog at the end of the four-week period of complete parenteral nutrition including fat emulsion. The caloric intake of this dog was 80 kcal/kg/day.[30]

The four dogs which received complete parenteral nutrition including the fat in the form of olive oil emulsion remained healthy and lively throughout. Their hair was smooth and shining (Fig 7). The fifth dog, which received no fat, appeared emaciated and apathetic. Its hair was very coarse and dry, and epilation was beginning on the hind legs (Fig 8). The animals receiving complete parenteral nutrition, including fat, maintained or slightly increased their body weight during the period of infusion; but the dog which did not receive fat lost 14% of its initial weight. The nitrogen balance of the four dogs receiving fat was slightly variable during the period of infusion. The nitrogen retention of the dog given no fat was much less than that during the control period with oral feeding.

A number of tests, which included rose bengal clearance, serum alkaline phosphatase, total plasma proteins and plasma NPN, RBC and WBC counts, blood hemoglobin, hematocrit, and water balance, did not reveal any abnormalities attributable to the procedure.

164

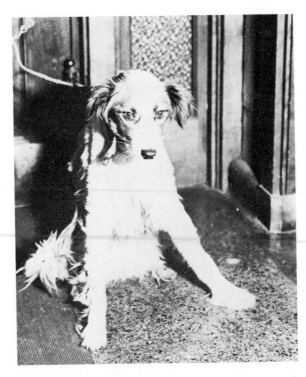

Fig 8. Photograph of the dog at the end of the four-week period of parenteral nutrition without fat emulsion. The caloric intake of this dog was 53 kcal/kg/day.[30]

The weight loss of the dog which did not receive fat in the above experiment, may have been due to insufficient caloric intake, deficiency of essential fatty acids (EFA), deficiency of triglyceride, or a combination of these factors.

The second part of the study was undertaken to investigate the cause of weight loss, or more specifically whether a diet furnishing adequate calories and EFA—but deficient in triglyceride—would maintain health, weight, and nitrogen balance.

As in the experiment described above, five healthy adult male dogs were fed a normal synthetic diet furnishing 80 kcal/kg/day for three weeks. Immediately following this period, one dog, which was the "control" animal, received the same caloric intake of protein, carbohydrate, and fat, administered by vein. Two dogs also received parenteral nutrition except that glucose was substituted isocalorically for fat, and a supplementation of EFA was given by mouth: methyl linoleate, methyl linolenate, and methyl arachidonate in amounts of 100 mg, 100 mg, and 10 mg/kg/day, respectively. The other two dogs received isocaloric parenteral nutrition with no fat or EFA supplementation. All five dogs received the same amount of protein, vitamins, and minerals. The period of parenteral nutrition lasted for four weeks.

The control dog receiving complete parenteral nutrition, including fat emulsion, remained healthy and lively throughout. The two dogs which re-

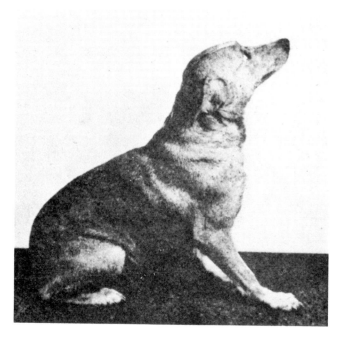

Fig 9. Photograph of a dog at the end of the four-week period of parenteral nutrition including fat emulsion. The caloric intake of this dog was 80 kcal/kg/day.[3]

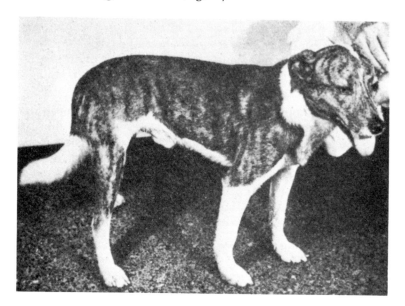

Fig 10. Photograph of a dog at the end of the four-week period of parenteral nutrition without fat. Essential fatty acids as methyl esters of linoleic, linolenic, and arachidonic acids were given daily. The caloric intake was 80 kcal/kg/day as a hypertonic solution of glucose.[3]

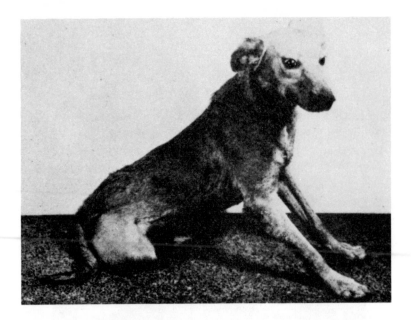

Fig 11. Photograph of a dog at the end of the four-week period of parenteral nutrition with neither fat nor essential fatty acids. The caloric intake was 80 kcal/kg/day as hypertonic solution of glucose.[3]

ceived only the EFA supplement were not as lively and alert as the control dog, but no abnormal changes were observed in their hair. The two dogs which received neither fat nor EFA appeared apathetic and emaciated. Their hair was coarse, dry, and fell out rapidly. Figures 9, 10, and 11 are photographs of dogs receiving parenteral nutrition with fat, with EFA, and with neither fat nor essential fatty acids.

The dog on complete parenteral nutrition with fat emulsion gained 7.6% of its initial weight during the four-week period. The other four dogs receiving the same total caloric intake but lacking fat emulsion lost 4.3% to 9.2% of their initial weights. Supplementation of EFA did not prevent weight loss. In no instance was the nitrogen balance negative in the dog given parenteral nutrition with fat emulsion, although nitrogen retention was less during the weeks of parenteral nutrition than in the period of oral feeding. The other dogs which received no fat showed little retention or negative nitrogen balance.

These results indicate that—without triglyceride—an adequate diet with respect to calories, protein, the known vitamins and minerals does not promote optimal body weight gain. The administration of EFA prevents certain specific pathologic changes but does not permit optimal weight gain and well-being in the absence of triglyceride. Also, intravenous infusion of a complete diet including adequate triglyceride is compatible with excellent health, weight gain, and positive nitrogen balance.

Admittedly, the results are by no means conclusive. Further work is required to substantiate or negate these findings.

How much fat or triglyceride should be given in parenteral nutrition?

Our experience with an adult patient receiving 2,700 kilocalories from non-protein sources suggests that 900 kilocalories or 100 gm of fat may be given. Hence, approximately one-third of the total caloric supply may come from fat, with the fat dosage about 1.5 gm/kg/day. Our usual practice is to start at 0.5 gm/kg/day in parenteral nutrition; the dosage is increased stepwise to 1.5 to 2.0 gm/kg/day. In infants and young children, fat may be given at a dosage as high as 3 to 4 gm/kg/day as suggested by Coran et al.[27-29] It is suggested that the rate of infusion of fat emulsion should not be more than 0.3 gm/kg/hr in adults and 0.5 gm/kg/hr in infants. Perhaps it may be given continuously during the 24-hour period. This reduces the rate of infusion considerably. Certain biochemical and physiological studies (eg, hemogram, including thrombocyte count, blood coagulation, liver function tests, and plasma lipid profile) should be monitored before each increment of fat dosage and at appropriate intervals in long-term administration of fat emulsion.

Removal of IV fat emulsion from circulation The rate of removal of the intravenously administered emulsion from the blood circulation depends on the dosage.[31] Figure 12 illustrates the removal of four fat emulsions given to rats at different dosages. Note that fat given at 300 mg/kg or less was removed at a faster rate, while doses higher than 500 mg/kg remained in the blood considerably longer. The T 1/2 (time taken to remove half of the initial

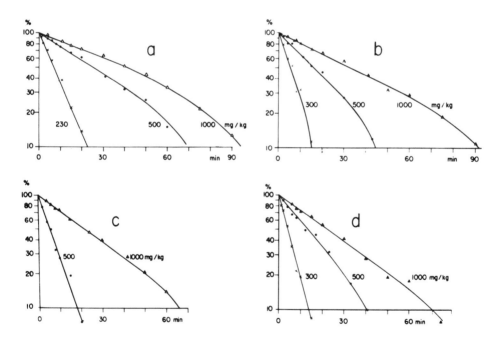

Fig 12. Removal from rat blood of chylomicrons and three different fat emulsions: (a) Chylomicrons, (b) cottonseed oil-soybean phosphatide emulsion (Infonutrol or Lipomul), (c) nonphosphatide-cottonseed oil emulsion (SR 695), (d) soybean oil-egg phosphatide emulsion (Intralipid).[31]

168

dose) removal of chylomicron and Intralipid triglyceride in dogs given 500 mg/kg was 13.8 and 15.3 min, respectively, while that of SR 695 (nonphosphatide emulsion) was 8.3, and that of Infonutrol (Lipomul) was 37.2 min (see Fig 13).[31] Similar findings were reported by Hallberg et al (see Fig 14).[20] Thus, the removal of a standard dose of chylomicron and Intralipid triglyceride seems quite similar.

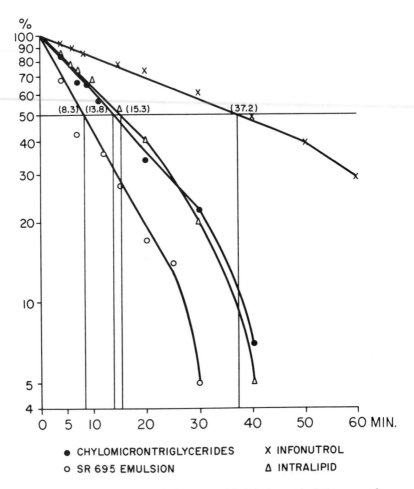

Fig 13. Disappearance of three artificial fat emulsions and washed dietary chylomicrons from the blood circulation of dogs. Dose: 500 mg triglycerides per kg; ●, chylomicra; O, nonphosphatide emulsion (SR 695); x, cottonseed oil emulsion, stabilized with phosphatides (Infonutrol); Δ, soybean oil emulsion, stabilized with egg phosphatides (Intralipid). Figures in parentheses are T 1/2 in minutes.[31]

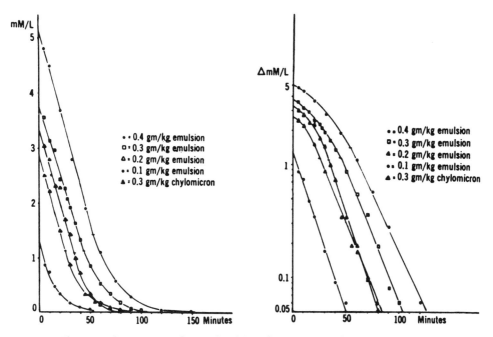

Fig 14. Elimination from the blood stream in dogs receiving a single injection of fat emulsion and chylomicrons. The triglyceride concentration is given for whole blood and represents the increase above the basal level. The intercept on the curves represents the critical concentration. The left diagram is a linear graph, and the right diagram is on a semilogarithmic scale.[16]

For an explanation of how intravenously administered emulsion is removed from the circulation, we have turned to a communication of Scow[32] and to Scow and associates.[33] At the moment we can say that removal of triglyceride, at least in part, requires prior lipolysis. Figure 15 shows that the plasma free fatty acid levels were progressively increased during intravenous infusion of a fat emulsion (Intralipid) in a dog given 1 gm/kg of triglyceride. This finding suggests an increase in lipolytic activity of lipemic plasma; and this proves to be the case. As shown in Table 2, we have isolated and partially purified a lipase from the lipemic plasma of a dog given a fat emulsion. Other investigators have also reported the increase in lipolytic activity of hyperlipemic plasma following intravenous infusion of fat emulsions.[34-36]

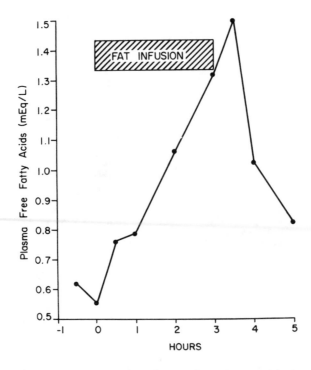

Fig 15. Progress increase in plasma free fatty acids in a dog during intravenous infusion of Intralipid. The dose of fat was 1.0 gm/kg; the infusion was completed in 3 hours.

The rate of removal of the intravenously infused fat emulsion is increased by the intravenous administration of heparin. This is because heparin injection releases clearing factor lipase or lipoprotein lipase which hydrolyzes triglyceride to free fatty acids, free glycerol, and lower glycerides. Free fatty acids and monoglycerides are removed from the blood circulation at a faster rate than triglyceride. Serum total fatty acids in dogs given fat emulsion plus heparin were lower (see Fig 16) than in those given the same amount of fat without heparin; even the total cholesterol was significantly lower in the animals receiving heparin than in those given no heparin.[37]

Table 2.—Lipolytic Activity of Lipemic Plasma and Partially Purified Hyperlipemia-Induced Lipase

Fraction	Total Protein Nitrogen (mg)	Total Activity (units)	Units/mg	Degree of Purification	Yield (%)
Lipemic plasma	6,500	120,000	18.4	0	100
Partially purified fraction	35	35,000	1,000	54.3	29.2

Heparin injection also produced an increase in plasma free fatty acid or unesterified fatty acid levels and increased the rate of removal of the infused triglyceride in man (see Table 3).[38]

Coran et al[28] reported that heparin increased the rate of disappearance of the intravenously injected Intralipid from the blood stream and increased the serum levels of free fatty acids.

In view of the heparin effect, I am compelled to question whether we should give heparin to patients receiving fat emulsion. If the answer is yes, how much heparin should be given? How should it be given? By continuous

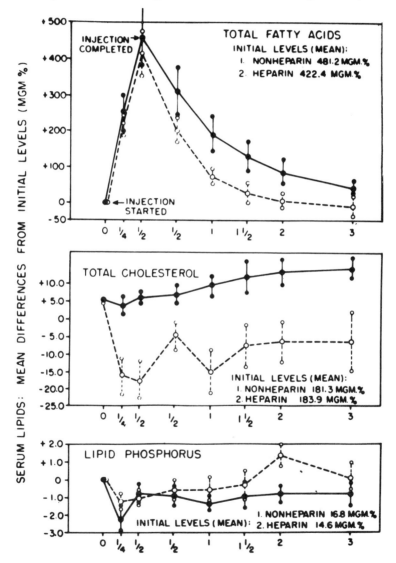

Fig 16. Changes in serum lipids: mean differences from initial levels. Solid lines indicate nonheparinized dogs (10 dogs). Broken lines indicate heparinized dogs (8 dogs). Vertical lines represent standard error of mean.[37]

Table 3.—Effects of Heparin on Changes of Plasma Unesterified Fatty Acids and Total Lipids Following Intravenous Infusion of Fat Emulsion

Analysis		Plasma Unesterified Fatty Acids (mEq/liter)		
	Time	Before Infusion	End of Infusion	3 Hours After Infusion
Mean	Nonheparin	0.493	1.464	0.612
	Heparin	0.543	4.136	0.812
Mean Difference* ±SE		0	2.607	0.188
	P		<0.001	>0.1

*Mean difference between heparinized and nonheparinized groups: For plasma unesterified fatty acids: Mean difference from preinfusion level of heparinized group; mean difference from preinfusion level of nonheparinized group.

infusion with fat emulsion or by injections at intervals? I must emphasize that the heparin required for "clearing" the triglyceride from the blood stream is much less than that necessary for preventing blood coagulation.

LONG-TERM DAILY ADMINISTRATION OF FAT EMULSION

Numerous investigations have been made on the effects of long-term infusions of fat emulsion in animals.[12, 16, 17, 21, 39] The long-term studies in humans have been conducted primarily with Lipomul[39-47, 49, 50] and Intralipid.[16, 21, 23, 24, 39, 48] The results are as follows:

Anemia After daily infusion of Lipomul (cottonseed oil emulsion) for two to three weeks or longer, a mild to moderate degree of anemia was observed.[49, 50] The cause of the anemia is not well understood.[51] Long-term infusion of Intralipid (soybean oil emulsion) produced a slight decrease in hemoglobin and red blood cell count; however, a large amount of fat was given.[52, 53]

Blood platelets and blood coagulation Daily infusion of Lipomul for four weeks produced a slight decrease in blood platelets (from an average control level of 230,000/cu mm to that of 185,000).[50] A mild decrease in thrombocytes was also observed in some patients given Intralipid (M.D. Caldwell, A. Otten, H.C. Meng, and J.A. O'Neill, Jr., unpublished data).

The blood coagulation time was shortened during infusion of Lipomul in the presence of hyperlipemia. The coagulation time was slightly to moderately prolonged after daily infusions for four weeks. Poor clot restriction was also observed after long-term infusions of Lipomul. Possible mechanisms of these changes have been discussed by Meng and Kaley.[50] Duckert and Hartmann[54] and Cronberg et al[55] have shown that infusion of Intralipid has no effect on the coagulation or on the fibrinolytic system. But the possibility of hypocoagulability after long-term daily infusion of any emulsion should be kept in mind, and blood coagulation time should be monitored when patients are given long-term fat infusion.

	Plasma Total Lipids (mg/100 ml)			
Before Infusion	1 Hour During Infusion	End of Infusion	After Infusion	
			1 hr.	3 hrs.
681	1199	1963	1579	1492
722	1043	1715	1254	922
0	172	329	396	587
	>0.1	=0.009	=0.004	<0.001

For plasma total lipids: Mean difference from preinfusion level of nonheparinized group; mean difference from preinfusion level of heparinized group.

Plasma fibrinogen was not significantly altered in concentration after long-term infusions of Lipomul. The oxalated plasma, however, remained fragile and jellylike after recalcification, and addition of thrombin did not correct the defect.[50]

Serum lipids In our study with Lipomul, we noted no significant increase in serum total fatty acids and neutral lipid fatty acids after long-term infusions at a dosage of 1 to 1.5 gm fat per kg. Serum total cholesterol and phospholipids were not altered. This is true even in patients in whom "overloading syndrome" was encountered.[45]

Liver functions Serum alkaline phosphatase was not increased after multiple daily infusions of Lipomul. In some patients, slight to moderate increase in bromosulfophthalein retention was noticed after two to four weeks of daily infusions. Prothrombin time (expressed as percent of normal) was also decreased in some patients after multiple infusions of Lipomul.[50] Some changes in liver function have also been observed after intravenous infusion of Intralipid.[24]

Overloading syndrome Overloading syndrome has been observed by several investigators in patients receiving multiple infusions of Lipomul.[38-43, 50] These patients experienced anorexia, fever, headache, abdominal pain, nausea, vomiting and sore throat and showed signs of impaired liver function, anemia, thrombocytopenia, and, at times, hepatosplenomegaly, spontaneous bleeding, and delayed blood clotting. The exact nature of this syndrome and the mechanism of its production remain unexplained. It does not appear to be due to accumulation of lipids in the blood circulation.[43, 44] Meng and Kaley reported that the only significant change which may correlate with this syndrome was the significant decrease in both urinary 17-ketosteroids and 17-hydroxycorticosteroids.[50] This syndrome has not been observed in patients given multiple infusion of Intralipid. Joint efforts should be made, nevertheless, by investigators conducting clinical studies of Intralipid to be certain that adverse effects do not occur.

Intravenous fat pigments IV fat pigments, also microgranulomas in the liver and spleen, have been observed in animals and patients after intravenous infusions of the fat emulsions studied.[56] While the significance of the pigment deposition is not known, it would be desirable to prevent the formation of microgranulomas. In collaboration with the US Army Medical Research and Nutrition Laboratory, we have investigated the possibility of preventing or minimizing these changes.[57] At dosages of 2.5 mg or 5.0 mg/day, vitamin E, with methionine, selenium, or choline was given to rats receiving 15 ml or 3.0 gm of fat per kg as 20% Intralipid. As predicted, Intralipid alone produced IV fat pigment deposition in the liver and spleen. Vitamin E at a dosage of 2.5 mg might have decreased the pigment deposition slightly. However, other agents given alone or in combination did not produce any beneficial changes (see Fig 17).

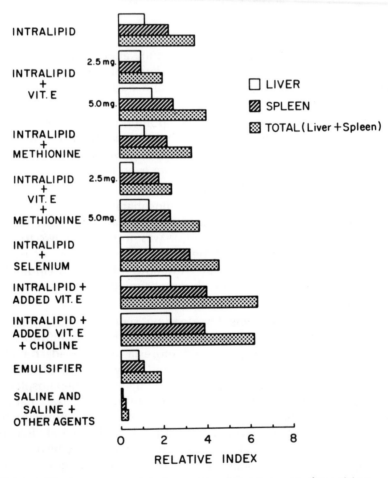

Fig 17. Mean scores of intravenous fat pigment deposition in the livers and spleens of rats given 30 consecutive daily injections of Intralipid alone or with oral administration of antioxidants and/or lipotropic agents.[56]

Injection of a 20% Intralipid solution at a dosage of 15 ml or 3.0 gm of fat per kg produced microgranuloma formation in the liver and spleen (Fig 18). This microgranuloma formation was much less than the pigment deposition. Administration of 2.5 mg of Vitamin E prevented the formation of microgranulomas in the liver and decreased that in the spleen. No microgranulomas were observed in the livers and spleens of rats given Intralipid along with Vitamin E (2.5 mg/day) and methionine. But 2.5 mg of Vitamin E were more effective than 5 mg in preventing the microgranuloma formation.

Gastric secretion In rats given 15 ml/kg (3.0 gm fat/kg) of a 20% Intralipid solution, a slight increase in acid secretion was observed. Increasing the dosage of Intralipid to 30 ml or 6 gm of fat per kg produced an inhibition of gastric secretion (Fig 19). The volume of gastric secretion did not change when 15 ml or 3.0 gm/kg of fat were given. A decrease in volume of gastric secretion occurred when 30 ml or 6.0 gm of fat per kg of Intralipid were administered (Fig 20).[58]

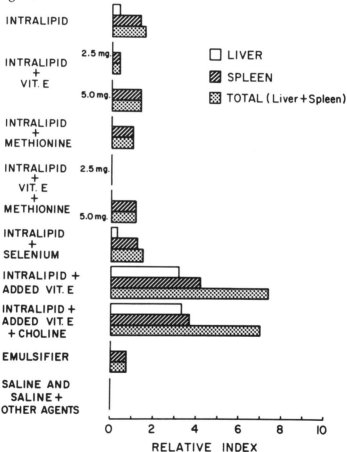

Fig 18. Mean scores of microgranuloma formation in the livers and spleens of rats given 30 consecutive daily injections of Intralipid alone or with oral administration of antioxidants and/or lipotropic agents.[57]

176

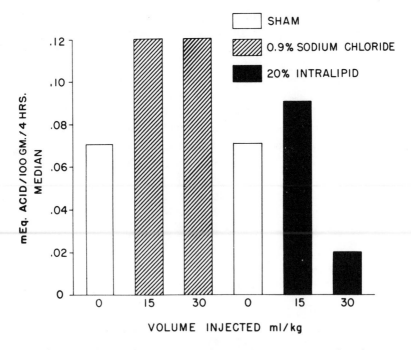

Fig 19. Gastric acid output from total gastric pouch of rats given 20% Intralipid (modified from Baume et al[58]).

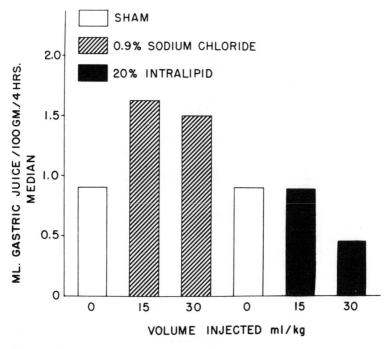

Fig 20. Volume of gastric secretion from rats given 20% Intralipid (modified from Baume et al[58]).

Cohn et al[59] and Meng (unpublished data) observed peptic ulcer formation in dogs receiving Lipomul. I am not aware of any study concerning the effect of fat emulsion on gastric secretion in man and would welcome investigation of the problem.

ESSENTIAL FATTY ACID REQUIREMENT IN TPN

Numerous observations suggest the multiple functions of the essential fatty acid(s).[60, 61] Before discussing these, I would like to bring up a few points pertinent to the use of fat emulsion in parenteral nutrition. First, let us look at some unsaturated fatty acids (Fig 21). Oleic acid (monoene), one of

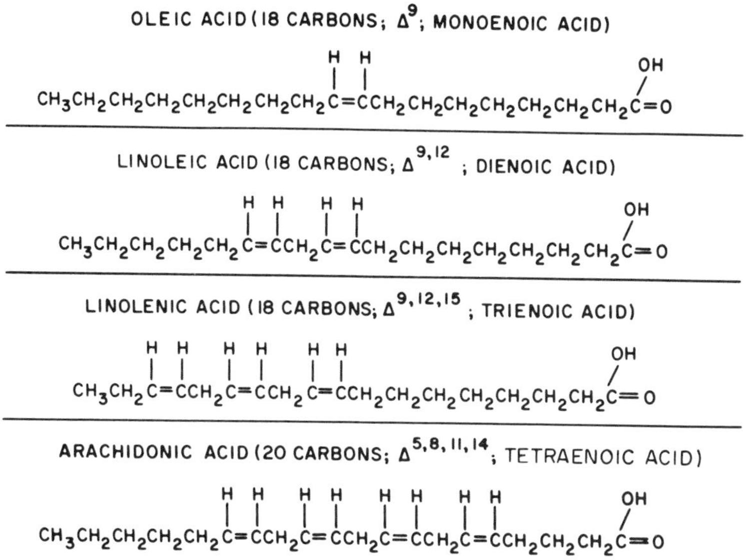

OLEIC ACID (18 CARBONS; Δ^9; MONOENOIC ACID)

$$CH_3CH_2CH_2CH_2CH_2CH_2CH_2CH_2\underset{|}{C}=\underset{|}{C}CH_2CH_2CH_2CH_2CH_2CH_2CH_2C=O$$

LINOLEIC ACID (18 CARBONS; $\Delta^{9,12}$; DIENOIC ACID)

$$CH_3CH_2CH_2CH_2CH_2C=CCH_2C=CCH_2CH_2CH_2CH_2CH_2CH_2C=O$$

LINOLENIC ACID (18 CARBONS; $\Delta^{9,12,15}$; TRIENOIC ACID)

$$CH_3CH_2C=CCH_2C=CCH_2C=CCH_2CH_2CH_2CH_2CH_2CH_2C=O$$

ARACHIDONIC ACID (20 CARBONS; $\Delta^{5,8,11,14}$; TETRAENOIC ACID)

$$CH_3CH_2CH_2CH_2CH_2C=CCH_2C=CCH_2C=CCH_2C=CCH_2CH_2CH_2C=O$$

Fig 21. Formulas of unsaturated fatty acids.

the commonly occurring fatty acids with one double bond, is not considered an essential fatty acid. Linoleic (diene), linolenic (triene), and arachidonic (tetraene) acids with two, three, and four double bonds at the specific positions of the carbon chain are polyunsaturated and are essential fatty acids.

18:1 (Δ^9) $\longrightarrow$ 18:2 ($\Delta^{6,9}$) $\longrightarrow$ 20:2 ($\Delta^{8,11}$) $\longrightarrow$ 20:3 ($\Delta^{5,8,11}$)
OLEIC ACID   EICOSATRIENOIC ACID

18:2 ($\Delta^{9,12}$) $\longrightarrow$ 18:3 ($\Delta^{6,9,12}$) $\longrightarrow$ 20:3 ($\Delta^{8,11,14}$) $\longrightarrow$ 20:4 ($\Delta^{5,8,11,14}$)
LINOLEIC ACID   ARACHIDONIC ACID

18:3 ($\Delta^{9,12,15}$) $\longrightarrow$ 18:4 ($\Delta^{6,9,12,15}$) $\longrightarrow$ 20:4 ($\Delta^{8,11,14,15}$) $\longrightarrow$ 20:5 ($\Delta^{5,8,11,14,17}$) $\longrightarrow$
LINOLENIC ACID
22:5 ($\Delta^{7,10,13,16,19}$) $\longrightarrow$ 22:6 ($\Delta^{4,7,10,13,16,19}$)

Fig 22. Desaturation and carbon chain elongation of unsaturated fatty acids.

In the absence of a dietary supply of the essential fatty acids, there will be a decrease of dienes and tetraenes and an increase in monoenes (oleic acid). These would lead to the failure of formation of arachidonic (tetraene) and other polyunsaturated fatty acids which may be necessary for maintenance of normal structure of cell membranes among other functions. The desaturation and carbon chain elongation of oleic acid will form a triene, eicosatrienoic acid, which is present in a minute amount in individuals with adequate intake of essential fatty acids (Fig 22).

With absence of essential fatty acids in the diet and increase in the formation of eicosatrienoic acid, a decrease in dienoic and tetraenoic acids will occur. These changes are observed by determining the serum fatty acid composition by gas liquid chromatography. Table 4 illustrates the changes in serum dienes, trienes, and tetraenes in infants of various ages on a milk mixture intake containing various amounts of linoleic acid.[62] Holman et al reported that the triene to tetraene ratio was increased in infants of two to four months of age when their intake of linoleic acid was less than 1% of the total caloric intake.[63] Figure 23 shows this relationship. Based on the evidence of serum fatty acid composition, the minimum requirement and optimum intake of linoleic acid in infants appear to be 1% and 4% of the total

Table 4.— Mean Dienoic, Trienoic and Tetraenoic Acids in Blood Serum in Relation to Age of Infant and Dietary Intake of Linoleate

Age (months)	Linoleic Acid in Milk Mixture (% of Calories)				
	<0.1	0.1	1.3	2.8	7.3
3					
dienoic	2.8	5.5	12.9	29.0	35.4
trienoic	5.5	3.7	2.5	1.8	1.4
tetraenoic	2.6	2.7	8.0	9.1	10.8
6					
dienoic	7.9	10.9	15.7	30.5	37.6
trienoic	4.4	3.5	2.2	1.7	1.3
tetraenoic	3.3	3.9	8.6	9.8	10.5
9					
dienoic	9.2	17.1	17.6	30.8	36.9
trienoic	3.1	3.4	2.3	1.8	1.4
tetraenoic	4.6	5.9	9.1	10.5	11.6
12					
dienoic	12.5	19.9	20.9	30.6	36.5
trienoic	3.1	2.5	2.0	1.8	1.8
tetraenoic	6.5	8.3	10.1	10.7	11.2

Note: Dienoic, trienoic, and tetraenoic acids are expressed as percent of the total fatty acids in serum.

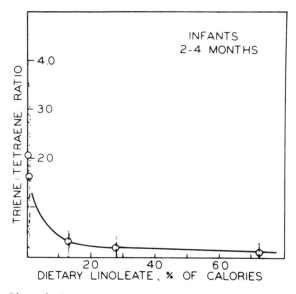

Fig 23. Plot of triene to tetraene ratio of total serum fatty acids versus the intake of linoleic acid of infants two to four months of age.[63]

calories, respectively. Soderhjelm et al compiled data of other investigators showing that essential fatty acid deficiency decreased the efficiency in calorie utilization.[61] Note in Table 5 that the optimum amount of linoleic acid intake appears to be 4% to 5% of the total calories.

Table 5.—Effect of Linoleic Acid Intake on Utilization of Calories

Investigator	Caloric Utilization Expressed As	Dietary Linoleic Acid % of Calories			
		<0.1	1.0-1.5	4-5	>5
Adam et al	Kcal/kg/day	155	106	85	85
Combes et al (prematures)	Kcal/kg gm gain/day	7.4*	. . .	6.5*	. . .
Hansen et al	Kcal/kg gm gain/day	6.3†	4.7†	3.9†	. . .

*P<0.02
†P<0.01

Essential fatty acid deficiency has also been reported by Collins et al in an adult patient given long-term parenteral nutrition without fat.[64] Data in Figure 24 show the eicosatrienoic acid in plasma phospholipid fatty acids to be increased. After infusions of Intralipid for a few days a marked decrease in eicosatrienoic acid was observed. The increase in eicosatrienoic acid was correlated with the clinical syndrome that could be induced by discontinuing Intralipid for about three weeks. It could be prevented by the administration of Intralipid. Biochemical and clinical observations of essential fatty acid deficiency in infants given long-term parenteral nutrition without fat have been reported.[65-68] We also observed EFA deficiency in our studies of adults (M.D. Caldwell, A. Otten, H.C. Meng, and J.A. O'Neill, Jr., unpublished data).

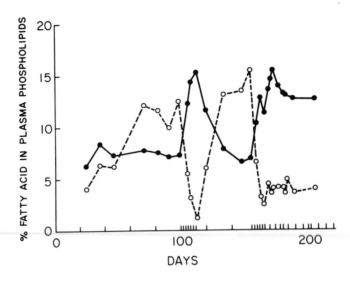

Fig 24. Patient P.P., placed on intravenous therapy on day 1, was maintained without fats except as shown by the vertical bars; each bar represents 500 ml of a 20% Intralipid containing 100 gm of soybean oil. At the times shown, samples of plasma were obtained, the lipids extracted and separated by thin layer chromatography, and the fatty acids from the phospholipids analyzed by gas chromatography. Arachidonic acid is shown as ●—●—●, and 5, 8, 11—eicosatrienoic acid is shown o----o.[64]

CONTRAINDICATIONS FOR CLINICAL USE OF FAT EMULSION

Waddell and Geyer[69] reported that removal of intravenously administered emulsion from the blood circulation was decreased in depancreatized dogs. Insulin corrected this defect. We do not know if the insulin effect is secondary to the improvement of glucose metabolism. Coran et al[70] reported that Intralipid infusion did not cause any increase in serum insulin levels. Apparently insulin control is necessary in diabetics receiving fat emulsion.

Intravenous administration of fat emulsion may be contraindicated in patients with certain types of hyperlipidemia. It is known that clearing factor lipase (lipoprotein lipase) release after heparin administration was greatly decreased in these patients.[71]

The liver functions in uptake and metabolism of chylomicron triglyceride fatty acids. Careful consideration should be given before fat emulsion is administered to patients with liver diseases. Kern et al[72] observed, however, that administration of Lipomul to patients with Laennec's cirrhosis did not produce toxic effects attributable to liver disease.

Since the intravenously administered fat emulsion will reach the heart and lung first, should a patient with pulmonary disease be given fat emulsion? Pulmonary membrane diffusion capacity was decreased after intravenous infusion of Intralipid, according to Greene and associates.[73]

Some physicians consider that the insertion of a catheter into a central vein may be difficult and subject to high probability of sepsis, that it would be more convenient and safer to administer all solutions for parenteral nutrition into a peripheral vein. The reasoning is that, if fat emulsion is given, concentrated carbohydrate solution is not necessary and peripheral vein delivery may be possible. Coran was able to achieve weight gain, positive nitrogen balance, positive potassium balance, and proper K/N ratio in infants receiving parenteral nutrition including fat emulsion administered via peripheral veins.[29]

SUMMARY

Infusion of the fat emulsions currently available for clinical use is not followed by the acute adverse reactions we encountered some years ago. We have found from experimental and clinical studies that the intravenously administered fat emulsion is being biologically utilized for energy and to meet the requirement for essential fatty acids. Some undesirable long-term effects are observed, however, as a result of intravenous administration of fat emulsions—eg, IV fat pigments and formation of microgranulomas. Their cause and significance are not well understood. Further work is necessary to improve our understanding of the technique of TPN so that we may obtain fat emulsions that are more ideal and expand our knowledge in fat transport and metabolism. Our goal: to eliminate all possible adverse effects.

References

1. Deuel HJ Jr, Greenberg SM, Calbert CE, et al: The effect of fat level of the diet on general nutrition. V. The relationship of the linoleic acid requirement to optimum fat level. *J Nutr* **40:**351-366, 1950.

2. Meng HC, Youmans JB: The indispensability of fat in parenteral alimentation in dogs. *J Clin Nutr* **1:**372-383, 1953.

3. Meng HC: Preparation, utilization and importance of neutral fat emulsion to intravenous alimentation, in Najjar V (ed): *Fat Metabolism*. Baltimore, Johns Hopkins Press, 1954, p 69.

4. Meyer CE, Fancher JA, Schurr PE, Webster HD: Composition, preparation and testing of an intravenous fat emulsion. *Metabolism* **6:**591-596, 1957.

5. Zilversmit DB, Salky NK, Trumbull ML, McCandless EL: The preparation and use of anhydrous fat emulsions for intravenous feeding and metabolic experiments. *J Lab Clin Med* **48:**386-391, 1956.

6. Wretlind A: Effect of tributyrin on circulation and respiration. *Acta Physiol Scand* **40:**59-74, 1957.

7. Wretlind A: The toxicity of low-molecular triglycerides. *Acta Physiol Scand* **40:**338-343, 1957.

8. Shafiroff BGP, Frank C: A homogenous emulsion of fat, protein and glucose for intravenous administration. *Science* **106:**474-475, 1947.

9. Shafiroff BGP, Baron HC, Roth E: Intravenous infusions of a combined fat emulsion into dogs. *Proc Soc Exp Biol Med* **69:**387-391, 1948.

10. Shafiroff BGP, Mulholland JH, Roth E, Baron HC: Intravenous infusions of a combined fat emulsion into human subjects. *Proc Soc Exp Biol Med* **70:**343-349, 1949.

11. Shafiroff BGP, Mulholland JH: Effects of intravenous infusion of experimental "instant" fat emulsion into volunteer subjects. *Proc Soc Exp Biol Med* **91:**111-113, 1956.

12. Geyer RP: Parenteral nutrition. *Physiol Rev* **40:**150-186, 1960.

13. Edgren B, Wretlind A: The theoretical background of the intravenous nutrition with fat emulsions. *Nutr Dieta* **5:**364-386, 1963.

14. Wretlind A: The pharmacological basis for the use of fat emulsions in intravenous nutrition. *Acta Chir Scand* (suppl) **325:**314, 1964.

15. Lawson LJ: Parenteral nutrition in surgery. *Br J Surg* **52:**795-800, 1965.

16. Hallberg D, Schuberth O, Wretlind A: Experimental and clinical studies with fat emulsion for intravenous nutrition. *Nutr Dieta* **8:**245-281, 1966.

17. Geyer RP: Parenteral emulsions: Formulation, preparation and use in animals, in Meng HC, Law DH (eds): *Proceedings of International Symposium on Parenteral Nutrition*. Springfield, Charles C. Thomas, 1970, p 339.

18. Krieger H, Abbott WE, Levey S, Holden WD: The use of fat emulsion as a source of calories in patients requiring intravenous alimentation. *Gastroenterology* **33:**807-816, 1957.

19. Artz CP: Newer concepts of nutrition by the intravenous route. *Ann Surg* **149:**841-849, 1959.

20. Scharli A: Praktische Gesichtspunkte bei der vollen parenteralen Ernährung. *Int Z Vitamin-Forsch* **35:**52-59, 1965.

21. Hallberg D, Schuberth O, Wretlind A: Experimental and clinical studies of fat emulsions for intravenous nutrition, in Meng HC, Law DH (eds): *Proceedings of International Symposium on Parenteral Nutrition.* Springfield, Charles C. Thomas, 1970, p 376.

22. Heller L: Problems of complete parenteral nutrition, in Meng HC, Law DH (eds): *Proceedings of International Symposium on Parenteral Nutrition.* Springfield, Charles C. Thomas, 1970, p 516.

23. Jacobson S, Wretlind A: The use of fat emulsions for complete intravenous nutrition, in Fox CL, Nahas GG (eds): *Body Fluid and Replacement in the Surgical Patient.* New York, Grune and Stratton, 1970, p 334.

24. Wretlind A: Complete intravenous nutrition: Theoretical and experimental background. *Nutr Metab* **14** (suppl): 57, 1972.

25. Zohrab WJ, McHattie JD, Jeejeebhoy KN: Total parenteral alimentation with lipid. *Gastroenterology* **64:**583-592, 1973.

26. Abbott WE, Krieger H, Holden WD, et al: Effect of intravenously administered fat on body weight and nitrogen balance in surgical patients. *Metabolism* **6:**691-702, 1957.

27. Coran AG, Nesbakken R: The metabolism of intravenously administered fat in adult and newborn dogs. *Surgery* **66:**922-928, 1969.

28. Børresen HC, Coran AG, Knutrud O: Metabolic results of parenteral feeding in neonatal surgery: A balanced parenteral feeding program based on a synthetic L-amino acid solution and a commercial fat emulsion. *Ann Surg* **172:**291-301, 1970.

29. Coran AG: The intravenous use of fat for the total parenteral nutrition of the infant. *Lipids* **7:**455-458, 1972.

30. Meng HC, Early F: Study of complete parenteral alimentation on dogs. *J Lab Clin Med* **34:**1121-1132, 1949.

31. Edgren B, Meng HC: The removal of dietary chylomicrons and artificial fat emulsions from the circulation of rats. *Acta Physiol Scand* **56:**237-243, 1962.

32. Scow RO: Transport of triglyceride: its removal from blood circulation and uptake by tissues, in Meng HC, Law DH (eds): *Proceedings of International Symposium on Parenteral Nutrition,* Springfield. Charles C. Thomas, 1970, p 294.

33. Scow RO, Hamosh M, Blanchette EJ, et al: Uptake of blood triglyceride by various tissues. *Lipids* **7:**497-505, 1972.

34. Edgren B: The lipolytic activity in dog plasma after intravenous fat emulsion. *Arch Int Pharmacodyn Ther* **126:**255-270, 1960.

35. Lever WF, Baskys B: Effects of intravenous administration of fat emulsions and their emulsifying agents: I. Effects on clearing factor and activity, electrophoretic pattern and clotting time of blood of dogs. *J Invest Dermatol* **28:**317-320, 1957.

36. Engelberg H: Human endogenous plasma lipemia clearing activity after intravenous fat emulsion (Lipomul). *J Appl Physiol* **12:**292-296, 1958.

37. Meng HC, Youmans JB: Effect of heparin on serum lipids following intravenous administration of fat emulsion in dogs. *Proc Soc Exp Biol Med* **97:**691-693, 1958.

184

38. Shoulders HH Jr, Meng HC, Tuggle S: Effects of heparin on body temperature and plasma lipids following intravenous administration of fat emulsion in man. *J Lab Clin Med* **52**:559-563, 1958.

39. Mueller JF, Canham JE (eds): Symposium on intravenous fat emulsions. *Am J Clin Nutr* **16**:1-4, 1965.

40. Levenson SM, Upjohn HL, Sheehy TW: Two severe reactions following the long-term infusion of large amounts of intravenous fat emulsion. *Metabolism* **6**:807-814, 1957.

41. Watkin DM: Clinical, chemical, hematologic and anatomic changes accompanying repeated intravenous administration of fat emulsion to man. *Metabolism* **6**:785-806, 1957.

42. Mueller JF: Recent advances in intravenous fat alimentation. *Am J Clin Nutr* **6:**472, 1958.

43. Mueller JF, Viteri FE: Clinical studies in patients receiving long-term infusions of fat emulsion. *J Okla State Med Assoc* **53:**367-373, 1960.

44. Alexander CS, Zieve L: Fat infusions: Toxic effects and alterations in fasting serum lipids following prolonged use. *Arch Intern Med* **107:**514-528, 1961.

45. Meng HC, Kaley JS, Shapiro JL: Serum lipids and electrophoretic patterns of proteins, lipoproteins and glycoproteins in patients receiving multiple infusions of fat emulsion. *Metabolism* **11:**315-328, 1962.

46. Kaley JS, Meng HC, Bingham C: Some hematologic changes in patients receiving multiple intravenous infusions of fat emulsion. *Am J Clin Nutr* **7:**652-656, 1959.

47. Preston CJ, Barnes AV, Mandel EE, et al: Effects of repeated infusions of a fat emulsion in surgical patients. *Metabolism* **6:**758-765, 1957.

48. Amris CJ, Brockner J, Larsen V: Changes in the coagulability of blood during the infusion of Intralipid. *Acta Chir Scand* (suppl) **325:**70-74, 1964.

49. Mueller JF, Viteri FV: Hematologic studies in patients receiving multiple infusions of Lipomul. *Am J Clin Nutr* **16:**151-155, 1965.

50. Meng HC, Kaley JS: Effects of multiple infusions on a fat emulsion on blood coagulation, liver function, and urinary excretion of steroids in schizophrenic patients. *Am J Clin Nutr* **16:**156-164, 1965.

51. Meng HC, Kuyama T, Kaley JS: Studies of anemia following multiple intravenous infusions of fat emulsions, in Hennig N, Berg G (eds): *Fette in der Medizin*, vol 6. Munich, Pallas Verlag, 1965, p 31.

52. Meng HC, Kuyama T, Thompson SW, Ferell JF: Toxicity testing of fat emulsion. I. Tolerance study of long-term intravenous administration of Intralipid in rats. *Am J Clin Nutr* **16:**29-36, 1956.

53. Hakansson I, et al: Studies of complete intravenous alimentation in dogs, in Henning N, Berg G (eds): *Symposium of the International Society on Parenteral Nutrition*. Munich, Pallas Verlag, 1967, p 11.

54. Duckert F, Hartmann G: Intravenöse Fett-infusion und Blutgerinnung. *Schweiz Med Wochenschr* **96:**1205, 1966.

55. Cronberg S, Nilsson JM: Coagulation studies after administration of a fat emulsion, Intralipid. *Thromb Diath Haemorrh* **18:**364-369, 1967.

56. Thompson SL: Histologic and ultrastructural changes following intravenous administration of fat emulsions, in Meng HC, Law DH (eds):

Proceedings of International Symposium on Parenteral Nutrition. Springfield, Charles C. Thomas, 1970, p 408.

57. Meng HC, et al: Effects of antioxidants and lipotropic agents in rats receiving long-term administration of a fat emulsion, Intralipid, in Berg G (ed): *Advances in Parenteral Nutrition.* Stuttgart, Georg Thieme Verlag, 1970, p 222.

58. Baume PE, Meng HC, Law DH: Intravenous fat emulsions and gastric acid secretion in the rat. *Am J Dig Dis* **11**:1-9, 1966.

59. Cohn I Jr, Atik M, Harlwig QL, et al: Experience with prolonged administration of intravenous fat emulsions: Behavior, course and laboratory findings in dogs. *J Lab Clin Med* **55**:917-928, 1960.

60. Holman RT: Biological activities of and requirements for polyunsaturated acids, in *Progress in the Chemistry of Fats and Other Lipids,* **9** (pt 5). Oxford, Pergamon Press, 1970, p 607.

61. Soderhjelm L, Wiese HF, Holman RT: The role of polyunsaturated acids in human nutrition and metabolism, in *Progress in the Chemistry of Fats and Other Lipids.* **9** (pt 4). Oxford, Pergamon Press, 1970, p 555.

62. Hansen AE, Wiese HF, Boelsche AN, et al: Role of linoleic acid in infant nutrition: Clinical and chemistry study of 428 infants fed on milk mixtures varying in kind and amount of fat. *Pediatrics* **31** (suppl 1, pt 2):171, 1963.

63. Holman RT, Caster WD, Wiese HF: The essential fatty acid requirement of infants and the assessment of their intake of linoleate by serum acid analysis. *Am J Clin Nutr* **14**:70-75, 1964.

64. Collins FD, et al: Linoleic deficiency in man, in *Proceedings of the Second International Symposium on Atherosclerosis.* Springer-Verlag, 1970, p 455.

65. Paulsrud JR, Pensler L, Whitten CF, et al: Essential fatty acid deficiency in infants induced by fat-free intravenous feeding. *Am J Clin Nutr* **25**:897-904, 1972.

66. Caldwell MD, Jonsson HT, Othersen HB: Essential fatty acid deficiency in an infant receiving prolonged parenteral alimentation. *J Pediatr* **81**:894-898, 1972.

67. Adam DJD, Hansen AE, Wiese HF: Essential fatty acids in infant nutrition. II. Effect of linoleic acid on caloric intake. *J Nutr* **66**:555-564, 1958.

68. Combes M, Pratt EL, Wiese HF: Essential fatty acids in premature infant feeding. *Pediatrics* **30**:136-144, 1962.

69. Waddell WR, Geyer RP: Effect of insulin on clearance of emulsified fat from the blood in depancreatized dogs. *Proc Soc Exp Biol Med* **96**:251-255, 1957.

70. Coran AG, Cryer PE, Horwitz DL: Effect of intravenously administered fat on serum insulin levels. *Am J Clin Nutr* **25**:131-134, 1972.

71. Fredrickson DS, Levy RI, Lee RS: Fat transport in lipoproteins: An integrated approach to mechanisms and disorders. *N Eng J Med* **276**:32, 94, 148, 215, 273, 1967.

72. Kern F, Jackson RG, Martin TE, Meuller JF: Some effects of a cottonseed oil emulsion in patients with laennec's cirrhosis of the liver. *Metabolism* **6**:743, 1957.

73. Greene HL, Hazlett D, Herman RH, et al: Effect of Intralipid on pulmonary membrane diffusion capacity and pulmonary capillary blood volume. *Clin Res* **19**:677, 1971.

Carbohydrates and Fats

Colloquium

Arvid Wretlind, M.D., chairman
William Schumer, M.D., rapporteur and editor

Dr. Schumer: We approached the problems attending the use of carbohydrates and fats in total parenteral nutrition as investigators and critics. First we looked into various studies in the field, then exposed them to critical evaluation. Our discussion covered the following topics:

    I. Glucose substitutes
        A. Fructose
        B. Sorbitol
        C. Xylitol
        D. Other carbohydrate sources (maltose)
        E. Ethyl alcohol
   II. Glucose and insulin
  III. Fat emulsions
        A. Essential fatty acid deficiency
        B. Intralipid and respiratory insufficiency

GLUCOSE SUBSTITUTES

Dr. Wretlind: Glucose is the carbohydrate of choice in nutritional formulas. However, glucose substitutes—among them, fructose, sorbitol, xylitol, maltose, and ethyl alcohol—have been the subject of much discussion and controversy.

Fructose

Dr. Wretlind: Fructose has been widely used in Europe. It is metabolized quickly and is to some extent insulin-independent. Also, it produces a lower incidence of thrombophlebitis when injected into the peripheral veins. Investigations have shown that the rate of glycogen formation in the liver is higher with fructose than with either glucose, sorbitol, or xylitol.[1]

Among the disadvantages in its use is increased formation of uric acid and lactate, which produces acidosis. In children, fructose should be given in small quantities, approximately 0.5 gm/kg/hr. Even this small dosage may cause increased uric acid production.

Dr. Schumer: We infused a 10% fructose solution with no added glucose at a rate of 550 mg/min in patients who had undergone gastric resection. Subsequently, we found that serum phosphate, amino acid, lactic acid, uric acid, SGOT, and bilirubin levels had increased.[2] Biopsies of these patients' liver tissues showed hepatocellular damage characterized by vacuolization of cells.

Förster, Mäenpää, and their coworkers postulated that, after infusion of fructose alone, an increase in uric acid is caused by the accelerated utilization of adenosine triphosphate (ATP) during phosphorylation.[3, 4] The cause of the bilirubin increase was unexplained. Increase in SGOT, however, is indicative of cellular injury.

The lactic acid increases—typical of the low-flow state—may rise to 4 mM/liter, which compounds the metabolic acidosis of shock. Consequently, we discontinued use of fructose in the treatment of shock.

Dr. Cahill: We administered fructose to normal subjects. At that time, we were unaware that it increased the uric acid level. In most subjects a large quantity of intravenous fructose produced pressing substernal pain, similar to the pain of a myocardial infarction. In fact, EKGs were taken to verify that it was not coronary pain. This pain is probably due to an acute enlargement of the liver. Infusion of 1 gm/kg of fructose for 15 to 30 minutes was followed by a significant but transient increase (one to three days) in some serum enzymes (eg, SGOT). This is reminiscent of the symptomatology of hereditary fructose intolerance, the only difference being that the hereditary defect produces these symptoms with a lower fructose dosage. Other sugars, including sorbose, can produce the same symptoms in normal subjects when given rapidly.

Dr. Schumer: Do you think that fructose is truly insulin-independent?

Dr. Cahill: The enzyme fructokinase is necessary for clearance of fructose from the blood and is not insulin-sensitive. It is a constitutive liver enzyme that does not change from the feeding state to the fasting. Since the disappearance rate of fructose is independent of the nutritional state, there is a maximum rate at which fructose can be cleared during refeeding. Conversely, glucose metabolism in the peripheral tissues of feeding or refeeding animals progressively improves with higher insulin concentration. Insulin not only increases the entry of glucose into peripheral tissues, it also stimulates the synthesis of the enzymes responsible for further glucose metabolism. In a certain sense, the utilization of fructose is limited by the amount of available fructokinase. With the use of glucose, the reserve capacity of this system is almost unlimited. The rate of glucose metabolism may be as high as 5 gm/min, which is much more than the rate of infusion in any conventional parenteral delivery system, including the central venous catheter.

Dr. Wretlind: Investigations in a Swedish hospital revealed that, with fructose infusion of less than 0.5 gm/kg/hr, there was no significant increase in lactic acid.[5] Does this agree with your findings?

Dr. Cahill: It does, but the amount of lactic acid increase does not concern me as much as the high susceptibility to intracellular liver damage of patients in low-flow states, those with anoxia, and those recovering from anesthesia.

Dr. Ali: Would a 50-50 mixture of glucose and fructose solve the problem?

Dr. Cahill: It would help because it would reduce the fructose load. However, since the liver of the fasting animal utilizes fatty and amino acids in its tricarboxylic acid (TCA) cycle to produce carbohydrates, I see no necessity for sending additional carbohydrate to the liver cell.

Dr. Broviac: Fructose may be preferable for patients with hepatocellular damage, since it is more easily utilized by the liver cell than is glucose.

Dr. Cahill: In the treatment of mild cirrhosis, the French go to the spa to get some baths and also a little fructose to *dégagé le foie*. However, neither current biochemical data nor careful clinical studies support the concept that fructose benefits the liver; as a matter of fact, it may even be detrimental. As fructose is utilized, the highest rate of lipid synthesis in the liver occurs. This lipid must be converted to very low-density lipoprotein and transported to adipose tissue. In mild liver disease, the capacity to synthesize and export lipoprotein is impaired, thus producing fatty liver. Therefore, in patients with predisposition to fatty liver, addition of a substrate such as fructose that uniquely augments fat synthesis can only be damaging. The logical treatment would be to avoid carbohydrates as far as the liver is concerned and to add a substrate—primarily glucose—to the periphery.

Fructose given to diabetics with ketoacidosis slightly accelerates the rate of ketone diminution, but the overall result is not particularly advantageous. Additionally, the capacity to measure reducing substance in the blood is lost, although this problem is now being minimized with glucose oxidase determinations. Most American clinicians have abandoned the use of fructose in diabetic ketoacidosis.

Dr. Beisbarth: Is there any advantage to the liver's utilization of amino acids instead of carbohydrate for gluconeogenesis to regulate blood sugar levels?

Dr. Cahill: I don't know whether amino acids are better for liver function than fatty acids, because I don't know which substrate the liver uses most of the time. But I suspect that fatty acids are the main substrate for the following reasons: Acetyl coenzyme-A, needed for the entrance of fuel into the TCA cycle, is mainly derived from fatty acids. How much of the amino acid in the normal individual is oxidized in the liver, and how much is oxidized peripherally, is still unknown. As Dr. Munro pointed out, essential amino acids are metabolized in the liver, except for the branched-chain amino acids which are metabolized in the periphery (see p 67). I believe that most nonessential amino acids are mainly metabolized in the periphery. Therefore, the main substrate of the liver would be fatty acids.

Dr. Beisbarth: I agree, especially in the immediate postoperative phase. It is known, however, that a high metabolic turnover of fatty acids in the liver favors gluconeogenesis from amino acids and that a high coenzyme-A level favors the turnover from alanine to glucose. Wouldn't this tend to increase protein catabolism?

Dr. Cahill: Biochemically, that is a valid point. But the factor that limits the rate of nitrogen metabolism in the liver is its capacity to trap amino acids going through it. Mallette, Park, and Exton have shown that high glucagon and low insulin concentrations induce the liver to trap amino acids for either oxidation or gluconeogenesis.[6] But if they are not trapped—which occurs with high glucose and good insulin levels—they are metabolized neither to glucose nor to oxygen via the TCA cycle. Thus, the limiting step is the trapping, not the metabolic direction of amino acids in the liver.

The point concerning protein catabolism is related to the direction the amino acids take inside the liver cell. High concentrations of fat force amino acids into glucose synthesis instead of oxidation. Apparently, the rate-limiting step occurs even before the amino acid is transported into the liver. Low glucagon and high insulin concentrations prevent the transport of amino acids into the liver.

In traumatized patients, my main concern is to protect the amino acid concentration in the muscles by maintaining a high insulin concentration. We should focus on the effect of insulin on peripheral nitrogen catabolism rather than on liver protein function, as long as the liver does not catabolize its own proteins.

Dr. Beisbarth: We are too concerned with the amino acid-producing proteins in the muscle rather than in the liver. At least some of the liver and mucosal enzymes have the shortest half-life of all body proteins; they will be readily utilized when gluconeogenesis is activated if other substrates are absent.[7] The breakdown of muscle protein is not as important as the expenditure of liver enzymes.

Dr. Cahill: This is true in rats, since their labile protein is in the skin and liver. However, man does not rely on skin and liver protein as a source of nitrogen; he relies mainly on muscle protein. Furthermore, death due to bronchopneumonia or almost any debilitating disease is death of peripheral protein due to loss of strength in the respiratory muscles.

Dr. Ausman: In considering fructose, we must evaluate its advantages and disadvantages in parenteral nutrition. It has been reported that uric acid levels rise with the use of fructose. It has also been reported that large infusions over short periods of time have not increased uric acid concentration. It has not been proved that fructose infusion will increase uric acid levels in all cases, nor has a toxic level of uric acid been established.

Chest pain, another untoward effect of fructose, was reported by Papper.[8] He stated that a dose of approximately 25 gm/hr of fructose, either alone or in combination with glucose (invert sugar), usually produced chest pain. An increased dosage rate of invert sugar produced symptoms such as increased SGPT and SGOT levels that, since they mimic myocardial infarction, further confuse the differential diagnosis.

Dr. Broviac: At the University of Washington we have seen the same symptoms with the use of glucose that you have seen with fructose.

Comment: In a taped presentation made before the American Society of Hospital Pharmacists in Houston, it was mentioned that fructose is not easily utilized by the central nervous system (CNS), but I could find no evidence for this in the literature.

Dr. Cahill: Fructose is used by the CNS minimally, if at all. Platt, at the Massachusetts Institute of Technology, is studying the effects of substrate infusions in dogs with acute hypoglycemia. His results indicate that fructose does not correct the electroencephalographic abnormality; but glucose, mannose, or beta-hydroxybutyrate will.

Dr. Wretlind: Obviously, there is little reason to substitute fructose for glucose. However, it might be possible to combine glucose with fructose without any harmful effect. A certain amount of fructose in total intravenous feeding may be correct, since the normal daily oral diet contains about 50 to 100 gm of fructose.

Sorbitol

Dr. Wretlind: The polyol sorbitol is used as a glucose substitute in Europe.

Dr. Carlo: Sorbitol, used in parenteral nutrition since 1953, is compatible with amino acids and better tolerated than glucose. Objections to its use are based on the claim that sorbitol is not adequately utilized because of its diuretic effect.

The initial studies on the diuretic effects of sorbitol were conducted with dogs. Generally, if the rate of sorbitol administration is about 150 gm in four hours, the urinary losses can be low, as little as 6%. A decisive advantage of sorbitol is its specific insulin-stimulating effect. This is desirable in inducing anabolic activity.

Sorbitol is converted to fructose and should present the same disadvantages as fructose, but the drop in ATP level is considerably less with sorbitol than with fructose.[9] Apparently the delay during conversion of sorbitol to fructose is critical to the prevention of an overload of fructose in the liver cell and its consequent side effects.

Dr. Broviac: When we substituted dialysate levels greater than 2 gm/100 ml of sorbitol for glucose in peritoneal dialysis, several patients became comatose. Mental obtundation and coma did not occur at serum sorbitol levels lower than 200 mg/100 ml. What serum levels of sorbitol will occur with the infusion of 150 gm over two hours?

Dr. Carlo: We have never observed such an effect when administering large amounts of sorbitol.

Dr. Ausman: Dr. Broviac has observed two causes for the problems. The first is an osmotic effect. As serum sorbitol is increased over 250 or 300 mg, the osmotic effect is directly proportional to that of glucose in peritoneal dialysis. The second is that coma appears to be related to an intracellular increase in the level of sorbitol. When the relative extracellular level of sorbitol is reduced, the osmotic gradient decreases, and edema occurs.

Dr. Wretlind: Dr. Cahill, do you find some advantage in using sorbitol instead of glucose?

Dr. Cahill: I can't find any. I do not understand Dr. Ausman's concept of the cause of cerebral edema with sorbitol administration. I doubt if cerebral edema occurs when sorbitol is administered alone, since sorbitol cannot pass into or out of the cell. However, it may occur when glucose infusion is followed at first by CNS dehydration. Then when glucose is lowered, a rapid shift of water back into the cell may produce edema.

Dr. Carlo: Sorbitol has been used as a calorie source in uremia at a dose of 150 to 300 gm/day without any adverse effects. Actually, 300 gm of sorbitol will disappear totally from the body in eight hours.

Dr. Ausman: One study attributes diabetic neuropathy to the accumulation of sorbitol at nerve endings and in the cataract. Dr. Cahill, can you explain or comment?

Dr. Cahill: The aldose reductase enzyme is almost ubiquitous. It is present in vascular intima, which is disturbing. Any cell or tissue that allows glucose to enter easily, such as the Schwann's cell of the peripheral nerve, the beta cells of the pancreas, the vascular intima, or the brain, will thus allow sorbitol synthesis and accumulation. The affinity of the sorbitol production enzyme (Km) is very high, so sorbitol is produced in tissues only when there is extreme hyperglycemia, that is, 200 to 600 mg/100 ml.

Gabbay has shown that peripheral nerve conduction times are changed in normal animals after accumulation of polyols such as sorbitol.[10] Thus, there are not only structural changes but also obvious physiologic changes due to the intracellular accumulation of sorbitol and other polyols.

Dr. Weston: I have been interested in the problem because of the difficulty with use of hypertonic sorbitol in peritoneal dialysis. We first suggested the use of sorbitol to achieve hypersorbitolemia in patients with uremia on chronic dialysis. We needed a substance that could restore osmolarity as the urea was removed, prevent complete anuria between dialyses, and be metabolized by patients in complete anuria and renal failure. The resultant impairment of sorbitol metabolism in uremia caused severe degrees of hypersorbitolemia and hyperosmotic coma.

Naturally, two questions follow: Why do uremic patients have greater impairment of sorbitol metabolism? Is this an aspect of the generalized ongoing impairment of carbohydrate metabolism?

Patients receiving nonhypertonic dialysis solutions of 1.5% or 1.8% sorbitol developed coma at a time when their blood sorbitol levels were only around 200 mg/100 ml. Dr. Cahill's discussion about the effect of fructose on liver ATP made me wonder, since two patients who died had elevated blood ammonias without any demonstrable organic liver disease. Could you comment on this, Dr. Cahill?

192

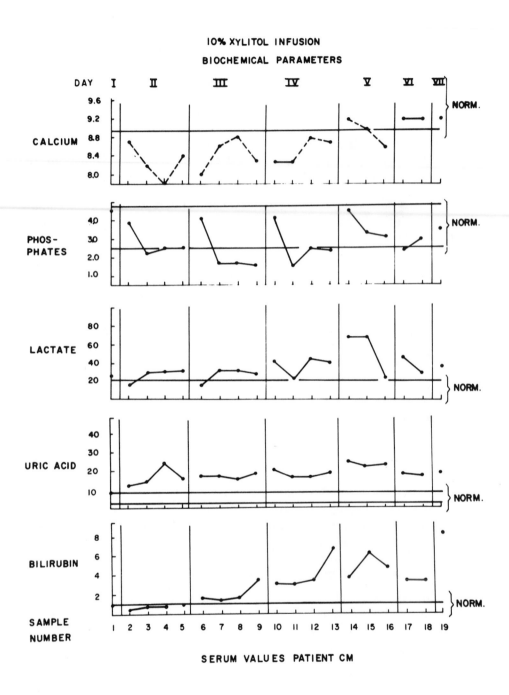

Fig 1. Ten percent xylitol infusion: biochemical parameters.

Dr. Cahill: One explanation is that, since sorbitol is mainly removed by the liver, anything that reduces hepatic flow will markedly prolong sorbitol clearance. If hepatic flow is reduced by half, the half-time clearance of sorbitol will double, and therefore the overall sorbitol level will be more or less doubled.

Dr. Wretlind: It is difficult to summarize this discussion, but, though there are few advantages to the use of sorbitol above glucose, the controversy seems to indicate that continued investigation is necessary.

Xylitol

Dr. Schumer: Our study of xylitol in both diabetic and nondiabetic patients was performed with a product imported from Japan. After receiving 1.0 to 1.5 gm/kg/hr, several patients developed threefold increases in lactic acid and uric acid and twofold increases in bilirubin and alkaline phosphatase toward the end of the infusion period, as compared to the control levels.[11]

Bassler and associates reported that xylitol was well tolerated.[12] We performed loading tests on normal subjects, who received as much as 4.4 gm/kg/day, but we had to stop after four days of testing. We found a continuing decrease in phosphates during xylitol infusion (see Fig 1). Lactate increased until at one point it reached 60 mg/100 ml; uric acid increased to 16 mg/100 ml; and bilirubin rose as high as 8 micrograms/100 ml. The situation was compounded as all these metabolite concentrations continued to increase. A sharp decrease followed cessation of the daily infusion, but by the end of each day the concentrations were still greater than on the previous day.

At the end of three to four days, the subjects receiving injections of fructose developed pain in the right upper quadrant, as Dr. Cahill described. Their livers were extremely tender. They had nausea and vertigo. The SGOT was approximately 5,700 units, lactic dehydrogenase (LDH) was 4,500 units, and alkaline phosphatase was 250 units. When this test was repeated on four normal subjects, biochemical signs of hepatocellular damage were evident.

In response to our publication of these studies, Coats (of Australia) wrote of 18 deaths following use of xylitol. Autopsies showed marked hepatocellular necrosis in all cases.

Dr. Beisbarth: I have a comment on Professor Coats' findings, based on personal communications. The compound 2-mercaptoimidazoline was used as a vulcanizing accelerator in the rubber stopper of the Japanese xylitol bottles and was extracted into the solutions. Coats succeeded in killing mice with a combination of xylitol and this compound, but he failed to do so using xylitol alone.

Dr. Schumer: Although the xylitol used in our first set of tests was of Japanese origin, it was bottled by an American pharmaceutical company. There was no rubber stopper in these containers, unless it was first bottled with such a stopper and later put into a different container.

Dr. Beisbarth: We must not confuse these two situations. What you have found is surely consistent with a special kind of carbohydrate therapy.

You gave your volunteers about 300 gm/day of single carbohydrates, and this could well produce an unfavorable effect. Coats' experiments, however, are consistent with intoxication by mercaptoimidazoline.

Other Carbohydrate Sources (Maltose)

Dr. Young: During our discussion of carbohydrate, no one mentioned maltose as a possible intravenous substrate. A maltose solution contains twice the calories of an isosmotic solution of glucose. Not much work has been done with intravenously administered disaccharides. Intravenously injected lactose or sucrose is almost quantitatively excreted in the urine, but this is not true of maltose. Studies on the recovery of CO_2 after maltose infusion showed that circulating maltose is as readily utilized as is glucose[13] (Fig 2).

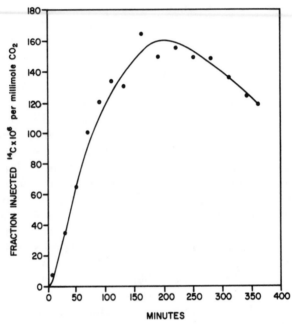

Fig 2. The fraction of injected ^{14}C recovered as expired $^{14}CO_2$ per millimol CO_2 for five subjects over a six-hour period following the intravenous administration of 10 grams of ^{14}C-labelled maltose.

The indications for parenteral feeding of maltose suggest the use of a 10% solution instead of the equimolar 5% solution of glucose. In effect you can give twice the kilocalories per unit of the glucose solution by giving the maltose solution.

Investigations with intravenously administered maltose are now being conducted in Japan, but I do not believe anything has been published.

Dr. Meng: The use of maltose should be investigated. With intravenous injections of starch or dextran, glucose is present in the urine, and there is increased blood sugar. Possibly, maltose would be utilized more completely.

195

Dr. Young: There is no maltose in human blood, so when maltose is given in a loading dose there is no increase in the blood glucose level. However, if the total reducing substances are measured, an increase of maltose in the blood is observed (Fig 3).

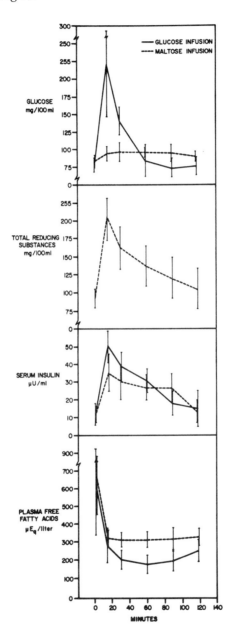

Fig 3. Mean concentrations of blood glucose, total reducing substances, insulin and free fatty acids for six subjects following the intravenous administration of 25 grams of maltose (----) or glucose (—).

Ethyl Alcohol

Dr. Wretlind: Ethyl alcohol was widely used before the introduction of hyperosmolar hyperalimentation and the availability of fat emulsions. Today it is used only rarely. Has anyone had experience with ethyl alcohol in intravenous feeding?

Dr. Sandstead: Use of ethyl alcohol as a calorie source in intravenous feeding is metabolically unwise, primarily because of its direct toxicity to such organs as the heart, muscle, and brain. It also impairs leukocyte migration and phagocytosis, which are important in resistance to infection and response to injury; it has a sedative effect on patients who then become lethargic and do not respond to pain. Hence, use of alcohol is contraindicated when a good calorie source such as glucose is available.

Dr. Wretlind: Dr. Beisbarth, could you give us some more detailed information?

Dr. Beisbarth: Four different parenteral postoperative regimens are shown in Figure 4, from which three principles can be drawn[14]: 1) Ethanol appears to be a better source of calories than fat as measured by nitrogen balance in a prestress state. 2) Infusion of ethanol instead of fat emulsion is unnecessary when there is no stress effect, but when stress exists—eg, during the first five days postoperatively—it should be used in preference to fat. 3) When ethanol is administered with fat, it is ineffective.

Dr. Broviac: When long-term parenteral feeding is a patient's only source of nutrition, a 12-hour overnight infusion of glucose must be administered to provide the necessary calories. Since it is almost impossible to administer a sufficient amount of calories in 12 hours using glucose, patients must be infused for 16 hours daily. In these cases, alcohol can be used partially as a caloric substitute for glucose to reduce the total infusion time.

Dr. Carlo: Ethanol's inhibition of the Krebs cycle may account for the reduced calorie utilization. When the Krebs cycle is inhibited, glucose utilization is directed toward the pentose pathway, which concurrently leads to an accumulation of the Krebs cycle intermediate, lactic acid, thus to an increase in the ratio of lactate to pyruvate.[15-20] Additionally, magnesium losses can increase by 160% in normal individuals after administration of only 30 ml of ethanol.

Dr. Schumer: Other points to be considered in the use of alcohol are: It should never be given when cirrhosis is present. Shulman and Westerfeld found that ^{14}C-labeled alcohol is exhaled mostly as acetylaldehyde, which is extremely irritating to the lung alveolar membrane.[21] In heavy smokers, alcohol increases pulmonary complications up to 20%.

Dr. Dudrick: Inflammatory diseases—gastritis, regional enteritis, or ulcerative colitis—can be aggravated by alcohol since it irritates the bowel mucosa, causing increased pain. In experimental pancreatitis, severe pain has been completely relieved with parenteral nutrition; the pain returns when alcohol is added and subsides when alcohol infusion is stopped.

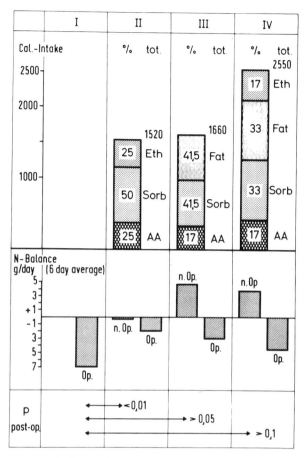

Fig 4. Groups I through IV represent collectives of patients after abdominal surgery (= Op) of moderate severity. Group I received only adequate water and electrolytes; Groups II through IV received different parenteral nutrition regimens (Eth = ethanol, Sorb = sorbitol, AA = amino acids, Fat = fat emulsion). The average nitrogen balances of the first six days postoperatively are compared with nitrogen balances of patients under the same nutrition who were not immediately operated upon (= n Op).

Dr. Sandstead: Alcohol suppresses the pulmonary toilet of the lung and impairs the function of its respiratory mucosal cilia.

Dr. Wretlind: Can we then say that ethyl alcohol has no place in modern intravenous nutrition?

Dr. Ausman: Some of the problems discussed here are not applicable to infants and neonates. Some pediatricians feel that ethyl alcohol is acceptable and, in fact, desirable as a carbohydrate and calorie source. The contraindications we have cited are true in adults, but I doubt that pediatricians are overly concerned about cirrhosis. On balance, alcohol may have some advantages.

Dr. Dudrick: Many pediatricians do not use alcohol because there may be irreversible damage to Betz's and other cerebral cells.

Dr. Vanamee: Alcohol depresses the platelet count and could indirectly affect clotting.[22]

Dr. Wretlind: Therefore, may I repeat what I just said? There seems to be no advantage to using ethyl alcohol in modern parenteral nutrition.

Dr. Beisbarth: Except for the existing contraindications, I must disagree.

Dr. Carlo: This issue could be resolved by referring to the papers of Rubin and Lieber in which all the drawbacks of alcohol are quite clearly described.[23-27]

GLUCOSE AND INSULIN

Dr. Carlo: Glucose is the carbohydrate of choice because it produces glucose-6-phosphate, the common substrate to the pentose and Embden-Meyerhof pathways. Determination as to which metabolic pathway will be used preferentially is made by the metabolic need of the body. A carbohydrate such as xylitol which is utilized exclusively in one metabolic pathway after oxidation to xylose may create a metabolic imbalance that causes these side effects.

Dr. Beisbarth: I agree. The best method of using carbohydrates in parenteral nutrition is in combination, alternating one bottle of glucose with one of fructose or xylitol. It may be advisable to eliminate glucose in the early postoperative period when glucose intolerance makes administration of large amounts of insulin necessary. In Germany doctors are warned to use insulin in these cases, because of a possible permanent insulin resistance developing from immunological events due to trauma.

Shipp at the Joslin Clinic has stated that 0.1% of diabetic patients are insulin-resistant for immunologic reasons.[28] He defines insulin resistance as a daily requirement of 200 units or more for two days. German researchers have found that the rate of insulin resistance increases to about 4% among diabetic patients when the definition is 100 units of insulin daily for two days.[29]

Dr. Cahill: Schichtkrull at the Novo Laboratories is working on the hypothesis that the main antigenic component of insulin is not in the insulin molecule itself but in other substances, which are either extracted from the pancreas with insulin or bound to the insulin molecule. Once a purified insulin is isolated, the immunologic problems should be eliminated.

Parenteral carbohydrates are given to increase weight by supplying sufficient calories. This can be done by administering either fats or carbohydrates that are utilized by adipose tissue. At present, only glucose can accomplish this: It is the sole substrate for peripheral fat synthesis other than lipid emulsions. Carbohydrate is given to stimulate insulin production for a nitrogen-sparing effect; therefore, the carbohydrate given must promote insulin production. Again, this can be produced only by sorbitol, which is converted to glucose, or to a lesser degree by xylitol. Insulin may be produced with administration of xylitol, but on a mole basis glucose produces more insulin. Therefore, the rationale for carbohydrate administration supports the use of glucose.

Dr. Wretlind: Our agreement on glucose as the most efficient carbohydrate prompts this practical question: should insulin be given with large amounts of glucose in parenteral hyperalimentation?

Dr. Cahill: The answer depends on the blood level of glucose; if this is 100 or 150, insulin is unnecessary. It is indicated when there is hyperglycemia. Most ill or traumatized individuals cannot produce enough insulin to metabolize glucose when it is given at any significant rate. Additionally, other unknown processes negate insulin's effectiveness peripherally. Combined, these two factors limit the patient's capacity to metabolize exogenous glucose, and insulin may be necessary if glucose is the calorie supplement.

Dr. Wretlind: Does this obviate the need to give insulin in a fixed combination with glucose?

Dr. Carlo: We observe insulin resistance after trauma, which is puzzling in patients in whom anabolic activity is needed. If insulin is an anabolic hormone that inhibits gluconeogenesis, why do posttraumatic or postoperative patients show insulin resistance? Is it because they need gluconeogenesis, and insulin is preventing it? In the absence of glycogen, massive gluconeogenesis is required to guarantee the survival of the central nervous system and the red blood cells. Hence, insulin activity must be curtailed. We can hypothesize that insulin resistance is a clinically induced condition due to an initial carbohydrate deficiency.

An increase in gluconeogenesis should not be allowed, particularly in preoperative patients. If the substrate supply is maintained, gluconeogenesis and its attendant catabolism is prevented.

Dr. Dudrick: We use insulin only when there is increased catabolic response or when the patient is in extremely poor nutritional condition. As an example, an elderly lady weighing 90 pounds fell and incurred fractures. She could assimilate only 1,500 kilocalories of glucose per day before spilling 4+ sugar into the urine. She had a low renal threshold, and the beta cells were unreactive—probably due to pancreatic fibrosis. In such cases we first add insulin subcutaneously to determine the extent to which glucose utilization can be improved. If the patient does well on 15 to 25 units per 1,000 kilocalories, we then give 2,500 kilocalories. With insulin, more sugar is utilized rather than spilled into the urine, so the patient is easier to manage.

This probably represents 7% to 10% of our patients. Another 5% to 10% are diabetic, so 80% or more do not receive insulin at all.

Insulin has no effect until the dosage reaches 150 to 200 units per 1,000 kilocalories. At this point something happens that allows an increase in glucose utilization. Hence, an efficient glucose-monitoring test would be invaluable in the parenteral force-feeding of patients.

Dr. Driscoll: There is similar intolerance in some premature infants. Generally, we start with a 10% glucose concentration at approximately 0.5 gm/kg/hr. In some infants an increase from 10% to 12% in glucose concentration over a 24-hour period is sufficient to raise the blood sugar from 100 mg/100 ml to 250 mg/100 ml. In these infants the ideal concentration is 20% to 25%, which may require 6 to 18 days of infusion. In a term infant this increase may be achieved within 48 to 72 hours.

Dr. Dudrick: We found that adding exogenous insulin does not decrease endogenous insulin production. At a high infusion concentration of glucose, the patient may have sugar in the urine. This does not deter us from adding calories; we simply add more insulin to the bottle. But if we are not careful, the patient may become hypoglycemic within five to ten days. In some patients the endogenous insulin output seems to rise in response to carbohydrate stimulation, and it does not matter whether we add insulin to the bottle or add it subcutaneously. A few patients have gone into hypoglycemic shock as a result. If insulin is used, the dosage should be carefully regulated rather than given at a fixed rate.

Dr. Vanamee: Secretion of growth hormone increases during trauma. Does this have an anti-insulin effect?

Dr. Cahill: In deep sleep, secretion of the growth hormone increases to a higher level than during stress. Malarkey and Daughaday followed metabolic concomitants, including glucose and fatty acid levels, after peak secretion of growth hormones and found no changes suggestive of an anti-insulin effect.[30] Only excessive concentrations of growth hormone over long periods produce an anti-insulin effect. Growth hormone in relation to carbohydrates and fats probably has very little, if anything, to do with normal homeostasis.[31]

Dr. Carlo: One of the best stimulants for insulin release is amino acid.

Dr. Wretlind: Yes, that is right. Concerning the dosage of glucose, the minimum daily amount under any circumstances is 100 gm to fulfill the brain requirements and to prevent ketogenesis. When only energy requirements exist, there is a dosage problem. Dr. Dudrick, what is your schedule for total parenteral nutrition with glucose?

Dr. Dudrick: In adults we give glucose at a rate anywhere between 0.4 and 0.9 gm/kg/hr, but in children this rate may be as high as 1.2 gm. We generally give about 500 to 600 gm of glucose in 24 hours, aiming for 2,500 to 3,500 kilocalories, which is the general requirement of major surgical or trauma patients. We try to meet these requirements with glucose, although we are limited by the rate at which the patient can metabolize sugar. The metabolic rate of glucose oxidation is adversely affected in renal failure and sepsis. On many occasions a postoperative wound infection has been detected by noting a 4+ sugar excretion in the urine in a patient who had been handling the glucose load well for several days.

Dr. Cahill: In that situation, would you continue glucose administration and add insulin or reduce the dosage of glucose?

Dr. Dudrick: Usually I reduce the dosage, since this is safer. The dosage can then be slowly increased if the patient requires more sugar. But in wound infection, glucose tolerance will return to its former level within a day after drainage.

Dr. Sandstead: We approach this problem empirically, treating these patients as if they were diabetics. For all practical purposes, we are able to abort the so-called obligatory catabolism of stress by giving enough calories. We give 2,700 kilocalories of intravenous glucose a day and are able to control glucose tolerance by giving insulin on a sliding scale according to urinary sugar measurements every four hours. In most of these patients, excluding diabetics, we are able to control tolerance, prevent glucosuria, and maintain a positive nitrogen balance. After a couple of days the patient will require less insulin, as his capacity to create endogenous insulin returns.

FAT EMULSIONS

Dr. Wretlind: The object of complete intravenous feeding is to supply the body with required amounts of energy. We may give carbohydrates as the energy source, according to Dr. Rhoads' and Dr. Dudrick's technique; or we may give carbohydrates in combination with fat emulsions. The carbohydrates should supply at least 20% of the calories or 100 gm of the volume, and fats should supply the remainder. The primary advantage of this type of solution is that large amounts of energy can be given in very small volumes of isotonic fluid. Fat emulsion may be given in the peripheral veins in contrast to concentrated glucose solution, which must be given through a central venous catheter to reduce the possibility of thrombophlebitis. Fat emulsion infusion causes neither high osmolarity of the blood nor diuresis. Furthermore, there is no loss of the infused fat in the urine or feces. These emulsions also supply the required amounts of essential fatty acids.

The fat emulsion we have used in Scandinavia and also in other parts of Europe is Intralipid, which contains soybean oil, egg yolk phospholipid as an emulsifying agent, and glycerol to make it isotonic.

Investigations have been performed to test the toxicity of Intralipid. In one series of studies, a dosage of 9 gm/kg/day was given to dogs for four weeks with no toxic reaction whatsoever.[32] The only effects were the presence of intravenous fat pigment in the reticuloendothelial cells and occasional proliferation of these cells. Dogs which were not killed immediately after the infusion period to determine the pathological changes survived for several years.

Hallberg showed that Intralipid disappears from the bloodstream at about the same speed as chylomicrons, or about 4 gm/kg/day of fat, or roughly 35 kcal/kg/day. Starvation increases the excretion rate, corresponding to roughly 100 kcal/kg/day.[33, 34] These excretion rates vary with the patient's age.

The effect of fat emulsions on the coagulation system has been investigated by Cronberg and Nilsson,[35] and by Duckert and Hartman.[36] Their findings indicate that fat emulsions like Intralipid do not affect the coagulation system. This may explain the low incidence of thrombophlebitis with these infusions.

We have investigated complete intravenous feeding with fat emulsions in dogs over a 12-week period. In some cases, 87% of the total energy requirement was supplied by fats, although the proportion of fat intake is generally limited to 40%, corresponding to the normal intake in man.

Data in Table 1 show the amounts of calories and nutrients supplied daily to a dog fed intravenously during gestation.[37]

Table 1.— Daily Supply of Energy and Nutrients During the Period of Gestation in a Dog on Complete Intravenous Nutrition

	Nutrients	Daily supply per kg body weight
	Water	39-72 ml
Energy and sources of energy	Energy	75-100 kcal
	Amino acids	1-3 gm = 0.134-0.402 gm N
	Glucose or fructose	10-10.9 gm
	Fat	3.3-4.0 gm
Minerals	Sodium	2.1-3.5 mmol
	Potassium	1.0-1.6 mmol
	Calcium	0.22-0.29 mmol
	Magnesium	0.05-0.09 mmol
	Iron	9.3-19.3 μmol
	Zinc	4.1 μmol
	Manganese	0.39 μmol
	Copper	0.1 μmol
	Chlorine	0.79-2.36 mmol
	Phosphorus	0.24-0.30 mmol
	Iodine	0.02 μmol
Water-soluble vitamins	Thiamin	0.024 mg
	Riboflavin	0.036 mg
	Niacin	0.2 mg
	Vitamin B_6	0.04 mg
	Folacin	0.004 mg
	Vitamin B_{12}	0.04 μg
	Pantothenic acid	0.2 mg
	Biotin	0.006 mg
	Ascorbic acid	0.6 mg
Fat-soluble vitamins	Vitamin A	0.015 mg Retinol = 50 IU
	Vitamin D	0.05 μg = 2 IU
	Vitamin K_1	0.002 mg
	Tocopherol	3.1-4 mg

This investigation proved that puppies of normal weight can develop during complete intravenous feeding, apparently without impairment. The dog was given the infusion in the superior caval vein through a catheter fixed to a small steel saddle on her back. During infusion, the infusion tube was connected to the catheter. Unlike Dudrick's 24-hour infusion, we infused for only 5 or 6 hours a day.

We probably gave too many calories since the weight increase was more than was necessary. Figure 5 illustrates the weight curve of the dog who was mated the day before and the day after the start of intravenous nutrition. The dog was in good condition for the entire gestation period with 40% of the calorie intake as fat (Intralipid) and the remainder as glucose, fructose, and amino acids. On the 61st day the dog delivered six puppies. One was a stillbirth, two died during parturition, and three survived. All puppies seemed anatomically normal. A complication due to vitamin K insufficiency during the last period of infusion caused the three deaths.

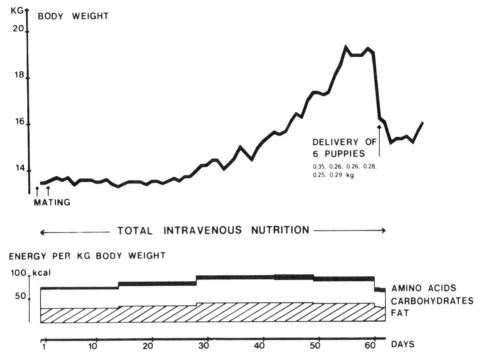

Fig 5. Supply of energy and change of body weight during pregnancy in a dog on complete intravenous nutrition. The amount of fat (Intralipid 20%) given corresponds to 40% of the total energy supply (from Wretlind[37]).

We have also studied complete intravenous feeding with fat over extended periods of time in man. Table 2 shows the daily supply of energy and nutrients to a 43-year-old female patient with brain damage secondary to carbon monoxide intoxication, who was fed fats intravenously for 7 months and 13 days.[38] The infusions contained 29 nutrients, including 1.8 gm/kg of fat per day. The patient's weight increased from 40 to 50 kg with a 0.5 kg increase in body water (Fig 6). Nitrogen equilibrium was maintained, indicating that most of this weight increase was from fat deposition. This is always a problem with bedridden patients. Body fat can be increased by infusion, but muscle tissue can be synthesized only by physical activity. Our calculations of energy balance were in agreement with the increase in body fat. Fat, carbohydrates, and amino acids were given in the amounts indicated in Table 2.

During the period when only carbohydrates and amino acids were given—approximately one month—there was no significant change in nitrogen balance (see Fig 7). We concluded, therefore, that whether the energy source was carbohydrate or a combination of carbohydrate and fat did not matter, as long as the energy requirement was met.

Data in Table 3 show the amount of nitrogen necessary to maintain equilibrium. In this case, positive nitrogen balance was maintained with 4 gm of nitrogen in the form of a complete crystalline amino acid mixture of about

204

the same composition as egg protein. The urinary loss of amino acid was small, about 2%.

A 70-year-old man with thrombosis in the superior mesenteric artery had most of his small intestine removed and was maintained on complete intravenous feeding for 69 days.[39] Table 4 is a summary of the nutrient supply kept constant during the last 35 days. He received 3.6 liters of water daily.

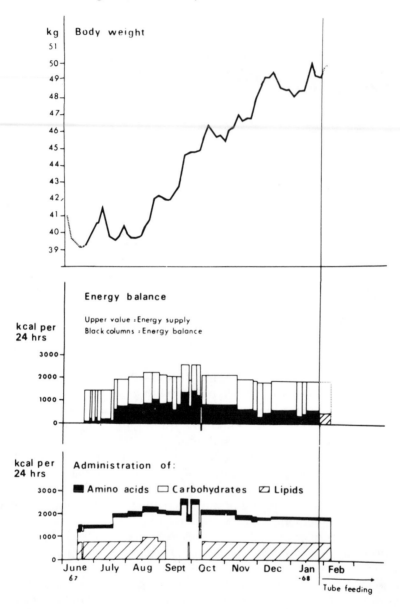

Fig 6. Change in a patient's body weight and energy balance during complete intravenous nutrition for 7 months and 13 days. The diagram also shows the intake of fat, carbohydrates and amino acids (from Bergström et al[38]).

Only 70 gm of amino acids were given; the amount of fat was the standard 100 gm; 12 minerals, 9 water-soluble vitamins, and 4 fat-soluble vitamins were included also. The crystalline amino acid solution contained all 8 essential and 10 nonessential amino acids (Table 5).

Table 2.— Daily Supply of Energy and Nutrients to a Patient on Complete Intravenous Nutrition for 7 Months and 13 Days (from Bergström et al[38])

	Nutrients	Average daily supply per kg body weight	
Energy and sources of energy	Water	42	ml
	Energy	43	kcal
	Amino acids*	1.3 gm = 0.18 gm N	
	Glucose or fructose	6.2 gm	
	Fat*	1.8 gm	
Minerals	Sodium	1.17	mmol
	Potassium	0.76	mmol
	Calcium	0.17	mmol
	Magnesium	0.038	mmol
	Iron	3.9	μmol
	Zinc	0.14	μmol
	Manganese	0.16	μmol
	Copper	0.0071	μmol
	Chlorine	1.48	mmol
	Phosphorus	0.19	mmol
	Fluoride	0.037	μmol
	Iodine	0.015	μmol
Water-soluble vitamins	Thiamin	0.22	mg
	Riboflavin	0.089	mg
	Niacin	0.89	mg
	Vitamin B_6	0.089	mg
	Folacin	0.068	mg
	Vitamin B_{12}	0.31	μg
	Pantothenic acid	0.31	mg
	Biotin	0.056	mg
	Ascorbic acid	2.2	mg
Fat-soluble vitamins	Vitamin A	111	IU
	Vitamin D	13	IU
	Tocopherol	0.022	mg

*See Table 4.

Table 3.— Average Nitrogen Balance and Urinary Excretion of α-Amino Nitrogen and Ammonium Nitrogen During Complete Intravenous Nutrition (from Bergström et al[38])

Period	Days	N Supply g/day	N Balance g/day	Urinary Excretion of α-amino N	
				mg/day	% of N supply
A	6	4.06	+0.51	120	3.0
B	29	5.36	+0.87	120	2.2
C	17	6.70	+1.07	180	2.7
D	14	8.04	+2.62	140	1.6
E	22	10.7	+2.25	220	2.1
F	10	10.7	+3.77	200	1.9
Mean:		7.6	+1.9	164	2.2

Note: Days without fever and with identical supply of nitrogen and energy are compiled to periods.

206

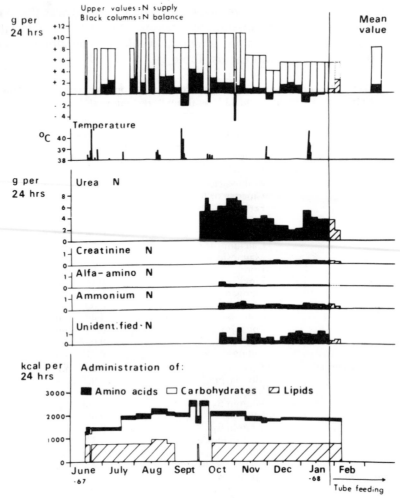

Fig 7. Effect on nitrogen balance and urinary excretion of some nitrogen compounds in a patient, during complete intravenous nutrition for 7 months and 13 days (from Bergström et al[38]).

All infusions were given during the night, starting at 6 PM with fructose and glucose. The amino acid mixture was added, followed by Intralipid and another mixture of glucose and fructose later with the electrolytes and vitamins.

For the first two or three weeks, very large amounts of energy—sometimes as many as 6,000 kcal—were necessary to maintain body weight (Fig 8). Interestingly, the potassium level decreased, indicating that the weight was maintained mostly from an increasing amount of body fat. Later, when the patient returned to oral feeding, his weight decreased, since only about 30 cm of the small intestine remained. He had a slight increase in cholesterol and little change in bilirubin (Fig 9). The hemoglobin value did not change substantially; vitamin B_{12} levels decreased despite administration of a reasonable amount (Fig 10). Perhaps vitamin B_{12} should be given in larger amounts in the postoperative period.

Table 4.— Daily Supply of Energy and Nutrients to a Patient Aged 70 on Complete Intravenous Nutrition After a Massive Intestinal Resection (from Jacobson[39])

	Nutrients	Average daily supply per kg body weight	
	Water	47.1	ml
Energy and sources of energy	Energy	37.5	kcal
	Amino acids*	0.9	gm = 0.12 gm N
	Glucose or fructose	5.33	gm
	Fat†	1.31	gm
Minerals	Sodium	1.88	mmol
	Potassium	1.05	mmol
	Calcium	0.17	mmol
	Magnesium	0.058	mmol
	Iron	‡	
	Zinc	0.13	μmol
	Manganese	0.13	μmol
	Copper	0.13	μmol
	Chlorine	2.37	mmol
	Phosphorus	0.32	mmol
	Fluoride	0.06	μmol
	Iodine	0.013	μmol
Water-soluble vitamins	Thiamin	0.395	mg
	Riboflavin	0.158	mg
	Niacin	1.58	mg
	Vitamin B_6	0.158	mg
	Folacin	0.026	mg
	Vitamin B_{12}	0.105	μg
	Pantothenic acid	0.237	mg
	Biotin	6.58	μg
	Ascorbic acid	5.26	mg
Fat-soluble vitamins	Vitamin A	263	IU
	Vitamin D	31.6	IU
	Vitamin K_1	0.13	mg
	Tocopherol	0.053	mg

*Crystalline amino acid mixture (Vamin®, Vitrum, Stockholm, Sweden).
†Soybean oil emulsion (Intralipid, Vitrum, Stockholm, Sweden).
‡Intermittent parenteral supply, when indicated.

We tested the hypothesis that in adults fat infusion can provide energy in the postoperative period.[40] After gastrectomy, one group of patients was given carbohydrates only, a second group received carbohydrates and amino acids, and a third group was given fats in addition to carbohydrates and amino acids (Fig 11). It was obvious that the loss of body protein decreased with increasing amounts of fats, indicating that fat was utilized but protein loss was never completely eliminated.[41, 42]

Fat emulsions have also been used in pediatrics by Børreson and his coworkers[41-43] and by Grotte[44] (Table 6). Both groups gave all infusions via a peripheral vein cannula kept at one location for three or four days. The types of solutions used are given in Table 7. The formula consisted of an amino acid mixture, a fat emulsion, and a glucose solution, to which two electrolyte solutions were added. This was infused during the day for 10 to 12 hours. Pediatric patients have been maintained for three or four weeks on this regimen.

208

Table 5.— Composition of the L-Amino Acids Solution, Vamin®,*
Used for Intravenous Nutrition

	mg	mmol/liter
L-Alanine	3,000	33.67
L-Arginine	3,300	18.94
L-Aspartic acid	4,050	30.43
L-Cysteine	1,400	11.56
L-Phenylalanine	5,450	32.99
L-Glutamic acid	9,000	61.17
Glycine	2,100	27.97
L-Histidine	2,400	15.47
L-Isoleucine	3,900	29.73
L-Leucine	5,250	40.02
L-Lysine	3,850	26.34
L-Methionine	1,900	12.73
L-Proline	8,100	70.36
L-Serine	7,500	71.37
L-Threonine	3,000	25.18
L-Tryptophan	1,000	4.90
L-Tyrosine	500	2.76
L-Valine	4,250	36.28
Fructose	100 gm	
	mEq/liter	
Sodium	60	
Potassium	20	
Calcium	5	
Magnesium (as sulphate)	3	
Chloride	55-60	
Sterile water to	1,000 ml	

*Vitrum, Stockholm, Sweden.

It is questionable whether fat emulsion is utilized similarly to carbohydrates. In our experiments, dogs received up to 80% of their energy requirement in fats for seven days, then in carbohydrates and amino acids for another seven days. During fat infusion, positive nitrogen balance was maintained; however, when carbohydrates were used alone, there was no significant change from the control group of dogs.

Correlative studies in man showed no difference in nitrogen balance between carbohydrate given alone and carbohydrate given with fat. The regular dosage of fat in adults is up to 2 gm/kg/day, unless there is a high requirement such as in patients with burns. In this case the dosage is increased to 3 or 4 gm/kg/day. Neonates and infants are given up to 4 gm/kg/day of fat.

In our human studies, we used a bottle of fat emulsion, a bottle of amino acids, and sometimes a third bottle of glucose. The infusions were given simultaneously by mixing the solutions immediately before entering the venous bloodstream by means of an ordinary y-type infusion set. In this way it was possible to reduce the incidence of thrombophlebitis considerably. We began with fat emulsion, adding amino acids or glucose solution after a few minutes. At the end of the infusion, glucose and amino acids were removed first, then the fat emulsion. The fat emulsion somehow prevents the formation of thrombophlebitis in the peripheral vein. This technique is used if the patient is expected to be fed intravenously for one or two weeks. But if the infusions are to be given over a period of several months, a central venous catheter might be more convenient.

Table 6.— Daily Supply of Energy and Nutrients to Neonates and Infants on Complete Intravenous Nutrition (according to Børresen et al[41-43] and Grotte[44])

Group of nutrients	Nutrients	Supply to neonates and infants per kg body weight and day
Energy and sources of energy	Water	130-136 ml
	Energy	86-100 kcal
	Amino acids	3gm = 0.4 gm N
	Glucose or fructose	11-12 gm
	Fat	3-4 gm*
Minerals	Sodium	1.05 mmol
	Potassium	2 mmol
	Calcium	0.5-1 mmol
	Magnesium	0.15 mmol
	Phosphorus	1.2-1.6 mmol
Water-soluble vitamins	Thiamin	2.5 mg
	Riboflavin	0.5 mg
	Niacin	5 mg
	Vitamin B_6	0.75 mg
	Pantothenic acid	0.75 mg
	Ascorbic acid	15 mg
Fat-soluble vitamins	Vitamin A	2.500 IU
	Vitamin D	250 IU
	Tocopherol	3.5-4.5 IU

*As Intralipid 20% with 500 IU of Heparin daily.

Table 7.— Solutions for Intravenous Nutrition in Neonates and Infants (According to Grotte[44])

Product	Volume ml per kg and 24 hours	kcal
Vamin "Vitrum"	40-50	26-32.5
10% glucose solution	80-70	32-28
KH_2PO_4 (1/ml)	1.5-2.0	
$MgSO_4$ (0.5/ml)	0.4	
Ca++ (Calcium,"Sandoz 10%", 0.25 mval CA++/ml)	6	
Intralipid 20%, "Vitrum"	15-20	30-40
Total volume and energy	143-148*	88-100

Note: 0.5-1ml "Pancebrin Lilly" and, if indicated, 1 mg vitamin K is added to a mixture of all solutions except for Intralipid.

*The volume should be reduced by about 20 ml per kg if the infants are placed in very humid atmosphere. The 10% glucose solution is then exchanged with a smaller volume of a 15% glucose solution.

210

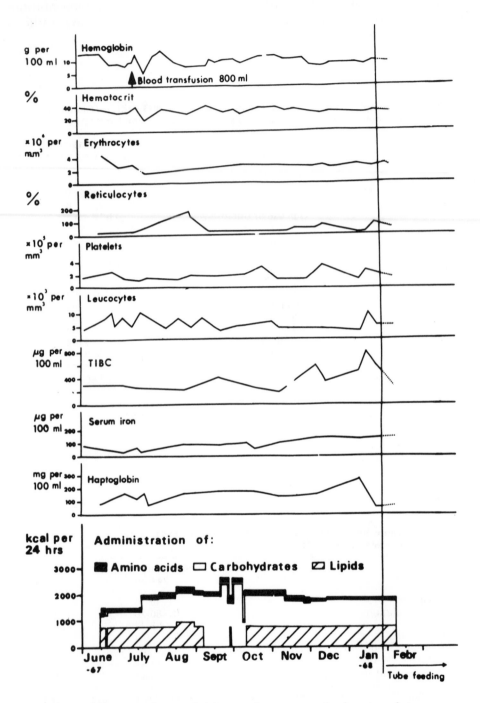

Fig 8. Effects on hemoglobin, erythrocyte, reticulocyte, platelet, leukocyte values and on the serum levels of TIBC, serum iron, and haptoglobin during complete intravenous nutrition (Bergström et al).

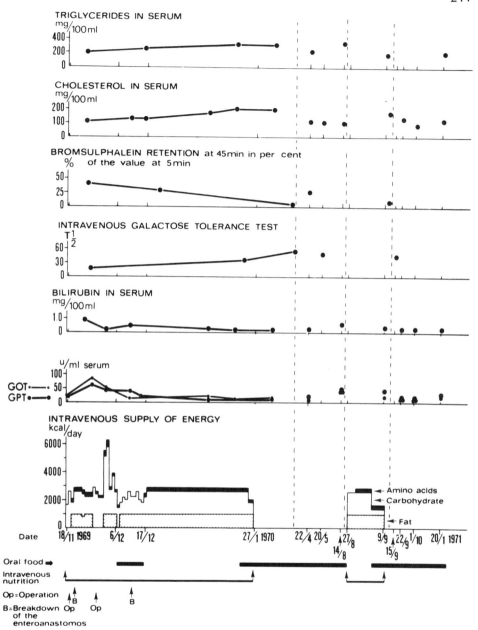

Fig 9. Changes in the serum triglycerides, serum cholesterol, bromsulphalein retention test, the intravenous galactose tolerance test, the serum values for bilirubin, SGOT, and SGPT during a period of intravenous nutrition, following a massive intestinal resection due to acute occlusion of the superior mesenteric artery in a 70-year-old man (Jacobson[39]). The figure also shows the development until January 1971, including the energy supply during a period of intravenous nutrition for 9 months and 14 days after the resection.

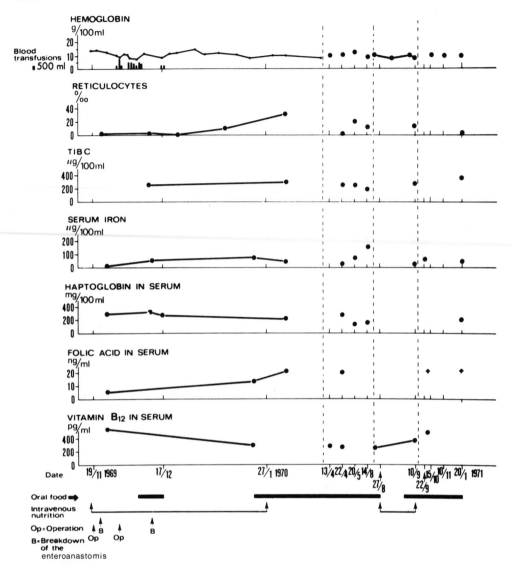

Fig 10. Changes in the serum values for total protein, gamma-globulin, and albumin during two periods of intravenous nutrition following a massive intestinal resection, in a 70-year-old man (Jacobson[39]). The resection was performed for acute occlusion of the superior mesenteric artery.

Dr. Otherson: Regarding your infusion technique, do both the fat and carbohydrates run simultaneously?

Dr. Wretlind: Yes, they run simultaneously.

Dr. Otherson: And there is no problem with degradation of the fat emulsion?

Dr. Wretlind: No.

Dr. Broviac: When will the Food and Drug Administration approve this technique?

Dr. Wretlind: I don't know that. These emulsions are now being tested in the United States, but I don't know how long FDA approval will take.

Dr. Victorin: I am not from FDA, but I have heard that the technique has been approved for clinical investigations.

Dr. Wretlind: Yes, but not for regular use.

Dr. Cahill: Dr. Wretlind, if you infuse a person for 8 hours a day, he will synthesize a certain amount of liver glycogen. This provides the brain with enough glucose for 6 to 8 hours. For the remaining 8 hours of the day, glucose is maintained by gluconeogenesis from body protein. This could be prevented by hyperalimentation for 8 hours a day and infusion of 5% glucose and water for the remaining 16 hours. This would provide just enough glucose for the brain's needs, therefore eliminating any need for gluconeogenesis from muscle protein.

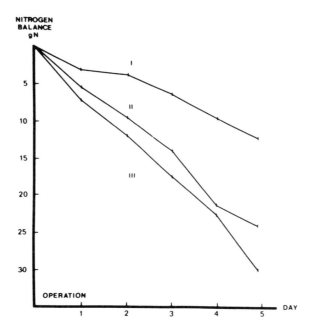

Fig 11. Cumulative nitrogen balance during the first five post-operative days after partial gastrectomy in patients with duo-denal ulcer. Group I (eight patients) received 36 kilocalories, 1.5 gm amino acids, 2 gm fat, and 3 gm glucose/kg body weight per day; Group II (eight patients) received 15 kilo-calories, 1.5 gm amino acids, and 2.2 gm glucose; Group III (four patients) received 16 kilocalories and 4.0 gm glucose (Hallberg et al[40]).

Wouldn't it be more advisable to infuse rapidly for perhaps eight hours? If the needle must be left in anyway, a solution of 5% or 10% dextrose in water could be infused gradually during the remainder of the day to conserve nitrogen as the weeks or months go by.

Dr. Wretlind: There are several reasons why we infuse only during the day. One reason is to follow the circadian physiological patterns and allow the patient to rest for 12 hours during the night. Another reason is to free the other 12-hour period for supplementary infusions in patients with increased energy and nutrient requirements.

Dr. Cahill: That is a philosophical reason.

Dr. Wretlind: Yes, but the old question is whether it is better for a man to eat for 24 hours or for 12 hours. This has not been settled for oral feeding and certainly not for parenteral. It is one of the physiological investigations that must be performed.

Dr. Broviac: Exactly how fast can 2,500 fat calories be infused in a patient weighing 60 kg?

Dr. Wretlind: We have given soybean oil emulsion with no problems at 30 gm of fat per hour.[40] We don't advise more than 25 gm of fat an hour however. This means that 2,500 fat calories may be given in about 11 hours.

Essential Fatty Acid Deficiency

Dr. Holman: The principal dietary EFA are linoleic, linolenic, and arachidonic. The linoleic acid molecule may be elongated by two carbon atoms and desaturated twice to form arachidonic acid, the major polyunsaturated acid of normal tissue. When EFA deficiency exists, an endogenous eicosatrienoic acid is synthesized from oleic acid and is substituted for arachidonic acid in tissue lipids. The normal arachidonic acid diminishes in proportion and the abnormal eicosatrienoic acid increases. The ratio of eicosatrienoic to arachidonic acid is normally 0.4; a ratio greater than this indicates EFA deficiency.

About two years ago, Whitten of Detroit's Children's Hospital asked for our cooperation in the analysis of the serum lipids of a child in whom he suspected EFA deficiency. The child had developed a volvulus at birth and, with nearly all of his small intestine subsequently removed, was maintained solely on fat-free intravenous feeding. We examined serial blood specimens over a period of 4½ months of intravenous feeding. Six other patients being fed intravenously were also included in the study.[45] Analyses were made of serum triglycerides, cholesterol esters, and phospholipids in all cases.

For each individual in the study, nonfat intravenous feeding caused shifts in fatty acid composition which have been well documented as being caused by EFA deficiency in animals[46] and in humans.[47] During prolonged intravenous feeding (Fig 12) the content of linoleic acid ($18:2\omega6$) in serum phospholipids decreased precipitously, and the content of arachidonic acid ($20:4\omega6$) also decreased markedly. These were offset by a dramatic increase in eicosatrienoic (20:3ω9) acid. These shifts in composition are biochemical evidence of EFA deficiency. There were also changes in triglycerides and in cholesterol esters. The severity of this deficiency can be measured by determining the ratio of arachidonic to eicosatrienoic acids. The most severe deficiency observed in animals or humans was a ratio of 6; after 100 days of nonfat infusion, the ratio in this patient was 18. The fatty acid compositions of several tissues were analyzed at autopsy and confirmed the deficiency. After three months of intravenous feeding, a scaliness of skin developed which was

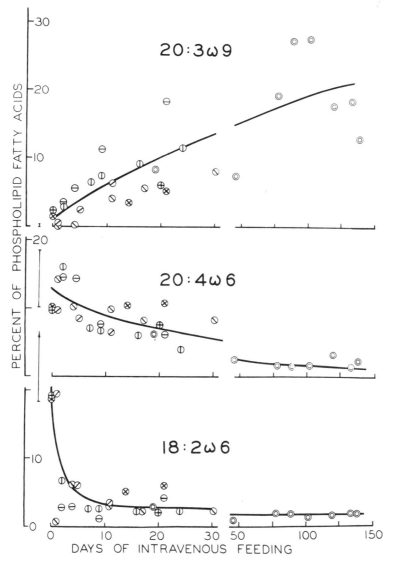

Fig 12. Content of linolenic acid (18:2ω6) in serum phospholipids during prolonged intravenous feeding. The double circles represent analyses on the volvulus patient with the small intestine removed.

216

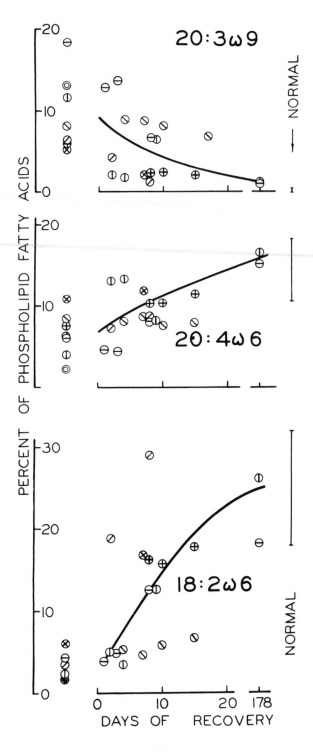

Fig 13. Patterns of fatty acid composition with oral feeding after prolonged intravenous feeding.

very similar to that previously observed by Hansen and coworkers in their studies of deficiency induced by low-quality formula preparations.[48]

Fortunately, these effects of prolonged nonfat intravenous alimentation are to some extent reversible. Six of the patients studied were eventually able to accept and utilize normal food. Serial analyses of the same serum lipids revealed that when food was taken by mouth, the patterns of fatty acid composition eventually returned to normal. For each individual, changes were toward normal composition (Fig 13).

In infants the development of the deficiency is quite rapid: significant changes in serum lipids are apparent within 10 days of fat-free total intravenous feeding. Collins and coworkers reported that EFA deficiency was induced in a 44-year-old man after 100 days and reversed by intravenous feeding of a fat emulsion.[49] In another case, a 77-year-old woman developed flakiness of skin after 7.5 months of fat-free intravenous feeding, but her ratio of eicosatrienoic to arachidonic acid never rose above 0.6, indicating that the deficiency was only marginal. These reports suggest that deficiency appears more rapidly in the young than in the old. Animal studies confirm this.

Septicemia is a common complication during long-term intravenous feeding regimens involving indwelling catheters. Increased rates of infection are also common during EFA deficiency in animals[50] and humans.[48] It is possible that depleted tissues are more easily invaded by microorganisms. If this is the case, the deficiency may enhance any inadvertent infection.

Fat-free intravenous feeding, a lifesaving practice now in common use in the United States, necessarily leads to EFA deficiency if it is prolonged. Hence, this deficiency, which was formerly thought to occur rarely, if at all, in humans, is now being induced in US hospitals. The medical community should be aware of this fact and take its consequences into consideration.

Dr. Caldwell: A six-month-old female developed EFA deficiency after 23 weeks of total parenteral alimentation. The nutritional problem resulted from midgut volvulus secondary to malrotation, which required resection of 50% of the small bowel on the tenth day of life. Multiple attempts to anastomose the remaining proximal small bowel to the duodenum failed, resulting in the creation of a duodenostomy and an ileostomy. Efforts to provide adequate caloric intake through ileostomy feedings were hampered by the development of an enterocutaneous fistula in the remaining small bowel. The only means of feeding was by total parenteral alimentation, which was begun on the 18th day of life and continued for six months. The formula used was similar to those used by Meng and Dudrick. During the parenteral alimentation, multiple attempts at closing this enterocutaneous fistula were unsuccessful due to inadequate healing. After 20 weeks of intravenous nutrition, which included weekly administration of plasma or whole blood, scaly skin lesions appeared over the anterior chest and on the arms (Fig 14). Sparse hair growth and thrombocytopenia were also noted. These changes, together with poor wound healing, suggested essential fatty acid deficiency. Plasma fatty acid levels confirmed the diagnosis (Table 8). The patient showed increased palmytoleic, oleic, and 5, 8, 11-eicosatrienoic acids and markedly decreased linoleic and arachidonic acids.

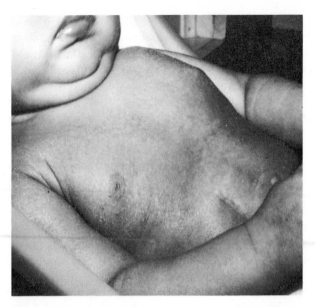

Fig 14. Scaly skin lesions are seen over the anterior chest and upper arm.

Table 8.—Relative % of Total Plasma Fatty Acids

	C16:1	C18:1	C18:2	C20:3ω9	C20:4ω6
Control	4.7	17.3	34.6	NSA	8.2
K W	13.3	37.8	4.0	9.8	NSA
K W after Intralipid	6.05	25.0	20.2	2.6	4.0

Note: NSA = no significant amount (<0.1%).

When the patient was 25 weeks of age, we began intravenous administration of 10% Intralipid to correct the EFA deficiency. Four percent of the daily caloric requirement was provided by linoleic acid in 60 cc of the emulsion, which was infused through a peripheral vein at 10 cc/hr. This dosage was based on studies by Hansen and Wiese, who stated that 4% of the daily caloric intake as linoleic acid produces optimal serum triene-tetraene ratios.[51] Also, this percentage of linoleic acid is similar to that in breast milk.

Skin lesions cleared after intravenous fat therapy (Fig 15). Correction of the thrombocytopenia following Intralipid administration was also seen (Table 9). A significant rise in linoleic and arachidonic acids and a significant decrease in the 5, 8, 11-eicosatrienoic acid occurred after Intralipid infusion (Table 8).

At 28 weeks of age, a duodenostomy, a duodenoileostomy, and a closure of the enterocutaneous fistula were performed with complete healing of all surgical wounds. The child was later discharged on an oral diet.

I emphasize Dr. Holman's statement that any patient on total parenteral alimentation for as few as 10 to 14 days may develop biochemical evidence of EFA deficiency. Unfortunately, the quantitative intravenous require-

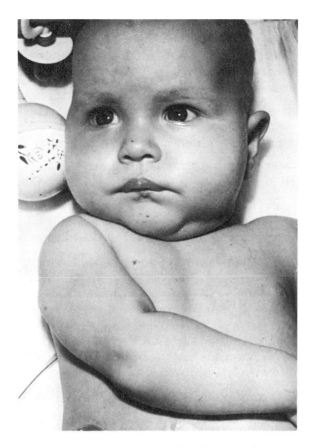

Fig 15. Complete clearing of the skin lesions after intravenous fat therapy.

Table 9.—Platelet Counts

Before administration of Intralipid	56,000/mm³
7th day of Intralipid infusions	158,000/mm³
14th and last day of Intralipid infusions	196,000/mm³

ment for essential fatty acids is unknown, and intravenous therapy must at present be governed by oral standards. Until better information is available, I believe that 4% of the daily calories as linoleic acid is sufficient.

Dr. Wilmore: Changes in the lipid pattern occur relatively early in fat-free intravenous diets, depending on the metabolic rate and metabolic turnover. The limits that really need definition are the physiologic changes: When will a decrease in EFA concentration appear in cell membranes? When will we see a change in cellular function or in skin regeneration?

Dr. Holman: This cannot be answered with the data available for humans, but animal experiments have shown that discernible physiologic and biochemical changes in the subcellular particles of the liver occur within two weeks.[46]

Human investigations indicate that wound healing does not proceed normally during fatty acid deficiency. This probably has something to do with a defense mechanism or cell multiplication. The literature indicates that both deficient animals[50] and deficient babies[51] show a higher than normal incidence of infectious diseases and respiratory problems.

Dr. Caldwell: A study by Decker and associates showed that tail wounds healed in normal mice but not in EFA-deficient mice, suggesting a correlation between wound healing and fatty acid deficiency.[52]

Dr. Schumer: Since we cannot use Intralipid in the United States, has plasma been used to replete any of these patients with EFA deficiency?

Dr. Holman: The normal plasma linoleic acid value is probably around 103 mg/100 ml. In a child, about 2.5 liters of plasma daily is needed to provide enough linoleic acid to prevent deficiency. This is an unfeasible approach.

Dr. Cahill: Children born with no β-lipoprotein may provide an excellent model. They have no transport of fat from the bowel into the blood stream. After two or three weeks they develop EFA deficiency, mental retardation, acanthocytosis, and poor wound healing. These infants are given plasma taken from specific donors who have eaten a quantity of soybeans. The children, who receive one infusion per week of this blood, purportedly lose their acanthocytosis, grow normally, and their skin lesions heal. It is an alternative to parenteral nutrition in EFA deficiency.

Dr. Broviac: Most of my patients on long-term home parenteral nutrition can eat some food but can't absorb all of it. By eating one or two patties of corn oil margarine on toast once a day they can absorb some fat, but does this prevent EFA deficiency?

Dr. Holman: I assume that corn oil margarine has some quantity of linoleic acid remaining in it. If 4% of calories can be provided as linoleic acid, the deficiency should be prevented or cured.

Dr. Schumer: What is the effect of fatty acid deficiency on the structure and function of the red cell membrane?

Dr. Wilmore: In patients with burns, abnormal concentrations of cations are found in the red blood cell, and there is a high level of intracellular sodium. With parenteral feedings, the sodium level returns toward normal. We have documented the deficiency of polyunsaturated fatty acids in the red cell membrane and are correlating this structural change with functional changes in membrane transport. Does the hypermetabolic patient who has burns, trauma, sepsis, peritonitis, or fracture catabolize essential fatty acids at a faster rate than the patient who is in a state of resting starvation? Our preliminary data suggest that this is the case and that these fatty acids are necessary for normal cellular membrane structure and function.

Dr. Cahill: I would like to see a practical bedside test to determine whether or not infusion of polyunsaturated fats is necessary at a given time. The physician could observe the red cells rather than wait for a blood sample to be separated and analyzed.

Intralipid and Respiratory Insufficiency

Dr. Greene: Intralipid can be administered in peripheral veins. It therefore appears to be a good calorie source for premature babies if used over a short period of time, perhaps one to two weeks. But many of these infants have some type of respiratory distress, so I felt it necessary to study the effects of this fat emulsion on pulmonary diffusion. Five normal adult volunteers received 500 cc of 10% Intralipid on the first day and 500 cc of saline on the second day; in some subjects this order of infusion was reversed. Each day, lung volume, flow rate, airway resistance, cardiac output, and steady state pulmonary function were measured using the technique standardized by Gilles Filley.[53] The technique was reproducible from one day to the next; 42 patients measured one week to one month apart showed similar values with a standard deviation as shown by the two lines forming a 45° angle in Figure 16. The only parameter that changed significantly was pulmonary membrane diffusion in 5 of the 10 subjects.[54]

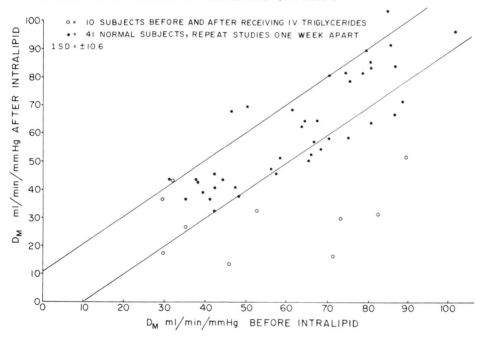

Fig 16. Membrane diffusion capacities in patients and subjects treated with Intralipid. Closed circles are measurements of membrane diffusion in 41 patients (ordinate) and in the same patients one week later (abscissa), illustrating the reproducibility of such measurements in a given patient. The parallel lines represent one standard deviation in the patient data. Open circles represent membrane diffusion values in ten subjects before and after Intralipid. By analysis of variance, six of the ten subjects showed a significant decrease in membrane diffusion following Intralipid.

222

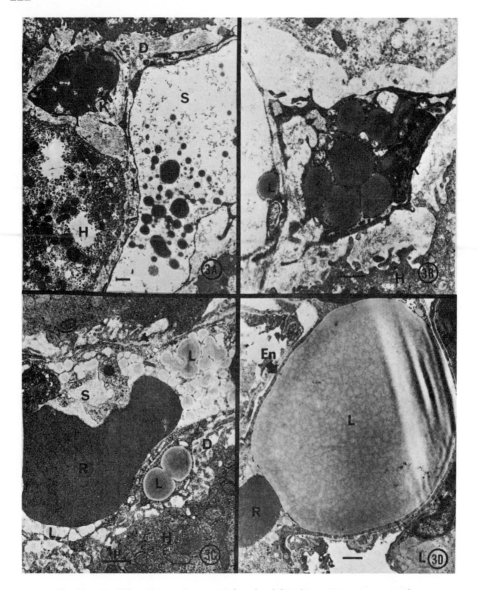

Fig 17. A. Electron micrograph of rabbit liver 30 minutes after Intralipid infusion. (S = sinusoid, L = lipid particles, K = Kupffer cell, D = space of Disse, H = hepatocyte, and all markers indicate 1 micron.)

B. Higher magnification of 18A showing lipid in the Kupffer cell and the transport of lipid across the sinusoidal membrane into the space of Disse.

C. One hour later Intralipid showing the increased amount of lipid in the liver sinusoid (= L).

D. One hour after Intralipid, a large lipid particle in lung tissue which had apparently coalesced and is seen to occlude a capillary. This was the only section in which this phenomenon was observed.

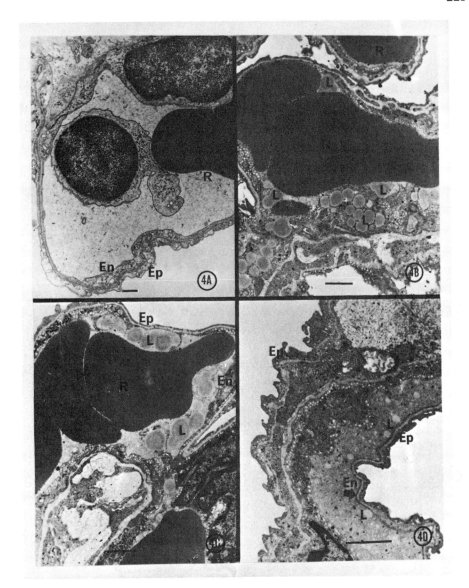

Fig 18. A. Electron micrograph of rabbit lung. Control lung showing the normal pulmonary structures before Intralipid. (Ep = alveolar epithelium, En = capillary endothelium, R = red blood cell, and all markers indicate 1 micron.)

B. Electron micrograph of rabbit lung 30 minutes after Intralipid infusion (L = lipid).

C. Electron micrograph of rabbit lung one hour after Intralipid infusion.

D. Electron micrograph of rabbit lung six hours after Intralipid infusion.

Tissues were fixed in 2.5% glutaraldehyde, postfixed with tetroxide osmium, and stained with uranyl acetate and lead citrate.

224

We also measured the capillary blood volume, and the subjects who showed decreases in capillary membrane diffusion also had a slight increase in the capillary blood volume following the infusion of Intralipid. These measurements were taken one hour after a four-hour infusion.

On the basis of these findings, six rabbits were infused with 10 cc/kg of body weight of Intralipid over a 30-minute period. The animals were then sacrificed after various periods of time. The electron microscopic findings in the liver are shown in Figure 17.

Figure 18 demonstrates the serial changes in the lung after infusion. If at 30 minutes one compares the number of lipid particles in the liver sinusoid (Fig 17) with that in the pulmonary capillary (Fig 18), there appears

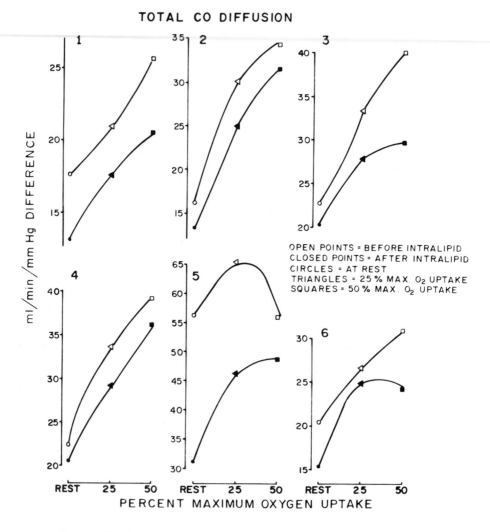

TOTAL CO DIFFUSION

OPEN POINTS = BEFORE INTRALIPID
CLOSED POINTS = AFTER INTRALIPID
CIRCLES = AT REST
TRIANGLES = 25 % MAX. O_2 UPTAKE
SQUARES = 50 % MAX. O_2 UPTAKE

ml/min/mm Hg DIFFERENCE

PERCENT MAXIMUM OXYGEN UPTAKE

Fig 19. Total carbon monoxide diffusion in the six subjects who showed a significant decrease in CO diffusion following Intralipid infusion at two levels of exercise.

to be more lipid retained in the lung during the early phase after the lipid infusion. This difference disappeared within one hour after the infusion. Figure 17 demonstrates that the lipid is transported into the space of Disse and taken up by the Kupffer cells.

Figure 18 shows the changes with time in the lungs. At 30 and 60 minutes after the infusion, a large amount of lipid appeared to be localized along the periphery of the vessel, but at no time was there any lipid deposition in the capillary endothelium or alveolar epithelium.

On the basis of these observations in the rabbit lung, one might speculate that, theoretically, a portion of the red blood cells is surrounded by lipid particles at various times during the brief period of gaseous exchange in the pulmonary capillaries, and the physiologic changes in carbon monoxide diffusion observed in humans may be due to the mechanical interference in movement of gases between the alveolar space and red blood cells.

To clarify the clinical significance of these findings, we repeated the human studies using exercise and arterial blood samples. Five subjects were given 500 ml of physiological saline over a two-hour period. Pulmonary diffusion was measured with exercise on a treadmill, at rest, and at 25% and 50% maximum oxygen uptake. Arterial gases, pO_2, and pCO_2, were measured at various levels of exercise. Only one subject showed a significant decrease in arterial pO_2 at rest and at 25% maximum oxygen uptake. This subject took six hours—longer than the others—to clear the triglycerides. But this slight pO_2 decrease did not prevent the pO_2 and membrane diffusion from increasing normally with exercise, and no symptoms were present.

The pulmonary diffusion measurements before Intralipid infusion yielded the predicted values—that is, pulmonary diffusion capacity increased normally with exercise. After Intralipid, six of the ten subjects showed some degree of change in pulmonary diffusion at each level of exercise. By analysis of variants, the differences were statistically significant in these six subjects (Fig 19). In the remaining four subjects, no statistical change could be demonstrated.

Next, we tested the effects of Intralipid plus heparin on pulmonary function. The two subjects who showed the greatest change in pulmonary diffusion were given Intralipid with 50 units of heparin per kilogram of body weight one hour before and four hours later (Fig 20). Results showed that in both patients, the carbon monoxide diffusion had increased above the base-line levels. Triglycerides and plasma optical density returned to base-line levels much sooner than when Intralipid was not given. Thus the pulmonary changes noted earlier were reversed by this small dose of heparin.

Dr. Wilmore: My information supplements Dr. Greene's data. We infused Intralipid into both normal convalescing patients and patients with acute thermal injury.[55] Five hundred milliliter doses were given over a four-hour period at a constant rate of infusion. Blood was drawn before and after infusion; temperature, pulse rate, blood pressure, and respiratory rate were monitored during infusion and for 12 hours afterward. There were no changes in any of these in 50 patients. Complete blood count and liver function studies were normal 24 hours after infusion (Table 10).

Table 10.— Studies Before and After Infusion of 500 ml Intralipid
(N = 15, Mean ± SD)

	Before	After
Hematocrit	41 ± 5	42 ± 4
WBC	7,900 ± 2,200	7,700 ± 2,200
Total proteins	7.3 ± 0.5	7.6 ± 0.4
Albumin	3.6 ± 0.6	3.7 ± 0.4
Alkaline phosphatase	13 ± 3	15 ± 4
SGOT	30 ± 11	34 ± 9
Total bilirubin	0.5 ± 0.3	0.5 ± 0.3
Direct bilirubin	0.1 ± 0.0	0.1 ± 0.0

RESTING PULMONARY DIFFUSION CHANGES WITH INTRALIPID

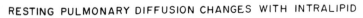

▭ AFTER 500 ml OF SALINE
▦ AFTER 500 ml OF 10% INTRALIPID
■ 3 DAYS(1) AND 10 HOURS (2) AFTER INTRALIPID
▨ AFTER 500 ml OF 10% INTRALIPID PLUS HEPARIN

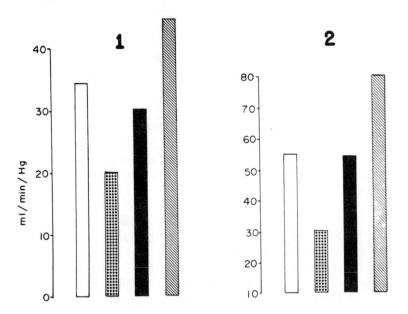

Fig 20. Total carbon monoxide diffusion in two resting subjects after saline, 10% Intralipid, and 10% Intralipid plus heparin.

Fat clearance studies were performed in both normal individuals and patients with burns. Serum optical density was measured at 700 millimicrons by a spectrophotometer. The peak level in these patients was only about one-fourth the normal level, demonstrating the rapid clearance of the fat emulsion following injury. The complications that Dr. Greene and his associates reported

227

occurring in normal individuals have not been seen in starved patients or patients with burns. These pulmonary complications may be associated with a slow lipid clearance rate in normal subjects and rapid clearance following injury or starvation (Fig 21).

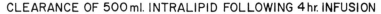

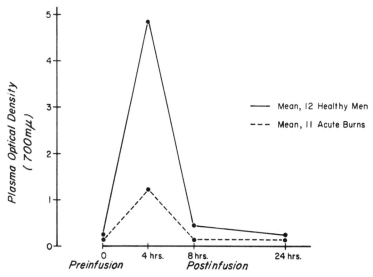

Fig 21. Clearance of 500 ml of Intralipid following a four-hour infusion.

Because pneumonia and other pulmonary complications represent some of the more common causes of death in patients with burns, we were cautious in administering fat emulsion to seriously burned patients before its safety and efficacy for ventilatory function was documented.

Total diffusion or total resistance equals membrane resistance plus red cell resistance. Red cell resistance is composed of the red cell volume in the pulmonary capillaries and the reaction rate of carbon monoxide with hemoglobin. The *Handbook of Physiology* expresses the formula as follows:[56]

$$\underbrace{\frac{1}{D_{L_{CO}}}}_{\text{Total Resistance}} = \underbrace{\frac{1}{D_M}}_{\text{Membrane Resistance}} + \underbrace{\frac{1}{\phi V_C}}_{\text{Blood Resistance}}$$

where $D_{L_{CO}}$ = total diffusing capacity
D_M = membrane diffusion capacity
ϕ = the combination rate of carbon monoxide with human blood
V_C = capillary blood volume

We measured total diffusing capacity, which is not the same as Dr. Greene's measurements of membrane resistance and red cell volume.

Table 11 demonstrates diffusing capacity with carbon monoxide expressed per minute per milliliter of mercury after a four-hour infusion of Intralipid in convalescing subjects. All values were within the predicted normal limits for height, weight, and size of each individual, and no significant changes in pulmonary diffusing capacity were demonstrated. Xenon-133, a soluble gas that diffuses across the alveolar membrane at a known rate, was given to seven patients before and after Intralipid administration. The rate of xenon clearance across the alveolar membrane was determined with a scintillation counter, and this highly sensitive technique showed no difference in clearance rate before or after Intralipid infusion.

Table 11.— Diffusion Capacity Before and After Infusion of 500 ml Soybean Emulsion in Four Normal Individuals (Mean ± SD)

Preinfusion	Immediately Postinfusion	4 Hours Postinfusion
33.88±2.42	33.78±2.58	34.49±3.01

Blood gases were analyzed on arterial samples of 20 severely burned patients before and after Intralipid infusion. In both samples from every patient, the pCO_2, pO_2, and pH were comparable, demonstrating no significant deviations (Table 12).

Table 12.—Effect of Intravenous Fat on Blood Gases (Mean ± SD)

	PO$_2$		PCO$_2$		pH	
	Before	After	Before	After	Before	After
1 gm/kg	91.6±9.5	86.0±9.4	26.9±6.1	27.8±4.4	7.448±0.072	7.466±0.066
2 gm/kg	86.0±22.9	89.7±20.1	28.1±6.5	30.6±7.1	7.454±0.040	7.460±0.060
3 gm/kg	75.2±10.7	78.4±12.5	32.3±3.2	32.1±4.3	7.444±0.046	7.448±0.037

Respiratory changes frequently accompany alterations in nutritional support. Keys stated that, during a period of partial starvation, changes in ventilatory function occur with decreases in vital capacity, respiratory, minute volume, and respiratory efficiency[57] (see Table 13). The respiratory changes following ingestion of 900 calories from carbohydrate have been carefully studied by Saltzman and Salzano.[58] They observed increases in minute ventilation, tidal volume, blood lactate production, and oxygen consumption (Table 14).

Working with Curreri and Spitzer, we demonstrated similar changes in response to a graded caloric intake in six thermally injured patients.[55] Patients had a daily intake of 600, 3,000, or 6,000 kilocalories during three consecutive two-day study periods. With supranormal caloric administration, there was a moderate increase in minute ventilation, a slight increase in respiratory rate, and a significant increase in carbon dioxide production and oxygen consumption (Table 15). Thus, it is obvious that, with either caloric support or starvation, alterations in pulmonary function occur. Further pulmonary function studies should be designed to determine whether respiratory changes are related to the method of nutritional support or to a secondary effect of the specific substrate on the respiratory system.

Table 13.—Respiratory Changes During Starvation[57]

	Control	Semi-Starved	
		12 Weeks	24 Weeks
Vital capacity, in liters	5.17	4.94	4.78
Respiratory rate, per min.	11.45	9.89	9.86
Minute volume, liters/min.	4.82	3.49	3.35
Tidal volume, cc/respiration	421	353	340
Respiratory efficiency	47.93	45.20	42.65

Table 14.—Respiratory Changes Following Carbohydrate Ingestion[58]

(Mean Values)		
	Fasting	Ingestion of 920 kcal
$\dot{V}_e$	6.91	9.57 *
F	11.2	12.4
$\dot{V}_t$	628	783 *
$\dot{V}CO_2$	196	280 *
$\dot{V}O_2$	234	265 *
RQ	0.84	1.05
pO_2	88.9	98.2 *
pCO_2	40.1	39.5
pH	7.400	7.378*

*Significant changes, $p < 0.01$

Table 15.— Respiratory Changes with Varied Daily Caloric Support (Mean values)

	600 kcal/day	3,000 kcal/day	6,000 kcal/day
$\dot{V}_{le}$	11.6	11.6	14.4
Frequency	15	17	18
$\dot{V}CO_2$	259	302	345
$\dot{V}O_2$	325	337	341
RQ	0.80	0.89	1.01
pCO_2	83	82	80
pCO_2	27	31	30
pH	7.47	7.44	7.47

Dr. Wretlind: Let us move to the problems of feeding fat emulsions to neonates and infants. Dr. Victorin and his associates have investigated the excretion rate of fat emulsion in these subjects.

Dr. Victorin: In small premature babies, oral feeding cannot provide sufficient caloric intake. We should distinguish here between prematures who are appropriate in size for the time they are born and those who are small-for-date babies. The small-for-date baby is generally considered to be a victim of intrauterine malnutrition or starvation and has, compared to the appropriate-size baby, minimal supplies of fat and glycogen.

We investigated the effect of single injections of 0.5 gm/kg of Intra-lipid® in the two types of infants and then calculated the elimination curve the same way as for adults.[59] The initial elimination capacity was compatible with that in adults. However, comparison of the two groups of infants showed that two hours after injection, the appropriate-size babies had eliminated nearly all fat given to them, while the small-for-date babies had not.

Lipid electrophoretic studies revealed that the prolonged high serum fat level in small-for-date babies could be attributed to two different fat fractions. First, the elimination rate of the injected fat, as chylomicrons, was markedly reduced. Second, a pronounced band was found at the place for pre-β-lipoproteins within the first half hour after the injection. This last fat fraction, considered as low-density-lipoprotein, constitutes a second generation of the infused fat that is partly metabolized in the liver.

Repeated lipid injections were given in a series of both appropriate-size and small-for-date infants. We divided the daily dosage of between 3 and 4 gm/kg into 24 doses and gave one dose every hour. During the first eight hours, we found a progressive increase in total lipids in small-for-date babies but not in the appropriate-size babies. While continuing the hourly lipid injections, we injected 50 IU/kg of heparin as a single dose into small-for-date babies with increased fat levels. In virtually every case we found, as expected, an acute and sustained normalization of serum fat despite the continuing fat injections. These results indicate some kind of defective lipoprotein-lipase activity in small-for-date babies, which was corrected by heparin injection.

In a limited number of cases, we observed the free fatty acid pattern with gas chromatography during hourly fat injections, especially after heparin was added. Invariably, total serum fat dropped while free fatty acids showed a marked increase of eight to ten times the initial value. Possible deleterious effects of this high free fatty acid level must be considered. For instance, these acids may be a mitochondrial uncoupling factor that could, among other things, increase bilirubin toxicity, a matter of prime concern with premature babies.

We still lack strong data to recommend administration of heparin with fat for the newborn. Pediatric surgeons in Scandinavia are using parenteral feeding with heparin according to the program by Børresen, Coran, and Knutrud,[42] reportedly without clinical side effects. The question is not settled; more investigations are necessary before we can recommend this form of hyperalimentation for widespread use among premature babies.

Dr. Wretlind: Administration of heparin with intravenous fat feeding is associated with controversy. Most infusions of Intralipid in adults are given without heparin to accelerate the elimination of fat particles from the bloodstream. Continued investigation of the use of heparin, especially in small-for-date children, is a necessity. In pediatrics most physicians use heparin in connection with infusions of Intralipid according to Børreson and associates.[42]

Dr. Greene, would you say that heparin should be used with fat?

Dr. Greene: It depends on the patient's condition, particularly on the desirability of rapidly clearing the plasma lipids. In traumatized patients or in others with good clearance rates, it makes little difference whether heparin is given or not. However, if Intralipid affects the blood gases, then a patient with a poor clearance rate would perhaps benefit from a small dose of heparin that would not produce an anticoagulant effect.

Dr. Wretlind: Dr. Victorin, would you recommend giving heparin in combination with fat in small infants or neonates, or do you prefer to investigate this further?

Dr. Victorin: More investigations are necessary. One must consider that surgical disease is less frequent in small infants and neonates.

Dr. Meng: Rapid clearing may or may not indicate utilization. This can only be determined when metabolic data are available.

Dr. Wretlind: That is an important point.

Dr. Otten: During infusion of Lipofundin and Intralipid in premature infants, we found decreases in triglycerides and glucose and increases in glycerol and ketone bodies. At the end of the infusion, there was a decrease in ketone bodies, an increase in glucose, and normal levels of triglycerides and glycerol. Whether the infusion rate was 0.5 gm/kg in 5 minutes, or 2 gm/kg in 4 hours, or 2 gm/kg in 6 hours, the results were the same.

Dr. Wretlind: Numbers of investigators have shown that fat emulsion can be used as an energy source. Very large dosages—up to 12 gm/kg/day—have been given to adults without adverse effects. Our recommendation is that fats should be used in about the same percentage as they occur in oral diets; that is, 40% of the total energy supply or about 2 gm/kg. Fat should be used in combination with a reasonable supply of carbohydrate. For infants, we need more information before recommending an amount corresponding to oral intake; however, as Dr. Greene suggested, the dosage should not be more than 4 gm/kg given with glucose.

The use of heparin with intravenous fat requires further investigation. With regard to the infusion techniques, a peripheral vein can be used for long-term infusion.

Contraindications to fat emulsions obviously include essential hyperlipemia and irreversible liver damage. Great care must be taken with patients with histories of allergies, who may react unfavorably to intravenous nutrition with fat emulsions. This kind of adverse reaction has been reported by Austrian researchers.[60]

References

1. Bergström J, Fürst P, Gallyas F, et al: Aspects of fructose metabolism in normal man. *Acta Med Scand,* suppl 542, pp 57-64, 1936.

2. Schumer W: High calorie solutions in traumatized patients, in Fox CL Jr, Nahas GG (eds): *Body Fluid Replacement in the Surgical Patient.* New York, Grune & Stratton, 1970, p 326.

3. Förster H, Mehnert H, Alhoug I: Anstieg der Serumharnsäure nach Verabreichung von Fructose. (Rise in uric acid serum levels following administration of fructose.) *Klin Wochenschr* **45:**436, 1967.

4. Mäenpää PH, Raivio KO, Kekomäki MP: Liver adenine nucleotides: Fructose-induced depletion and its effect on protein synthesis. *Science* **161:** 1253-1254, 1968.

5. Andersson G, Brohult J, Sterner G: Increasing metabolic acidosis following fructose infusion in two children. *Acta Paediatr Scand* **58:**301-304, 1969.

6. Mallette LE, Exton JH, Park CR: Control of gluconeogenesis from amino acids in the perfused rat liver. *J Biol Chem* **244:**5713-5723, 1969.

7. Maurer W: Die Grösse des Umsatzes von Organ—und Plasmaeiweiss, in *Colloquium No. 10 of the Gesellschaft für Biologische Chemie, Dynamik des Eiweisses.* Berlin, Springer Verlag, 1960, p 1.

8. Saxon L, Papper S: Abdominal pain occurring in the rapid administration of fructose solutions. *N Eng J Med* **256:**132-133, 1957.

9. Raivio KO, Kekomäki MP, Mäenpää PH: Depletion of liver adenine nucleotides induced by D-fructose: Dose-dependence and specificity of the fructose effect. *Biochem Pharmacol* **18:**2615-2624, 1969.

10. Gabbay KH, Snider JJ: Nerve conduction defect in galactose-fed rats. *Diabetes* **21:**295-300, 1972.

11. Schumer W: Preliminary report: Adverse effects of xylitol in parenteral alimentation. *Metabolism* **20:**345-347, 1971.

12. Bassler KH, Prellwitz W, Unbehaun V, Lang K: Xylitstoffwechsel beim Menschen zur Frage der Eignung von Xylit als Zucker-ersatz beim Diabetiker. (Xylitol metabolism in man: On the value of xylitol as sugar substitute for diabetic patients.) *Klin Wochenschr* **40:**791, 1962.

13. Young JM, Weser E: The metabolism of circulating maltose in man. *J Clin Invest* **50:**986-991, 1971.

14. Beisbarth H, Schultis K: The role of fat as calorie source in parenteral nutrition. *Med Ernähr* **13:**141, 1972.

15. Bode C, Kono H, Goebell H, Bode C, Martini GA: Zur Pathogenese der Fetteinlagerung in die Leber durch Alkohol. III. Effekt von Athanol auf Metabolite und Coenzyme des energieliefernden Stoffwechsels in der Leber und im Blut bei Standardkost und proteinarmer Ernährung. *Klin Wochenschr* **48:**1180-1188, 1970.

16. Carey MA, Jones JD, Gastineau CF: Effects of moderate alcohol intake on blood chemistry values. *JAMA* **216:**1766-1769, 1971.

17. Forsander OA: Alkoholabbau und Leber Stoffwechsel des Aethylalkohols. *Therapiewoche* **20:**2261, 1970.

18. Williamson JR, Scholz R, Browning ET, et al: Metabolic effects of ethanol in perfused rat liver. *J Biol Chem* **244:**5044, 1969.

19. Kreisberg RA, Owen WC, Siegal AM: Ethanol-induced hyper-lactacidemia: Inhibition of lactate utilization. *J Clin Invest* **50:**166-174, 1971.

20. Rinaldi F, Mancuso L, Canonico A, et al: Variazioni del Lattato e Piruvato Arteriosi in Soggetti Normali e in Cirrotici durante e dopo Infusione di Etanolo. *Boll Soc Ital Biol Sper* **45:**1491-1494, 1969.

21. Schulman MP, Westerfield WW: A new pathway for the metabolism of ethanol. *Fed Proc* **16:**244, 1957.

22. Sahud MA: Platelet size and number in alcohol thrombocytopenia. *N Eng J Med* **286:**355, 1972.

23. Lieber CS, Rubin E: Ethanol—a hepatotoxic drug. *Gastroenterology* **54:**642, 1968.

24. Rubin E, Lieber CS: Experimental alcoholic hepatic injury in man: Ultrastructural changes. *Fed Proc* **26:**1458-1467, 1967.

25. Rubin E, Lieber CS: Effects of alcohol on the normal human liver. *Am J Pathol* **52:**55a, 1968 (abstract #114).

26. Rubin E, Lieber CS: Alcohol-induced hepatic injury in nonalcoholic volunteers. *N Eng J Med* **278:**869-876, 1968.

27. Rubin E, Lieber CS: Alcoholism, alcohol, and drugs. *Science* **172:** 1097-1102, 1971.

28. Shipp JC, Cunningham RW, Russell RO, Marble A: Insulin resistance: Clinical features, natural course, and effect of adrenal steroid treatment. *Medicine* **44:**165-186, 1965.

29. Daweke H: Klinik der insulinresistenz. *Dtsch Med Wochenschr* **91:**974-978, 1966.

30. Malarkey WB, Daughaday WH: Variable response of plasma GH in acromegalic patients treated with medroxyprogesterone acetate. *J Clin Endocrinol Metab* **33:**424-431, 1971.

31. Felig P, Marliss EB, Cahill GF Jr: Metabolic response to human growth hormone during prolonged starvation. *J Clin Invest* **50:**411-421, 1971.

32. Hååkonsson I: Experience in long-term studies on nine intravenous fat emulsions in dogs. *Nutr Dieta* **10:**54-76, 1968.

33. Hallberg D: Studies on the elimination of exogenous lipids from the blood stream: The kinetics for the elimination of a fat emulsion studied by single injection technique in man. *Acta Physiol Scand* **64:**306-313, 1965.

34. Hallberg D: Elimination of exogenous lipids from the bloodstream: An experimental methodological and clinical study in dog and man. *Acta Physiol Scand*, suppl 65, p 254, 1965.

35. Cronberg S, Nilsson IM: Coagulation studies after administration of a fat emulsion, Intralipid. *Thromb Diath Haemorrh* **18:**664-669, 1967.

36. Duckert F, Hartmann G: Intravenöse Fettinfusion und Blutgerinung. *Schweiz Med Wochenschr* **96:**1205-1206, 1966.

37. Wretlind A: Complete intravenous nutrition. Theoretical and experimental background. *Nutr Metab* **14:** Suppl: 1-57, 1972.

38. Bergström K, Blomstrand R, Jacobson S: Long-term complete intravenous nutrition in man. *Nutr Metab* **14:** Suppl: 118-149, 1972.

234

39. Jacobson S: Long-term parenteral nutrition following massive intestinal resection. *Nutr Metab* **14:** Suppl: 150-161, 1972.

40. Hallberg D, Holm I, Obel A-L, et al: Fat emulsions for complete intravenous nutrition. *Postgrad Med J* **42:** A71, A87, A99, A149-152, 1967.

41. Børresen HC, Knutrud O: Parenteral feeding of neonates undergoing major surgery. *Acta Paediatr Scand* **58:** 420, 1969.

42. Børresen HC, Coran AG, Knutrud O: Metabolic results of parenteral feeding in neonatal surgery: A balanced parenteral feeding program based on a synthetic L-amino acid solution and a commercial fat solution. *Ann Surg* **172:** 291-301, 1970.

43. Børresen HC, Coran AG, Knutrud O: Parenteral feeding of newborns undergoing major surgery, in Berg G (ed): *Advances in Parenteral Nutrition:* Symposium of the International Society of Parenteral Nutrition, Prague, September 3-4, 1969. Stuttgart, Georg Thieme Verlag, 1970.

44. Grotte G: Les Solutés de Substition Réequilibration Métabolique. Paris, Libraire Arnette, 1971, p 509.

45. Paulsrud JR, Pensler L, Whitten CF, et al: Essential fatty acid deficiency in infants induced by fat-free intravenous feeding. *Am J Clin Nutr* **25:** 877-904, 1972.

46. Holman RT (ed): Essential fatty acid deficiency: A long, scaly tale, in *Progress in the Chemistry of Fats and Other Lipids,* vol IX. Oxford, Pergamon Press, 1968, p 279.

47. Söderhjelm J, Wiese HF, Holman RT: The role of polyunsaturated acid in human nutrition and metabolism, in Holman RT (ed): *Progress in the Chemistry of Fats and Other Lipids,* vol IX. Oxford, Pergamon Press, 1968, p 555.

48. Hansen AE, Wiese HF, Boelsche AN, et al: Role of linoleic acid in infant nutrition. *Pediatrics* **31:** Suppl 1, Part 2: 171, 1963.

49. Collins FD, Sinclair AJ, Royle JP, et al: Plasma lipids in human linoleic acid deficiency. *Nutr Metab* **13:** 150-167, 1971.

50. Hansen AE, Beck O, Wiese HF: Susceptibility to infection manifested by dogs on a low fat diet. *Fed Proc* **7:** 289, 1948.

51. Wiese HF, Hansen AE, Adam DJD: Essential fatty acids in infant nutrition. *J Nutr* **66:** 345-360, 1958.

52. Decker AB, Fillerup DL, Mead JF: Chronic essential fatty acid deficiency in mice. *J Nutr* **41:** 507-521, 1950.

53. Filley GF, McIntosh DJ, Wright GW: Carbon monoxide uptake and pulmonary diffusing capacity in normal subjects at rest and during exercise. *J Clin Invest* **33:** 530-539, 1954.

54. Linderholm H: On the significance of CO tension in pulmonary diffusing capacity with the steady state CO method. *Acta Med Scand* **156:** 413-427, 1957.

55. Wilmore DW, Curreri PW, Spitzer KW, et al: Supranormal dietary intake in thermally injured hypermetabolic patients. *Surg Gynecol Obstet* **132:** 881-886, 1971.

56. Förster RE: Diffusion of gases, in Field J (editor-in-chief): *Handbook of Physiology,* vol I, section 3. Fenn WO, Rahn H (eds): *Respiration.* Baltimore, Williams & Wilkins, 1963, p 857.

57. Keys A (ed): Respiration, in *The Biology of Human Starvation,* vol I. Minneapolis, University of Minnesota Press, 1950, p 601.

58. Saltzman HA, Salzano JV: Effects of carbohydrate metabolism upon respiratory gas exchange in normal men. *J Appl Physiol* **38:**228-231, 1971.

59. Gustafson A, Kjellmer I, Olegard R, Victorin L: Nutrition in low-birth-weight infants. I. Intravenous injection of fat emulsion. *Acta Paediatr Scand* **61:**149-158, 1972.

60. Depish D: Bedrohliche Hyperlipämie im Rahmen eines allergischen Schocks bei parenteraler Ernährung einer Tetanuspatientin. *Anaesthesist* **20:**437-441, 1971.

Digest of Colloquium

CARBOHYDRATES

The participants opened the discussion by asking, "What is the best and most efficient carbohydrate for parenteral alimentation?" Fructose, sorbitol, xylitol, maltose, ethyl alcohol, and glucose were considered.

Fructose A 10% fructose solution given at the rate of 0.5 gm/min decreased serum phosphates. Lactic acid, uric acid, and bilirubin concentrations increased. Uric acid increase after fructose infusion was reported by Förster and coworkers, who attributed it to the utilization of adenosine triphosphate (ATP) in the phosphorylation of fructose by the cell. Reports of increased serum glutamic oxaloacetic transaminase (SGOT) indicate hepatocellular dysfunction. Clinical reports associate fructose infusion with right upper quadrant epigastric pain and liver enlargement.

The consensus was that the disadvantages of fructose outweighed its advantages, and its use as the primary carbohydrate in the intravenous alimentation was not recommended. If used at all, it should be given with glucose, since fructose is not well utilized by the brain. Fructose is partly insulin-independent and has a protein-sparing effect.

Sorbitol Sorbitol is compatible with amino acid solutions and apparently produces fewer adverse effects than either glucose or fructose, but adverse effects—severe complications, coma, and death—have been reported with its use. These were attributed to an osmotic effect on the brain, producing cerebral edema when sorbitol was used in peritoneal dialysis. Other side effects have been said to include neuritis and cataracts. One participant claimed these data on toxicity of sorbitol to be a misinterpretation and mentioned its consistent use in Europe over long periods of time without toxic reaction. The reported toxic effect on lenses has nothing to do with sorbitol administration, but is a diabetic disturbance, he said, emphasizing that sorbitol does not penetrate the lens. He would not recommend massive administration of either glucose or sorbitol without careful monitoring, however.

Successful use in Germany of high concentrations of sorbitol in treating cerebral spinal hypertension was cited, although another participant recalled that sorbitol can cause swelling of the liver and decrease of hepatic blood flow; hence it might elevate blood ammonia, causing some toxicity.

Sorbitol is metabolized to fructose and produces sequelae similar to those of fructose. It was difficult to cite any advantages of sorbitol over glucose; therefore, it was not advised as a component in hyperalimentation solutions.

Xylitol Xylitol is a pentitol alcohol described by McCormick and Touster (*J Biol Chem* **229**:451, 1952) as an intermediate metabolite of carbohydrate metabolism in animals and man. Reports have indicated that xylitol is effective as an energy sugar substitute since it can be metabolized partly by an insulin-independent pathway. Workers in Japan, Germany, and South Africa have suggested that xylitol could be a useful source of calories in conditions of carbohydrate intolerance and insulin resistance.

Xylitol tests in this country, however, have indicated a dose-related alteration of liver function characterized by increased bilirubin and liver enzymes, lactic acidemia, uric acidemia, and solute diuresis. Deaths after xylitol infusion have been reported by Coats in Australia, but there is a question of whether these might be related to chemical contamination of the xylitol.

In view of these clinical and biochemical findings, the use of xylitol as a calorific solution in humans is contraindicated. Further controlled investigations should be meticulously performed before it is made available for intravenous alimentation formulas in the United States.

Other carbohydrate sources (Maltose) One participant reported on maltose as a calorie source in parenteral alimentation. The absence of the enzyme maltase in the serum allows the administration of the disaccharide maltose at higher concentrations without untoward osmotic effects. Maltose is probably metabolized in the tissues, yielding glucose units. Further investigations with this substance may be productive.

Ethyl alcohol Ethyl alcohol produces about 7 kcal/gm, but its use as a hyperalimentation component has serious drawbacks: It is toxic to the liver, muscle, and brain. Also, it has been implicated in the decrease of leukocyte migration and phagocytosis and in platelet derangements. It is metabolically degraded to acetaldehyde and partially excreted through the lung. Acetaldehyde is irritating to the pulmonary alveoli and produces a significant increase in pulmonary complications. Among other factors mitigating against the use of alcohol are its excessive sedative and inebriating effects; both are undesirable in patients who need specific physical activity. Despite some reports of beneficial effects of alcohol, its use was not recommended by the group for intravenous alimentation formulas, especially in patients with previous pulmonary disease, pancreatitis, or cirrhosis.

Glucose Apparently the most effective substrate for parenteral alimentation is glucose. The hourly glucose supply in parenteral hyperalimentation should be 0.4 to 0.9 gm/kg. If the patient has a higher requirement, this dose can be increased to 1.2 gm/kg.

Insulin Although required for diabetic patients, insulin should be administered only as needed in nondiabetic patients and should be carefully monitored by the urinary excretion of glucose. Use of continuous in-line monitoring of serum glucose could elicit more accurate information by measurement of existing sugar concentrations.

FAT EMULSIONS

Among the fat emulsions discussed were Intralipid, a soybean oil emulsion containing egg yolk phospholipid as an emulsifying agent and glycerol to obtain isotonicity, also fat emulsions containing cottonseed oil.

There are several advantages to the use of fat emulsions:

A large amount of energy can be given in a small volume of isotonic fluid.

Because of their isotonicity, the fat emulsions may be given via a peripheral vein in contrast to concentrated glucose solutions, which must be given via a central vein.

Thrombophlebitis occurs infrequently in isotonic fat emulsions.

Infusion of fat emulsions causes neither hyperosmolarity of the blood nor diuresis.

No fat losses have been observed either in the urine or in the feces.

Fat emulsions supply the body with essential fatty acids and triglycerides.

Toxicity studies of Intralipid in dogs have shown that a daily dose of 9 gm of fat per kg for four weeks produce no abnormal reactions. Total intravenous nutrition with 40% of the energy supplied from fat has been maintained in dogs throughout the gestation period.

That long-term complete intravenous nutrition can be achieved in man by using fat emulsion as part of the energy supply has been illustrated in many publications and reports. Some of the subjects received up to 60% to 80% of their calories as fat for several weeks with good results. Observations also indicate that the infused fat is readily utilized in the same way as the fat in food.

In one subject who received complete intravenous nutrition for 7 months and 15 days, the amount of the fat emulsion (Intralipid) corresponded to about 40% of the total energy given. The remaining calories (60%) were derived from carbohydrates (glucose and fructose) and amino acids. The patient gained weight and remained in good nutritional condition. Liver biopsies showed some pigmentation of the reticuloendothelial cells, with proliferation in some places. Liver biopsies one and two years afterward revealed no abnormal changes. No effect on blood coagulation, liver function, or on various other parameters was reported. In the postoperative period, intravenous fat emulsions have been shown to reduce losses of nitrogen and body protein.

The suggested daily dose for adults is 2 gm/kg of fat, with the infusion rate limited to 25 gm/hour. It should be given simultaneously with amino acids and glucose, but from a separate flask. The parenteral solutions including fat emulsions have generally been given during only 12 hours of the day.

A syndrome produced by essential fatty acid (EFA) deficiency in children and adults was discussed. This deficiency is characterized by a high ratio of the triene and tetraene fatty acids in the phospholipid fraction of the blood. Holman's investigations emphasized that the deficiency of essential fatty acids occurs within a few weeks of fat-free intravenous feeding. Clinically, EFA deficiency produces scaling skin, sparse hair growth, thrombocytopenia, and poor wound healing. These abnormalities can be reversed by infusion of a fat emulsion.

One participant illustrated a specific reversion of essential fatty acid levels to normal values with administration of fat emulsions. These biochemical changes were correlated with clinical improvement. If these EFA deficiency syndromes are diagnosed, and if fat emulsion cannot be obtained, the use of post high-fat-meal plasma may be helpful.

Another participant reported finding a pulmonary diffusion abnormality in rabbits with Intralipid infusion. He maintained that there was a significant inhibition of the diffusion of oxygen across the alveolar membrane. He supported these physiologic observations with ultramicroscopic studies of the capillary alveolar membrane, which revealed marked deposition of fat in the capillary and endothelial cells and some deposits deeper in the alveolar membrane. He found similar depositions in Kupffer and liver cells. He indicated that heparin helps to decrease this diffusion inhibition when administered prior to Intralipid.

No change in diffusion capacity, blood gases, blood coagulation, or level of liver enzymes was found in patients with burns who were infused with Intralipid. Xenon clearance was found to be normal. Some significant improvement in the overall respiratory function after infusion of Intralipid was reported.

Studies of the metabolism of Intralipid in premature and small-for-date infants revealed that the elimination curves were similar to those in adults. Chylomicron or pre-β-lipoprotein fraction elimination was delayed in small-for-date infants, but this was reversed by heparin administration, indicating a deficient lipoprotein lipase activity. After heparin administration free fatty acids increased in the serum. There was doubt concerning the effect of this increase in free fatty acids on bilirubin metabolism since these acids can be uncoupling factors.

Heparin should not be given to patients receiving fat emulsions who are suffering from trauma or burns, since their fat clearance rates are high. If low clearance rates are found, heparin should be administered. It was emphasized that the clearance rate of fat from plasma does not indicate the oxidation rate of the fat infused.

Contraindications to the use of fat emulsions are pathological hyperlipidemia, hepatocellular injury, coagulation disturbance, and allergies.

PART TWO

Section Three

Vitamins and Minerals

6 Vitamins
   Harry L. Greene, M.D.
7 Minerals
   Maurice E. Shils, M.D., Sc.D.

   Colloquium: Vitamins and Minerals
   Digest of Colloquium
   Theodore B. Van Itallie, M.D., and Harold H. Sandstead, M.D.

NUTRITIONAL COMPOSITION

Chapter 6

Vitamins

Harry L. Greene, M.D.

Vitamins are a necessary ingredient in the metabolism of carbohydrates, proteins, and fats and should be included in a complete parenteral nutrition program. The intravenous requirements of the vitamins are not known. Two methods of determining adequacy (urinary excretion and red cell transketolase activity) give conflicting results; therefore, further studies are required to determine the specific intravenous vitamin requirements. Since several diseases may improve with pharmacological doses of vitamins, the complete role of vitamins in intermediary metabolism is not yet understood.

The vitamin "requirements" given for adequate oral alimentation are, for the most part, based upon studies performed with healthy individuals and are not necessarily appropriate for a program designed for total intravenous nutrition or for a patient who may be either chronically or acutely ill. Furthermore, it is difficult to determine the actual requirements for every patient who is to receive total parenteral nutrition since these may be different in any given patient due to biological variability, vitamin intake prior to hospitalization, protein-calorie intake, catabolic rate, or route of administration.

In an effort to compensate for these variables, the present tendency is to give excessive amounts of the water-soluble vitamins with the idea that once the needs are met the remainder will be catabolized and/or excreted. We are now better able to judge at least the catabolic rate and the protein-calorie requirements of most patients; therefore, we should develop precise data that will assist us in defining more accurately the vitamin requirements in a total parenteral nutrition program.

WATER-SOLUBLE VITAMINS

Depletion times for the water-soluble vitamins reportedly have a wide range. Normal subjects who were studied in a metabolic ward have shown evidence of vitamin deficiency in much shorter periods of time than expected.

Pyridoxine The biological half-life of ^{14}C-labeled pyridoxine was studied in two subjects. One subject received an *ad libitum* diet providing between 1.75 and 2 mg of vitamin B_6 per day. The biological half-life of the vitamin was approximately 15 days. Another subject was maintained on a constant intake of 1.73 mg of vitamin B_6 per day and the biological half-life of the labeled vitamin was approximately 20 days. Further studies demonstrated that when young, healthy subjects were placed upon a vitamin B_6-deficient diet, biochemical evidence of deficiency could be detected as early as seven days.

242

Significant abnormalities in the electroencephalograms and electrocardio-grams occurred within less than three weeks on a vitamin B_6-deficient diet.[1]

Thiamin The biological half-life of thiamin labeled with ^{14}C in the thiazole moiety of the vitamin molecule was studied in three young men on a controlled diet providing a constant thiamin intake. One subject received 1.35 mg of thiamin in his daily diet. The half excretion time of thiamin was 18½ days. The second subject had an intake of 1.8 mg of thiamin per day and showed a half excretion time of 13 days. The third subject received 2.1 mg of dietary thiamin per day and the half excretion time was 9½ days.[2]

Considering that parenteral nutrition programs in this country depend mainly upon carbohydrates to provide the calories, one should be reminded of the effect of carbohydrates on the requirement for thiamin. In a study conducted by Sauberlich et al, subjects were placed upon a thiamin-deficient liquid formula which provided 15% of calories as protein, 40% as fat, and 45% as carbohydrate, with a total of 2,800 kcal/day.[3] At the end of period 1, the subjects were divided into two groups. Group A continued to receive the same diet but with supplemental thiamin. Group B subjects received the same thiamin supplement and, during periods 2 through 5, received the same amount of fat and protein as during the control period; but the carbohydrate was increased so that the diet provided 3,600 kcal/day. Figure 1 shows that the

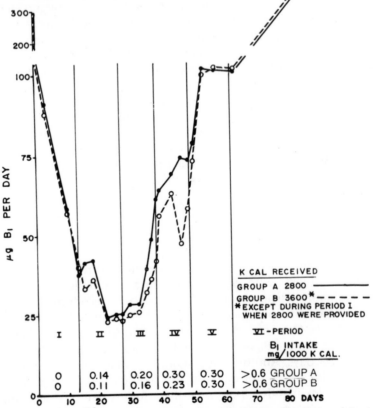

Fig 1. Average urinary thiamin excretion in normal subjects given varying amounts of calories and dietary thiamin.

urinary excretion of thiamin was inversely proportional to the amount of carbohydrate given and any differences in the amount excreted disappeared when the thiamin intake was made the same in terms of milligrams of thiamin per thousand kilocalories. Changes in red blood cell transketolase activity also reflected differences in thiamin needs during the various periods as seen in the percent of thiamin pyrophosphate stimulation (see page 250 for details of test). This confirmed in man what had previously been reported in animals and helps to emphasize the need for an adequate thiamin intake during a complete parenteral program which is primarily dependent upon carbohydrates for calories.

Vitamin C Two studies of vitamin C depletion were performed.[4, 5] Initial evidence of scurvy—as manifested by petechial hemorrhages—appeared as early as the 29th day of depletion. In both studies this sign disappeared only to reappear with other evidence of scurvy at variable times, dependent upon the rate of utilization of existing body stores (Table 1). Biological variation in the calculated average daily need for vitamin C was between 1.1 and 2.2 mg/day. The scurvy produced varied from mild to a marked degree at the end of approximately three months of depletion.

Folic acid Folic acid deficiency in the adult as demonstrated by abnormal excretion of formiminoglutamic acid (FIGLU) was reported to occur after four to five weeks of depletion.[6] On the other hand, Herbert required 4½ months to produce evidence of megaloblastic hematological changes, and these changes preceded an increase in the urinary excretion of FIGLU.[7] In animal studies, Herman et al have demonstrated that significant alteration of the jejunal glycolytic enzymes can be produced in rats on a folacin-deficient diet within a period of three weeks.[8]

Table 1.—Vitamin C Depletion

Subject	Rate of Catabolism of Existing Body Pool (percent)	Calculated Average* Daily Need (mg/day)
Study 1		
K	2.5	22.5
L	2.2	
N	2.7	25.0
S	2.4	20.0
Study 2		
H	4.1	26.0
M	3.2	21.4
P	3.5	24.0
R	2.8	21.3
S	2.6	25.0
Average	2.9 ± 0.6	

Source: Data given with permission of E. M. Baker and J. E. Canham.
*To supply metabolic needs and maintain pools.

Riboflavin Riboflavin deficiency has been studied by Tillotson and Baker.[9] A group of normal subjects was fed a synthetic riboflavin-free diet. Riboflavin status was evaluated by determining riboflavin urinary excretion and by measuring the activity of glutathione reductase of red blood cells with and without the stimulation of the reaction mixture by the addition of flavin adenine dinucleotide (FAD). Details of this measurement are given on page 250. Statistically significant changes in the glutathione reductase activity after the addition of FAD could be demonstrated as early as seven days on this deficient diet.

The conditions under which the foregoing studies were conducted are different from the conditions that prevail for the adult patient who requires complete parenteral nutrition. However, these studies help to bring into better perspective the relatively brief period of time required to produce biochemical, physiological, or clinical evidence of a deficiency of some water-soluble vitamins. Other vitamins have not been studied as extensively in our laboratory and include vitamin B_{12}, niacin, pantothenate, and biotin. These vitamins should also be considered when designing a complete parenteral nutrition program.

Vitamin B_{12} Vitamin B_{12} is unique among vitamins in being synthesized almost exclusively by microorganisms. These organisms grow well in the rumen or intestine of animals, but man derives little benefit since B_{12} is absorbed almost exclusively in the ileum. A value of $1\mu g$/day has been given as the parenteral requirement and is based on the minimal parenteral dosage required to keep patients with pernicious anemia in remission. However, the remission is incomplete and depleted liver stores may take several years to become repleted on this dose.[10] Therefore, a dose somewhat greater than this may be necessary during total parenteral nutrition.

Niacin The body obtains niacin not only directly from the diet, but indirectly from the conversion of tryptophan and possibly from that synthesized from intestinal microorganisms. It has been estimated that 60 mg of tryptophan gives rise to 1 mg of niacin. The amount of niacin available from intestinal bacterial synthesis is not known; thus, this vitamin probably should be given with total parenteral nutrition until further studies are completed.

Pantothenic acid Symptoms in man attributable to deficiency of this vitamin have not been substantiated. Clinical and biochemical abnormalities suggestive of adrenocortical insufficiency and peripheral neuropathy produced in volunteers by a deficient diet and omegamethyl pantothenic acid were not immediately relieved by pantothenic acid, but responded to a good diet that supplied multiple vitamins.[11] Its inclusion in a parenteral nutrition program may not be necessary, but further studies must be done in patients receiving TPN before a conclusion of this nature can be made.

Biotin Since biotin is readily made by intestinal bacteria, deficiency is unlikely to arise except when intestinal bacterial growth is severely depressed or when diets are excessive in raw egg white. This would suggest that supplementation of this vitamin may not be necessary in some patients receiving parenteral nutrition. However, the intestinal flora may be altered in patients who receive TPN, and sufficient amounts of biotin may not be made by the intestinal organism to supply the needs of the patient. Studies must be done with this vitamin, therefore, to determine its place in parenteral nutrition.

Choline and inositol These two compounds are not generally considered as vitamins. Their nutritional significance in man has been based largely on (1) occurrence and known functions of these substances in mammalian tissues, (2) experimental production of deficiencies in animals, and (3) occurrence of significant amounts of these compounds in conventional diets, especially in foods used to support early growth of young animals (eg, milk and eggs).

Deficiency symptoms have never been demonstrated in man, and whether the two compounds are essential nutrients for man is not known. Therefore, recommendations concerning their inclusion as part of a complete parenteral nutrition solution cannot be made until more studies are done with choline and inositol in elemental diets and parenteral nutrition.

Most observations concerning vitamin half-life and requirements apply primarily to normal young adult males and not to the young, rapidly growing infant who might be expected to have greater vitamin requirements.

Toxicity Toxic manifestations attributed to excessive quantities of the water-soluble vitamins in children or adults are thought to be rare. In fact, patients with renal insufficiency seem to tolerate extremely high serum levels of the water-soluble vitamins without symptoms attributable to the intravenously administered vitamins; premature and newborn infants are frequently given excessive amounts of vitamins intravenously. It is doubtful that this practice has caused any detrimental effect on the infant's rapidly growing central nervous system, but studies are in progress to estimate more closely the intravenous needs of the water-soluble vitamins in the rapidly growing neonate.

FAT-SOLUBLE VITAMINS

Vitamin A Time is required to deplete the adult of fat-soluble vitamins. Data on depletion periods were collected in a joint study at the University of Iowa and the US Army Medical Research and Nutrition Laboratory, Denver, on eight adult males given labeled ^{14}C-retinol acetate.[12] Table 2 demonstrates the biological variability of their vitamin A depletion times. In the first column, the biological half-life of the labeled vitamin A is given. The half-life varied from 101 to 597 days. The period of depletion is equally variable. Subject 5, who was the first to develop significant abnormalities of his electroretinogram and impairment of dark adaptation, required 360 days. Subject 4, who developed equally severe impairment, required 773 days.

The prolonged period required to produce significant vitamin A deficiency does not, however, permit us to ignore the fat-soluble vitamins in parenteral nutrition. If an individual has been on a deficient intake of vitamin A for a prolonged period of time, his liver stores may be relatively depleted. In fact, liver specimens from 41 individuals who died accidentally in five sections of the country were analyzed for vitamin A content, and 29% showed deficient vitamin A concentrations. Furthermore, the addition of a high quality protein

246

Table 2.—Vitamin A Depletion Time*

Subject	T 1/2	Period of Depletion (days)
1	295	678
2	355	360
3	101	420
4	597	773
5	212	360
6	275	588
7	147	505
8	205	596

*Preliminary results.

to the diet of an individual with deficient liver stores of vitamin A may stimulate release of the remainder of liver vitamin A and thus precipitate an acute vitamin A deficiency. Newborn infants also have relatively low vitamin A stores and therefore would be expected to show signs of deficiency earlier than adults if supplemental vitamin A were not given.

Vitamin D There are two principal sources of vitamin D in man: dietary absorption of preformed vitamin D and conversion of the sterols in the skin by sunlight to form active vitamin D. Dietary vitamin D or that released from the skin is initially trapped in the liver. This vitamin D_3 is then converted enzymatically to its various active hydroxylated compounds. This process has been studied extensively by DeLuca and coworkers.[13] Their studies indicate that vitamin D is actually a hormone and the rates of synthesis and turnover have not yet been determined. Although significant amounts of vitamin D may be synthesized normally, under the conditions imposed during total parenteral nutrition, it appears that supplemental vitamin D must be administered to maintain normal calcium homeostasis.

Vitamin E or tocopherol The requirement for vitamin E is related to the tissue content of polyunsaturated fatty acids, which may not necessarily reflect current consumption. The vitamin plays an important role in maintaining the stability of the erythrocyte and of membranes such as those of lysosomes in liver and muscle, but the role of the vitamin at the molecular level is not understood. For this reason it has been difficult to demonstrate that vitamin E deficiency is responsible for any clinical disorder in man. Infants are more prone to the development of symptoms attributable to vitamin E deficiency (anemia, edema, skin changes, and increased hemolysis of red cells). Some infants reportedly responded to the administration of vitamin E.[14] When fat is available for intravenous use in this country, supplemental vitamin E should be included as part of a complete parenteral nutrition program.

Vitamin K Vitamin K is readily synthesized by bacteria of the type usually found in the human intestinal tract. Deficiency is, therefore, rare unless absorption is interfered with. During the newborn period deficiency may develop, however, as a result of the sterility of the gastrointestinal tract. During periods of prolonged total parenteral nutrition, it appears unlikely that additional vitamin K is required in most patients; yet no studies have been done in patients with prolonged absence of dietary substrates regarding changes in intestinal flora and possible depletion of vitamin K stores. It has been found, however, that prolonged fasting and antibiotic therapy will cause vitamin K depletion.[15] For this reason, until further studies are done, it seems wise to give supplemental vitamin K periodically to patients who require prolonged parenteral nutrition.

Toxicity Toxicity to vitamins A, D, and synthetic vitamin K is well known. In our own experience we have had two patients who were given total parenteral nutrition and received excessive amounts of vitamin A. Only one developed symptoms attributable to vitamin A toxicity. This patient was an infant weighing 2,100 gm who required total parenteral alimentation for 18 weeks. During this period she received vitamins in the form of MVI (multiple vitamin infusion) with a total dose of 91,000 IU or a daily dose of 722 IU. After cessation of intravenous alimentation, she was inadvertently given oral multiple vitamin drops four times a day. Her vitamin A intake suddenly increased to 12,000 IU per day. The following week, her liver size increased to 4 cm below the costal margin, and her fontanelle was noted to be bulging and without pulsations. Her white blood count was 3,000/cu ml with 30% neutrophils, and her hemoglobin was 8.4 gm/100 ml. The spinal fluid was normal. She had several episodes of projectile vomiting over the subsequent eight days. Because the findings and symptoms resembled those of acute vitamin A toxicity, all supplementary vitamins were discontinued. During the succeeding four weeks, the fontanelle returned to normal, and her liver gradually returned to normal size. A blood vitamin A determination was not performed. However, the symptoms fit well with those described for acute vitamin A toxicity despite the fact that her actual intake of vitamin A during the 18 weeks of parenteral alimentation was only about twice that advocated for infants and approximately the same as that administered by Dudrick to a child who was carried for a more prolonged period of time. Our patient is now doing quite well and appears to be a normal two-year-old child.

According to an oral communication from B. Pruitt, MD, in January 1972, he observed one adult male patient who inadvertently received excessive amounts of vitamins in the form of MVI. The patient developed a markedly elevated serum calcium concentration with multiple areas of tissue calcification secondary to vitamin D toxicity at a dose of approximately 4,000 IU/day for three weeks.[15]

STUDIES RELATED TO THE INTRAVENOUS VITAMIN REQUIREMENTS

We measured the urinary excretion of vitamins B_6 and B_2 in a 48-year-old woman who received total parenteral nutrition for three months. Initially, she received Aminosol as the protein source, glucose as the calorie source, and MVI with added folate, also vitamins B_{12} and K. After 37 days of intravenous feedings, her outlook improved, but glycosuria and proteinuria developed. Her liver enlarged to 8 cm below the costal margin and was firm and tender. She experienced intermittent episodes of nausea and vomiting, and her serum glutamic oxaloacetic transaminase (SGOT) rose from normal to over 260 units/ml. Because she had received relatively large amounts of vitamin A intravenously, there was concern that vitamin A toxicity had been induced. However, the plasma vitamin A was 65μg/100 ml, and the liver vitamin A was 113μg/gm of tissue. Both of these values are normal. Histopathological examination of a liver specimen obtained by needle biopsy revealed a marked fatty infiltrate with some evidence of hepatocellular damage.

Immediately after the liver biopsy, the same nutrients were continued intravenously except that an 8% L-amino acid solution was substituted for the fibrin hydrolysate. The total amount of protein equivalent was decreased by 20% for five days, then increased back to the protein equivalent she had been receiving as fibrin hydrolysate. By the seventh day her liver decreased almost to normal size. However, the fibrin hydrolysate had to be readministered for 48 hours. During this period she again became nauseated, and her liver enlarged to 5 cm below the right costal margin. The L-amino acid solution was begun again, and, after four weeks of total parenteral nutrition with the L-amino acids as the protein source, her liver size returned to normal, as did her SGOT activity. Examination of a liver biopsy specimen four months later showed a mild degree of periportal fibrosis with complete disappearance of the fatty infiltrate.

Figure 2 depicts the percent of vitamin B$_6$ intake that was excreted at various times during her hospitalization. The percent of total B$_6$ excretion during the period when she was receiving the Aminosol ranged from between 31% to 57% of the intake. Free vitamin B$_6$ excretion varied from 14% to 30% of that infused. Once the source of nitrogen was changed to an L-amino acid solution, however, excretion of both total and free vitamin B$_6$ decreased, even though the total intake of vitamin B$_6$ was relatively the same as that in the first 25 days of her course.

The role of vitamin B$_6$ in the various metabolic pathways of the amino acids is well known. If there were an increased utilization of the nitrogenous material from the L-amino acid solution as compared to the hydrolysate, there should be an increase in the utilization of vitamin B$_6$. In Aminosol we found between 40% and 55% of the nitrogenous material in the form of peptides. With a copper-impregnated Sephadex column we determined that her utilization of these peptides varied between 60% and 80%.[16] However, when she was receiving the L-amino acid solution, we were only able to recover 3% of the amino acids in the urine. Hence, she utilized more of the nitrogenous products from the L-amino acid solution per day than from the Aminosol or peptide solution. This may explain the decreased excretion of vitamin B$_6$ during the amino acid infusion.

Riboflavin excretion was qualitatively similar, but not as dramatic as that seen with vitamin B$_6$. The reasons for the intolerance to carbohydrate and the liver enlargement in the early therapy are not completely explained. They may be related to her apparent intolerance or inability to handle the peptides, to the ammonia present in the hydrolysate solution, or perhaps to an inappropriate ratio of carbohydrate to utilizable protein.

Further observations on the urinary excretion of vitamins B$_6$ and B$_2$ in a second patient, who received all the vitamins orally in conjunction with total intravenous protein-calorie nutrition, suggest that the water-soluble vitamins are more efficiently utilized when administered orally than when given intravenously. When the vitamins were given intravenously the amount of pyri-

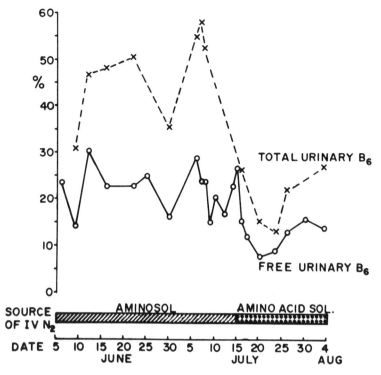

Fig 2. Percent pyridoxine excretion in a patient receiving total parenteral nutrition.

doxine excreted in the unbound form was between 58% and 67%. But when the vitamins were given orally, the amount of pyridoxine excreted in the unbound form was between 16% and 35%. Previous studies in normal subjects using ^{14}C-labeled pyridoxine have shown that over 95% is absorbed from the gastro-intestinal tract.[1] Therefore a larger portion of the intravenously administered vitamin B_6 was excreted by the kidneys.

An infant treated with TPN received 2.85 mg vitamin B_6 (approximate oral requirement: 0.2 mg/day) and 2.9 mg vitamin B_2 (approximate oral requirement: 0.4 mg/day). During the first nine days urinary excretion of the vitamins increased progressively from 0.1 mg to 1.4 mg for vitamin B_6 and from 0.1 mg to 2.3 mg for vitamin B_2. The same doses of the vitamins were then given orally 4 times a day from the 10th to the 16th day of TPN. Urinary excretion of both vitamins decreased progressively to approximately 0.1 mg by the 16th day.

These studies suggest that the liver and intestine may have a role— bypassed during intravenous administration—in conservation of these vita-mins when they are administered orally. Since the intravenous infusions of the vitamins were given over a 24-hour period as compared to the inter-mittent oral doses and the vitamins were given in pharmacological amounts, further studies are necessary for accurate interpretation of these data.

Another technique of measuring vitamin adequacy is to measure the activities of certain red blood cell enzyme activities which require specific vitamin cofactors for maximum activity. For example, the transketolase reaction requires thiamin as a cofactor. The red cell transketolase activity is measured before and after preincubation of red cells with added thiamin-pyrophosphate. If the patient is deficient in thiamin, the enzyme preincubated with thiamin will show a higher activity than the cells not incubated with thiamin. Another red cell enzyme which shows similar changes is glutathione reductase which is riboflavin-dependent.

The above techniques of determining vitamins B_1 and B_2 adequacy were utilized as a measure of vitamin adequacy in two infants receiving TPN. The infants were given vitamin supplements for five days prior to initiation of the study. Vitamins B_1 and B_2 were omitted from the TPN solution and red cell enzyme assays were performed every third day. By the 14th day of depletion, the red cell enzyme activities indicated deficient levels of B_1 and B_2 (Fig 3). The transketolase activity was corrected to normal within 24 hours by a constant infusion of thiamin, which was approximately two to three times the oral recommended dose of B_1. About the same daily recommended allowance of riboflavin corrected the glutathione reductase activity, but the infusion was required for 72 hours before activity was completely normal.

Obviously no firm conclusions can be drawn from these few studies, but they suggest that the intravenous requirements for vitamins B_1, B_2 and possibly B_6 may be similar to the oral requirements. On the other hand, the observed changes in red cell enzyme activities and urine concentration do not necessarily reflect adequate tissue levels during the intravenous administration of the vitamins. Further studies are needed to determine this relationship. A table listing approximate amounts of vitamins for intravenous use is given on page 458.

ENZYMATIC TRANSFORMATIONS OF VITAMINS

Although a great deal is known about the oral requirements of vitamins and their functions as cofactors in certain enzymatic reactions, much still remains unknown in terms of the enzymatic transformations of many vitamins. During recent years several clinical syndromes have been successfully treated with pharmacologic doses of specific vitamins. Examples of some of these conditions which require pharmacologic doses of vitamins are listed in Table 3. In some cases these inborn errors have led to a better understanding of the normal metabolism of vitamins. A more complete understanding of the active metabolites of vitamin D was found in the studies of vitamin D-resistant rickets, and the metabolites of vitamin B_{12} were better understood after studies related to the effect of B_{12} administration in certain patients with methylmalonicaciduria and homocystinuria.

We have studied the effect of pharmacologic doses of folic acid on certain jejunal epithelial glycolytic enzymes in normal individuals.[23, 24] Figure 4 demonstrates the effect of fasting, fasting plus folic acid, and diet plus folic acid on hexokinase, pyruvate kinase, fructose-1, 6-phosphate aldolase, fructokinase, and fructose-1-phosphate aldolase. Similar changes occurred in phosphofructokinase and the gluconeogenic enzyme fructose-1, 6-diphosphatase. The dose-response studies indicated that 15 mg/day gave the maximum in-

RBC TRANSKETOLASE ACTIVITY

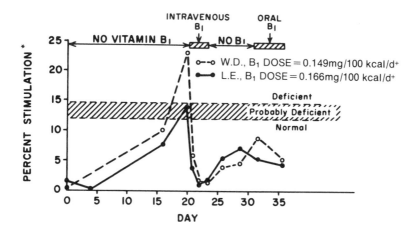

RBC GLUTATHIONE REDUCTASE ACTIVITY

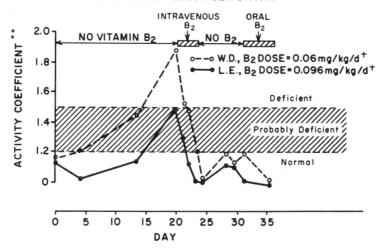

*Percent increase in transketolase activity with added thiamin pyrophosphate.

$$\text{**Activity Coefficient} = \frac{\text{glutathione reductase activity with added FAD}}{\text{glutathione reductase activity without added FAD}}$$

†Thiamin RDA = 0.025 mg/100 kcal per day; riboflavin RDA = 0.06 mg/100 kcal per day.

Fig 3. Changes in red blood cell transketolase and glutathione reductase activities in two infants receiving a constant amount of calories and protein during 35 days of TPN. These studies were performed in collaboration with Dr. Howard Sauberlich.

crease in enzyme activity, and the time-response studies showed that these changes were detectable within 1 hour and reached a maximum by 12 to 24 hours after 15 mg of oral folate.

The mechanism whereby folate causes these changes is not known. It does not appear to function as a cofactor or substrate for any of the glycolytic

Table 3.—Diseases That May Improve With Vitamin Treatment[15, 17-22]

Disease	Apoenzyme Implicated	Vitamin Treatment
B_6 dependent convulsions	?Glutamate decarboxylase	B_6
Cystathioninuria	Cystathioninase	B_6
"Iron loading" anemia with defective heme synthesis	Aminolevulinic acid synthetase	B_6
Xanthurenic aciduria	Kynureninase	B_6
Homocystinuria		B_6, B_{12}
Methylmalonicaciduria	Methylmalonyl CoA mutase	B_{12}
Hyperalaninemia and hyperpyruvic acidemia	Pyruvate decarboxylase	Thiamin
Maple syrup urine disease	Branched-chain decarboxylase	Thiamin
Leigh's subacute necrotizing encephalopathy	?Pyruvate carboxylase	Lipoic acid
Vitamin D-resistant rickets	?25-hydroxylase deficiency	Vitamin D 25-OH cholecalciferol
Propionic acidemia	?Propionyl-CoA carboxylase ?Biotin ligase	Biotin

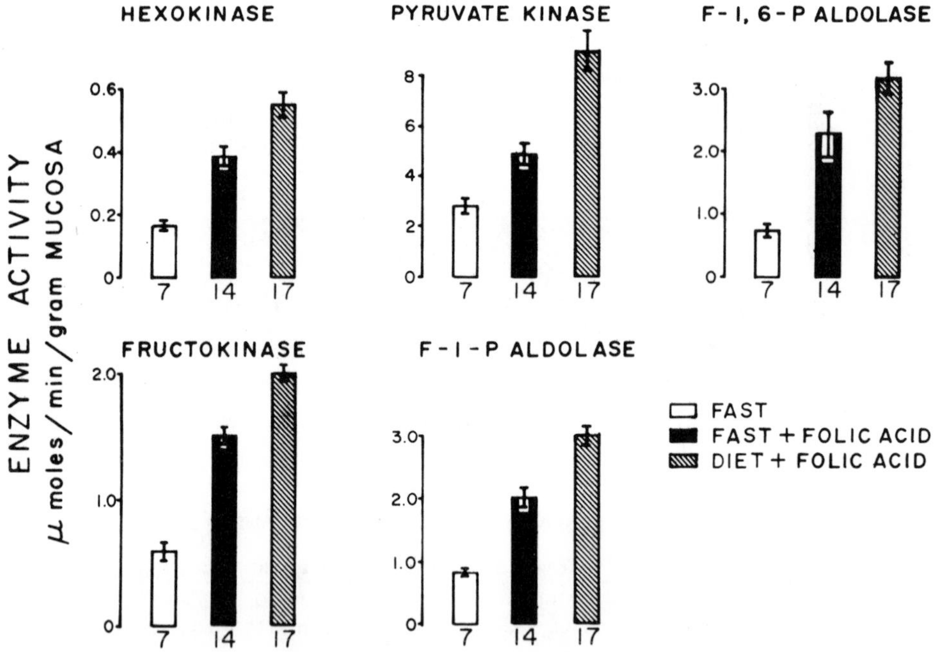

Fig 4. Diet and folate induced changes in intestinal glycolytic enzyme activities. Biopsies were performed on days 7, 14 and 17 of the study. The periods of fasting and fasting plus folate were seven days, and the period of diet plus folic acid was three days.

enzymes and it was hypothesized that it functions as an initiator of protein synthesis of some enzymes.[25]

We have extended these findings in the normal adult jejunum to the treatment of three patients with hepatic enzyme deficiencies. The first was a five-year-old patient with history of failure to thrive and intermittent episodes of hepatomegaly and jaundice. Fructose-1-phosphate aldolase (F-1-PA) deficiency or hereditary fructose intolerance was diagnosed three months before the study was begun, but, despite a fructose-free diet, she continued to have hepatomegaly, intermittent nausea and vomiting, and an elevation in SGOT. A liver biopsy specimen showed a periportal fatty infiltrate. Table 4 demonstrates the changes in hepatic F-1-PA and other glycolytic enzyme activities before and after folate therapy was begun. There was also some clinical improvement. Her liver size decreased to normal, nausea and vomiting ceased, and a hepatic fatty infiltrate resolved after folate treatment. She has remained asymptomatic for six months with continuous folate treatment.[26]

Table 4.—Effect of Folate on Liver and Jejunum Enzymes

Tissue	Pyruvate Kinase*	Fructose-1-P Aldolase	Fructose-1,6-P$_2$ Aldolase
Jejunum			
Normal†	202-771	43-153	44-171
Patient			
No folate	435.2	15.5	108.4
After folate	661.7	29.4	154.4
Liver			
Normal‡	54.9-108.4	39.2-98.0	46.4-100.1
Patient			
No folate	96.1	7.5	28.1
After folate	201.6	21.8	51.2

*Activities expressed as μmol/min/mg protein.
†Range of values from 9 normal adults and 3 normal children.
‡Range of values from 2 normal adults and 3 normal children.

Two patients with fasting hypoglycemia and ketoacidosis were found to have a hepatic deficiency of the gluconeogenic enzyme fructose-1, 6-diphosphatase. The enzyme activity increased by 60% in both patients (Table 5). Further studies indicated clinical improvement and an increased ability to convert glycerol to glucose (Fig 5).[27, 28] Similar changes occurred with fructose and alanine tolerance tests.

Table 5.—Effect of Folate on Liver Enzymes

Tissue	Pyruvate Kinase	Fructose-1-P Aldolase	Fructose-1,6-P$_2$ Aldolase	Fructose-1,6-Di-phosphatase
Normal	54-108	39-98	46-100	47-66
Patient #1				
Before folate	87.6	80.2	85.7	9.2
After folate	157.2	127.2	133.1	15.0
Patient #2				
Before folate	93.3	71.0	75.6	6.2
After folate	116.7	89.3	100.8	10.7

I have commented on these findings to further illustrate the vast amount of research still needed to satisfactorily complete the work of many investigators who in the first half of this century discovered, identified, synthesized, and developed tests for the measurement of these vitamins.

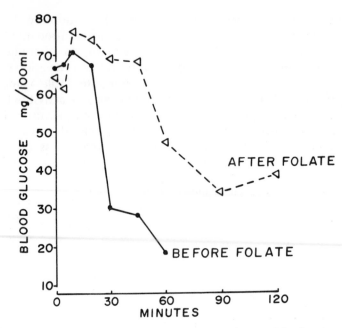

Fig 5. Glycerol tolerance tests in a patient with fructose-1, 6-diphosphatase deficiency. Hypoglycemic symptoms occurred after 60 minutes before folate treatment. No symptoms occurred after folate treatment.

In summary, vitamins are intimately involved in the metabolism of carbohydrate, protein, and fat; hence, they have a definite role in a complete parenteral nutrition program.

Because of the rapidity with which biochemical evidence of deficiency of many of the water-soluble vitamins develops, these should be included with the initiation of any total parenteral nutrition program.

From the studies performed on two patients, it would appear that the intravenous requirements of water-soluble vitamins are greater than the oral requirements, because, when given intravenously, a larger portion of these vitamins is excreted by the kidneys. Yet further studies in other patients suggest that the intravenous requirements may be less than the oral requirements during complete parenteral nutrition.

Significant toxic effects from large amounts of the water-soluble vitamins in adults are not apparent. Appropriate studies to determine the effect of excessive vitamins in the rapidly growing neonate are needed.

With MVI use, care should be taken to insure that the intake is rigidly controlled to prevent excessive administration of the fat-soluble vitamins.

The fact that some clinical diseases improve with pharmacologic amounts of certain of the vitamins demonstrates that considerable work must be done before we understand the complete role of vitamins in intermediary metabolism.

References

1. Tillotson JA, Sauberlich HE, Canham JE: Use of carbon-14 labeled vitamins in human nutrition studies: Pyridoxine, in *Proceedings, 7th International Congress of Nutrition,* vol 5, Physiology and Biochemistry of Food Components, New York, Pergamon Press, 1966, p 556.

2. Ariaey-Nejad MR, Balaghi M, Baker EM, Sauberlich HE: Thiamin metabolism in man. *Am J Clin Nutr* **23:**764, 1970.

3. Sauberlich HE, Herman YF, Stevens CO, and Herman RH: Thiamin requirement of the adult human, abstracted *Am J Clin Nutr* **23:**671-672, 1970.

4. Hodges RE, Hood J, Canham JE, et al: Clinical manifestations of ascorbic acid deficiency in man. *Am J Clin Nutr* **24:**432-443, 1971.

5. Baker EM, Hodges RE, Hood J, et al: Metabolism of ^{14}C- and ^{3}H-labeled L-ascorbic acid in human scurvy. *Am J Clin Nutr* **24:**444-454, 1971.

6. Eichner ER, Buergel N, Hillman RS: Experience with an appetizing high protein, low folate diet in man. *Am J Clin Nutr* **24:**1337-1345, 1971.

7. Herbert V: A palatable diet for producing experimental folate deficiency in man. *Am J Clin Nutr* **12:**17-20, 1963.

8. Herman RH, Stifel B, Herman YF, and Rosensweig NS: The response of jejunal glycolytic enzymes to a folate deficient diet in germ-free and pathogen-free diets, abstracted. *Fed Proc* **28:**628, 1969.

9. Tillotson JA, Baker EM: An enzymatic measurement of the riboflavin status in man. *Am J Clin Nutr* (in press).

10. National Research Council, Food and Nutrition Board: *Recommended Dietary Allowances,* ed 8, Publication 2216, Washington, DC, National Academy of Sciences, 1974.

11. Hodges RE, Ohlson MA, Bean WB: Pantothenic acid deficiency in man. *J Clin Invest* **37:**1642-1657, 1958.

12. Canham JE, Baker EM, Wallace DL, et al: Aspects of vitamin A nutrition in man. Read before the American Chemical Society of Agricultural and Food Chemistry, Los Angeles, Calif, 1971.

13. DeLuca HF: Recent advances in the metabolism and function of vitamin D. *Fed Proc* **28:**1678-1689, 1969.

14. Majaj AS, Dinning JS, Azzam SA and Darby WJ: Vitamin E responsive megaloblastic anemia in infants with protein-calorie malnutrition. *Am J Clin Nutr* **12:**374-379, 1963.

15. McLaren DS: The vitamins, in Bondy K (ed): *Duncan's Diseases of Metabolism,* ed 6, Philadelphia, WB Saunders, 1969, p 1316.

16. Buist RM, O'Brien D: The separation of peptides from amino acids in urine by ligand exchange chromatography. *J Chromatog* **29:**398-402, 1967.

17. Brunette MG, Hazel B, Scriver CR, et al: Thiamine-dependent neonatal lactic acidosis with hyperalaninemia, in *Proc Soc Ped Res, 40th Annual Meeting,* 1970, p 49.

18. Clayton BE, Dobbs RH, Patrick AD: Leigh's subacute necrotizing encephalopathy: Clinical and biochemical study, with special reference to therapy with lipoate. *Arch Dis Child* **42:**467-478, 1967.

19. Barnes ND, Hull D, Balgobin L, Bompertz D: Biotin-responsive propionicacidaemia. *Lancet* **2:**244-245, 1970.

20. DeLuca HF: 25-hydroxycholecalciferol, the probable metabolically active form of vitamin D. *Am J Clin Nutr* **22:**412-424, 1969.

21. Norman AW: Evidence for a new kidney-produced hormone, 1, 25-dihydroxycholecalciferol, The proposed biologically active form of vitamin D. *Am J Clin Nutr* **24:**1346-1351, 1971.

22. Mahoney MJ, Rosenberg LE: Inherited defects of B_{12} metabolism. *Am J Med* **48:**584-593, 1970.

23. Rosensweig NS, Herman RH, Stifel FB, et al: Regulation of human jejunal glycolytic enzymes by oral folic acid, *J Clin Invest* **48:**2038-2045, 1969.

24. Rosensweig NS, Stifel FB, Herman YF, Herman RH: Regulation of human jejunal glycolytic enzymes by oral folic acid: Time and dose response, abstracted. *Am J Clin Nutr* **22:**677-678, 1969.

25. Herman RH, Rosensweig NS: The initiation of protein synthesis. *Am J Clin Nutr* **22:**806-812, 1969.

26. Greene HL, Stifel FB, Herman RH: Hereditary fructose intolerance. Treatment with pharmacologic doses of folic acid. *Clin Res* **20:**275, 1972.

27. Greene HL, Stifel FB, Herman RH: Hypoglycemia due to fructose-1, 6-diphosphatose deficiency and treatment of two patients with folate abstracted. *Pediatric Res* **6:**432, 1972.

28. Greene HL, Stifel FB, Herman RH: "Ketotic hypoglycemia" due to hepatic fructose-1, 6-diphosphatase deficiency. Treatment with folic acid. *Am J Dis Child* **124:**415-418, 1972.

Chapter 7

Minerals

Maurice E. Shils, M.D., Sc.D.

Current practice is reviewed concerning the addition of various minerals to total parenteral nutrition solutions. Requirements and recommendations for these minerals, including trace elements, are discussed, with emphasis on the fact that relatively little is known about the quantitative needs for a number of inorganic nutrients by the intravenous route.

Recent developments in the field of minerals in human nutrition direct attention to this area as one of basic importance and of potential benefit to patients. Among these developments are:

• Increasing concern about the long-term effects of depletion or surplus of these nutrients as increasing numbers of patients are being maintained on protracted intravenous feeding,

• Increasing information on the effects of deficiency in man of certain mineral elements such as magnesium and phosphorus, and

• Increasing awareness of the potential importance of trace elements.

On the basis of quantitative requirements we may divide mineral nutrients into two broad groups: macrominerals (Table 1) and microminerals or trace elements (Table 2).

MACROMINERALS

Sodium, Potassium, and Chloride

Probably the most critical aspect on a day-to-day basis concerns the requirements for water and electrolytes. A formula for total parenteral nutri-

Table 1. Macrominerals of Interest (200 mg or 5 mmol/day)

1. Sodium	5. Calcium
2. Chloride	6. Magnesium
3. Bicarbonate	7. Phosphorus
4. Potassium	8. Sulfur (?)

Table 2.— Microminerals of Interest (5 mg/day)

1. Iron*	7. Cobalt (-B_{12})†
2. Zinc*	8. Manganese
3. Copper*	9. Molybdenum
4. Iodide*	10. Selenium
5. Fluoride*	11. Vanadium
6. Chromium	

*Human requirement established.
†Cobalt other than that in vitamin B_{12}.

tion—no matter how well it is constructed in calories, amino acids, and vitamins—must be reviewed daily, sometimes more frequently, when administered to patients with serious problems in fluid and electrolyte balance. No single value or limited range can be given for the requirements for certain mineral ions because these will depend on cardiovascular, renal, gastrointestinal, and endocrine status of the patient. When these systems are determined to be within normal limits, the sodium, potassium, and chloride contents may vary appreciably. This fact is demonstrated in the wide range of these nutrients which have been added by various workers to the nutrient solutions for infants (Table 3) and for adults (Table 4). Regulation of sodium and potassium content for infants is more critical than for adults. It is known that human milk may vary in its sodium and potassium content and that cow's milk has three to four times higher concentrations. Taking the figure derived from Slater[1] of 2.4 mEq of sodium per 100 kilocalories for human milk with 91% absorption, most of the concentrations listed in Table 3 are in a reasonable range for infants without significant sodium losses.

Most of the solutions listed in Table 3 supply somewhat more potassium per 100 kilocalories than that occurring in human milk (approximately 2.0 to 2.3 mEq/100 kcal). The absolute requirement for potassium and other important intracellular ions will depend on losses and on the rate at which caloric and nitrogen intakes and retention permit new tissue growth. A minimum of 3 mEq K/gm of N deposited in muscle is indicated on the basis of analyses. K/N ratios of 5.6 and 6.7 have been found for infants on breast or

Table 3.— Composition of TPN Solutions, I (neonates and infants)

Ref	Year	Kilocalories	Na (mEq)	K (mEq)	Cl (mEq)	U*
2	1969	122	5.8	4.9	9.1	+
3	1968	128	8.0	4.0	10.8	+
4	1970†	86-100	1.05	1.75-2.75	?	+
5	1971	115	3.7	2.75	5.2	+
6	1971	120-140	3-5	1-2	?	+
7	1971	130	4.0	6.0	4.0	+

*U = Uniform formulation per unit bottle.
†With Intralipid.

Table 4.—Composition of TPN Solutions, II (adults)

Ref	Year	Kilocalories	Na (mEq)	K (mEq)	Cl (mEq)	U*
8	1969	1,000 (unit)	50	40	90	+
		2,500	125	100	225	
9	1970	900 (unit)	23	20	?	+
		2,500	64	56	?	
10	1970	2,500	90	80	130	−
11†	1970	2,500	68	44	86	+
7	1971	1,000 (unit)	53	48	72	+
		2,500	133	120	180	

*U = Uniform formulation per unit bottle.
†With Intralipid.

bottle feeding.[1] Any significant gastrointestinal losses must be measured and taken into account in estimating requirements for these and other ions. During periods of dysfunction or instability or when a patient is started initially on parenteral nutrition, daily measurements of serum electrolyte levels and of weight are necessary to arrive at the proper amounts. Where fluid losses are large, periodic checks on urinary sodium and potassium are useful guides.

Magnesium

Since the late sixties, new information has been gained in clinical medicine about magnesium deficiency. It is now recognized to produce significant symptomatology.[12] No competent hormonal homeostatic mechanism for controlling serum magnesium levels is evident as there is for calcium. As a result, the serum levels are dependent upon the balance between intake and output with renal mechanisms playing a key role. In adults, the magnesium present in large amounts in bones and cells is not sufficiently available to maintain serum levels. I gather that this is true, but perhaps to a lesser degree, in children. In periods as short as three to four weeks of acute deficiency, a series of events may occur in adults, including hypomagnesemia, hypomagnesuria, hypocalcemia, hypocalciuria, and hypokalemia. In our experience, the fall in serum calcium secondary to magnesium depletion is associated with the occurrence of neurological signs. As depletion develops, gastrointestinal dysfunction may occur characterized by anorexia, nausea, and vomiting.

Magnesium requirements are not known with certainty and this is especially true for IV requirements. There is evidence that the absorptive efficiency of magnesium, like that of calcium[13] is related to previous and current intakes and other constituents of the diet.[14] Human milk contains approximately 0.45 mEq/100 kcal (0.6 mEq per 130 kcal). Assuming that approximately one-half of this oral source of magnesium is absorbed, 0.3 mEq/kg/day should be adequate for infants when given slowly by the IV route. Comparison with this level may be made with Table 5, which indicates that various workers have tended to give widely differing amounts. The lowest figure of 0.15 mEq was considered by these investigators to be somewhat low on the basis of Mg/N retention ratios. They recommended 0.3 mEq/100 kcal/kg/day.[15] The ratio of Mg (in mEq) to N (in grams) in infant muscle is approximately 0.7;[16] this means that an acceptable rate of N deposition (ie, 250 mg/kg in the first week of life) would require net retention of about 0.2 mEq of Mg. In pediatric practice, minerals are added at a standard level per unit; therefore, the amounts given will depend on total fluid and caloric provision (Table 5).

In surveying the amounts prescribed for adults, it is apparent from Table 6 that the approach differs. A fixed amount of ion per unit is added by some physicians, an optional administration of magnesium is given by others, and one group gives a fixed amount per total daily intake. The NRC Recommended Dietary Allowance[13] (RDA) of magnesium for adults is approximately 25 mEq (see p 466). Absorption of one-third of this oral dosage would result in 8 mEq entering the circulation. As with infants, the range of administration varies widely, from 4 to 25 mEq/2,500 kcal (Table 6). One patient receiving approximately 4 mEq/day was stated to be in electrolyte balance over many

Table 5.—Composition of TPN Solutions, III
    (neonates and infants)

Ref	Year	Ca (mg)	P (mg)	Mg (mEq)	Trace Elements (Source)‡	U*
2	1969	25	9	0.3	P, B, Fe	+
3	1968	38	30	2	P, Fe	+
4†	1970	20	36–48	0.15	P	+
5	1971	?	?	0.9§	?	+
6	1971	?	?	?	P, B, Fe	+
7	1971	80	5 mEq	2.0	P, B, Fe	+

*U = Uniform solution per unit bottle.
†With Intralipid.
‡P, B, Fe—plasma, blood or parenteral iron periodically.
§Estimated from data.

months. Reducing the dosage to 2 mEq resulted in negative balance.[17] This patient had normal absorption and presumably was losing very little from the GI tract. Whether the majority of adult patients can be sustained on this relatively low level is unknown. With intravenous alimentation, urinary losses are related to the rapidity of the infusion and the level of circulating magnesium in relation to renal threshold level, approximately 1.3 mEq/liter in the normal kidney. Loss of magnesium in diverted gastrointestinal secretions or as the result of renal tubular dysfunction should be replaced. Where glomerular filtration is seriously impaired, the amount of magnesium should be reduced appropriately to prevent hypermagnesemia.

With the exception of patients who are having significant and persistent breakdown of lean tissue or who have renal insufficiency, the maintenance of serum magnesium within the normal range indicates adequate administration. Because of the importance of this ion in metabolism, hypomagnesemia should be avoided. Periodic determinations of serum and urine levels will give the information needed to make appropriate adjustments in the supply of this ion.

It has been reported that magnesium administration retards or prevents calcium stone formation.[18] This brings up the question: Is an excess of mag-

Table 6.—Composition of TPN Solutions, IV
    (adults)

Ref	Year	Kilocalories	Ca (mg)	P (mg)	Mg (mEq)	Trace** Elements	U*
8	1969	1,000 (unit)	ai‡	ai	1.5	P, B, or Fe	+
		2,500	ai	ai	4		
9	1970	900 (unit)	ai	ai	3.3	?	+
		2,500	ai	ai	9.2		
10	1970	2,500	215	310	17	Solution	−
11†	1970	2,500	396	344	4	?	+
7	1971	1,000 (unit)	100§	4 mEq§	4–10§	P	+
		2,500	250	10	10–25		

*U = Uniform solution per unit bottle.
†With Intralipid.
‡ai = as indicated.
§Optional.
**P, B, Fe—plasma, blood or parenteral iron periodically.

nesium beneficial in patients who are either in negative calcium balance because of immobilization or trauma, or who are being given intravenous calcium salts? Would such an excess of magnesium minimize calcium deposition in the tubules or other soft tissues? Note should be taken of an opposite finding in animals getting large amounts of vitamin D where administration of excessive magnesium increased soft tissue calcification over and above that seen without the extra magnesium.[19]

Calcium and Phosphorus

These ions have been added routinely to infusions given to infants as indicated in Table 5. It will be noted that the amounts given per kilogram per day vary widely. Published data on serum levels or balances of these ions are meager, but growth rates have been reported to be good. Neonates on breast feeding ingest approximately 34 to 44 mg of calcium and 21 to 24 mg of phosphorus per kg per day with absorptions of 55% and 89%, respectively.[1, 16] Most investigators have given significantly more of these ions intravenously. With adults, some investigators have given these ions optionally "as indicated" (Table 6), while others have added calcium at 200 to 400 mg/ 250 kcal/day, and phosphorus at 300 to 350 mg/day.

Orthophosphate ion The phosphorus of interest in this discussion is the orthophosphate ion. In this era of millimols and milliequivalents it may seem fashionable to express phosphate in these terms. However, phosphate, unlike sodium, potassium, calcium, and magnesium, exists biologically in both the monovalent and divalent forms. In extracellular fluid at pH 7.4 the ratio of divalent $HPO_4^=$ to monovalent $H_2PO_4^-$ is 4 to 1. To express concentrations as milliequivalents would require knowledge of this ratio and the performance of some arithmetic with every change in pH. This is obviously undesirable. If one tries to express balance, the problem is compounded because the ratios of these two ions also vary in the urine depending upon pH. At pH 5.4 the ratio, instead of being 4 to 1, is 4 to 100. Thus, while 80% of the phosphate in plasma exists as $HPO_4^=$ (divalent), virtually all the phosphate in acidic urine exists as $H_2PO_4^-$ (monovalent). Furthermore, the forms in which phosphorus enters the plasma from the IV solution may be complex. One can avoid this problem by expressing phosphate in millimols where valence is of no concern, or perhaps better by stating phosphorus values in old-fashioned milligrams. One advantage of the latter terminology is that it has no connotation of the form in which phosphorus enters and leaves the body. For conversion purposes, one millimol of phosphorus equals 31 mg.

Phosphorus and other minerals present in protein hydrolysates and other amino acid sources In this country two types of protein hydrolysates are used: one from blood fibrin, the other from casein, which is a phospho-protein. In the course of hydrolysis of casein, some bound phosphate is liberated. Calcium is then added. Table 7 summarizes analyses made in my laboratory on these two types of hydrolysate and on FreAmine. Casein hydrolysate has approximately six times as much calcium as fibrin hydrolysate with the calcium content of the former varying between 100 to 125 mg/liter. The fibrin hydrolysate contains approximately 10 mg of phosphorus per liter as

262

inorganic phosphate compared to approximately 220 mg of phosphorus per liter as free inorganic phosphate in the casein hydrolysate. An additional 240 mg of phosphorus becomes apparent on ashing the organic matter and heating for 10 minutes at 100 C in 0.1N hydrochloric acid to convert to orthophosphate any pyrophosphate formed in the ashing process. This latter amount presumably represents residual organically-bound phosphate. I am not aware of published data pertaining to the efficiency of utilization of this bound phosphate in various clinical states. There are significant amounts of sodium per liter in the casein hydrolysate in contrast to that in fibrin hydrolysate. Magnesium and potassium values are approximately the same in both hydrolysates. If protein hydrolysate is the only source of magnesium or if the amount of hydrolysate given is not large or if there is a rapid deposition of new tissue or an obligatory loss of magnesium, the amount of magnesium may be inadequate to sustain serum levels. FreAmine provides essentially no calcium, phosphorus, magnesium, or potassium.

Table 7.—Average Composition of Protein Hydrolysates

		Fibrin Hydrolysate 5% (Aminosol) (per liter)	Casein Hydrolysate 5% (Amigen) (per liter)§	Fre Amine 8.5%** (per liter)
Na	mEq	2.5	33.0	11.0
Cl	mEq	10.2	17.0	45.0
K	mEq	17.0	19.0	0.0
Ca	mg	20.0	115 *	3.0
P Free†	mg	10.0	220	3.0
P total‡	mg	10.0	460	6.0
Mg	mEq	2.5	2.2	0
Nitrogen	gm	7.4	6.8	12.2

*Range of 100-125 mg/liter.
†As free inorganic orthophosphate.
‡As determined after dry ashing and heating with 0.1N HCl.
§Amigen 10% has twice these values per liter.
Heird et al (New Eng J Med **287:944, 1972) noted the occurrence of hyperchloremic metabolic acidosis in infants receiving FreAmine. This is explained by the presence of an excess of cationic amino acids; their metabolism results in a net excess of hydrogen and chloride ions.

Parenteral Calcium and Phosphorus Requirements

There have been two points of view about addition of these two ions to intravenous solutions for this group. One position has been to add them routinely. The other was to omit them while following their serum levels, adding one or both as the levels indicated. In the individual whose kidneys, bone mineralization, and endocrine system are normal, parathyroid hormone will act to insure that serum levels of calcium are maintained through resorption of bone mineral. However, in individuals who are depleted of magnesium, serum calcium will fall despite adequate calcium and vitamin D administration, and this type of hypocalcemia should be treated with magnesium rather than with calcium.

Individuals who undergo prolonged periods of bed rest develop disuse osteoporosis accompanied by an increase in urinary and fecal calcium.[20, 21]

Hypercalcemia may develop. Since many patients requiring TPN spend all or a major portion of their day in bed, the question must be raised as to whether calcium infusion is useful, detrimental, or without significant effect in adults. We have few published data on this. Jacobson, when he gave approximately 300 to 400 mg/day to a patient over many months, noted intermittent but fairly prolonged periods of either positive or negative balance.[17] I found a small but persistent negative calcium balance in a patient followed for more than a year while receiving about 200 mg/day;[22] various studies indicated good bone mineralization and no soft tissue calcification. More data are needed on these points.

Some physicians feel that it is desirable or even necessary to administer calcium when phosphate is infused to prevent the occurrence of hypocalcemia. Some patients who previously were hypercalcemic developed hypocalcemia when given phosphate for the purpose of lowering the elevated calcium.[23] It is my impression that these episodes occurred when very large amounts of phosphate (ie, 1,500 mg or more) were infused within several hours; it is reportedly not observed with slower infusion of larger amounts.[24] These quantities and such a rapid rate are not required in TPN. In my experience, the infusion of 310 mg (10 millimols) of phosphorus without calcium over eight hours in normophosphatemic individuals is not accompanied by any significant fall in serum calcium. However, Dudrick and his coworkers have reported "intense hypocalcemia" in some hypophosphatemic patients given phosphorus in doses of 4 to 8 mEq over eight hours.[25] These apparent differences in calcium response to phosphate require further study.

The importance of inorganic phosphate for the synthesis of high energy organic phosphates would *a priori* suggest the need for adequate supply of this ion. Evidence obtained within the past few years amply confirms this point of view. Lotz et al reported a clinical syndrome including weakness, anorexia, malaise, and bone pain in hypoparathyroid and normal subjects in whom hypophosphatemia was induced by oral aluminum hydroxide and magnesium-aluminum gels.[26] After prolonged periods of phosphate depletion, osteomalacia may occur.[27, 28] In 1969, Lichtman et al noted hypophosphatemia, anorexia, nausea, malaise, muscle weakness, and mental depression developing in a patient with chronic renal disease and uremia who was under treatment with a low-protein diet, hemodialysis, and aluminum hydroxide gel.[29] Erythrocyte ATP concentration was markedly reduced during the period of hypophosphatemia. Discontinuance of the aluminum hydroxide gel completely reduced the biochemical abnormalities and clinical symptoms. The restoration of erythrocyte ATP and serum inorganic phosphate were highly correlated.

Anaerobic glycolysis is the sole pathway for net ATP synthesis in the mature human red cell and is essential for cell integrity. It has been known that mammalian red cells contain considerable quantities of 2,3-diphosphoglycerate (2,3-DPG), but it was not until 1967 that Benesch and Benesch reported this compound to be a powerful regulator of oxygen affinity for hemoglobin.[30] This and other studies provided evidence for the interdependence of red cell glycolytic rate, concentrations of 2,3-DPG and ATP, red cell survival, and the delivery of oxygen. The rate of red cell glycolysis and the passage of 1,3-diphosphoglycerate through a side cycle allows for the regula-

264

tion of 2,3-DPG concentration. The organic phosphates 2,3-DPG and ATP have been shown to bind specifically with deoxyhemoglobin, and this results in a marked lowering of its oxygen affinity. Since there is approximately 3½ times as much 2,3-DPG as ATP in a normal red cell,[31] the former is appreciably more important in this connection.

Lichtman et al studied a patient with marked malabsorption who had been maintained on intravenous feedings with 12% glucose and 4% casein hydrolysate.[32] Four days after institution of parenteral nutrition, the plasma phosphorus was less than 0.5 mg/100 ml (Fig 1), with urinary phosphate falling to undetectable amounts. During this period of hypophosphatemia a 60% reduction from their preinfusion levels occurred in red cell glucose utilization and lactate production. These returned to normal following phosphate repletion. Figure 2, also taken from Lichtman et al,[32] indicates that following the fall in plasma phosphate and in association with the decreased glycolytic rate, the concentration of red cell 2-3 DPG fell to 45% and that of ATP to 52% of their preinfusion levels. The return to previous values following phosphate repletion is clearly demonstrated. During a period of protracted hypophosphatemia induced by parenteral feeding, refrigeration of blood at 4°C for 24 hours resulted in spontaneous autohemolysis. Phase contrast microscopic examination of red cells showed that over 50% of the cells were spherocytes.

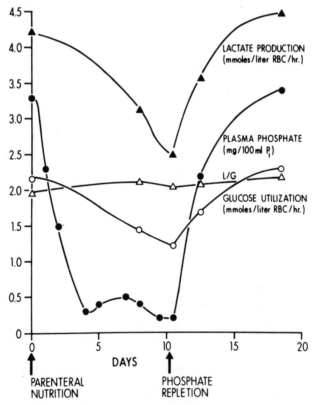

Fig 1. Relation of hypophosphatemia and its repletion to erythrocyte lactate production and glucose utilization.[32]

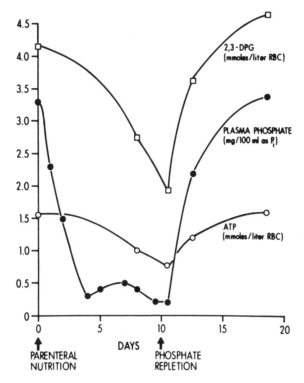

Fig 2. Plasma phosphate, red cell adenosine triphosphate (ATP), and 2,3-diphosphoglycerate (DPG) during parenteral nutrition, and phosphate repletion in vivo.[32]

Figure 3, also taken from Lichtman, shows the relationship between blood pO_2 and O_2 saturation and the effect of phosphate levels. During periods of normal phosphatemia, the percentage of hemoglobin saturation with oxygen at partial pressures from 25 to 85 mm of mercury was decreased. At this time the sum of 2,3-DPG and ATP was greater than normal, in keeping with the reduced hemoglobin concentration noted in the patient. During protracted hypophosphatemia, during which time the 2-3 DPG and ATP concentrations were less than half the expected value, the oxygen affinity of hemoglobin was increased. The estimated $P_{50}O_2$ was approximately 16 mm of mercury in the hypophosphatemic period in contrast to the value of 30 mm of mercury during the normal phosphatemic period. Thus, we have the first biochemical evidence for a metabolic disturbance resulting from hypophosphatemia in man. The authors outlined the steps in the glycolytic cycle where phosphate depletion could be expected to exert an effect.

These observations were confirmed and extended by Travis et al.[33] They found that, within seven to ten days after initiation of total intravenous hyperalimentation with solutions without supplemental inorganic phosphate, five of eight adults were found to be significantly hypophosphatemic (ie, having serum levels of less than 1 mg/100 ml of phosphorus as inorganic phosphate). The hypophosphatemia was associated with a decrease in red cell glucose-6-

266

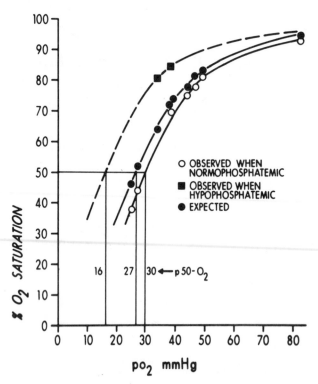

Fig 3. Oxygen saturation curves of hemoglobin in patient during period of normophosphatemia as contrasted with that during hypophosphatemia (see text).[32]

phosphate, fructose-6-phosphate, 3-phosphoglycerate, 2-phosphoglycerate, phosphoenolpyruvate, 2,3-DPG and ATP (Fig 4), and a marked increase in the concentration of "total triose-phosphates," (ie, fructose diphosphate, glyceraldehyde-3-phosphate and dihydroxyacetone phosphate). Reduction in 2,3-DPG and ATP was accompanied by an increase in red cell affinity for oxygen.

The investigators interpreted the results as follows: The reduced inorganic phosphate level decreases the activity of glyceraldehyde-3-phosphate dehydrogenase, of which it is a cofactor; as a result of this relative block in glycolysis, there are decreases in 2,3-DPG and the other intermediates below the glyceraldehyde-3-phosphate dehydrogenase step leading to an obligatory fall in the red cell ATP concentration. This decline in ATP causes a decrease in red cell hexokinase activity but with a concomitant increase in phosphofructokinase activity. These enzyme changes result in the lowering of red cell concentration of glucose-6-phosphate and an increase in triosephosphates.

Of the eight patients with hypophosphatemia, three manifested paresthesias about the mouth and in extremities, mental obtundation, and hyperventilation, and these had the lowest $p_{50}O_2$ values for hemoglobin. The two patients with the lowest $p_{50}O_2$ values demonstrated diffuse slowing of the EEG. Although no measurements of tissue ATP were performed in the patients, these investigators suggested that decreased oxygen delivery to tissues may be the

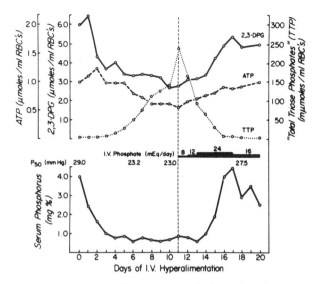

Fig 4. Changes in red cell ATP, 2,3-diphosphoglycerate (2,3-DPG) and "total triose-phosphates" in patient on total parenteral nutrition during periods of normophosphatemia and hypophosphatemia.[33]

primary etiological factor in the development of muscle weakness, anorexia, and malaise seen with phosphate depletion. Serum phosphate returned to normal rapidly after termination of the intravenous nutrition, suggesting that hypophosphatemia reflected massive shifts in phosphate partition as the result of the IV feeding.

Severe but reversible hemolytic anemia has been reported in a patient with marked hypophosphatemia (0.1 mg/100 ml).[34]

Several papers indicate that severe hypokalemia from a variety of causes may lead to severe hypophosphatemia, presumably secondary to tubular damage with failure to reabsorb phosphate properly.[35, 36] These facts again demonstrate the important interrelationships of these ions. We and other investigators find that 300 mg/day of phosphorus as inorganic phosphate is an amount usually adequate to restore and maintain normal serum phosphate. For debilitated patients given large amounts of glucose, however, larger amounts may be required for some days.

Another matter to consider is whether the administration of phosphate —especially when given with calcium separately or together in the course of a 24-hour period as a routine daily measure—is likely to lead to soft tissue calcification. It is well established that phosphate ingestion or infusion can decrease calcium excretion in the urine. [21, 37, 38] It has been variously suggested that the decreased serum and urinary calcium following phosphate administration is attributable to inhibition of bone reabsorption or stimulation of bone formation or to deposition of calcium phosphate in soft tissues, but no firm agreement has been reached on this.[39] With administration of large amounts of phosphate over fairly short periods of time to hypercalcemic patients, soft tissue calcification is seen. Whether this is due to the preexisting hypercalcemia

268

antedating the phosphate is often unclear because of a lack of pretreatment data. Kahil et al have demonstrated metastatic calcification in hypercalcemic patients independent of preceding phosphate therapy.[40] When large amounts of phosphate were given orally over long periods of time, calcification was demonstrated in serial studies by Dudley and Blackburn in extraskeletal areas of both normocalcemic and hypercalcemic patients.[41] The normocalcemic patients received the phosphate for approximately 15 months. In a postmortem examination of my patient[22] some 16 months after daily intravenous phosphate and calcium infusions were started, the pathologist found no evidence of nephrocalcinosis. Nor was there other soft tissue calcification. Further observations of this type are needed to give reassurance on this point.

Sulfur

Sulfur is present in methionine, cysteine, taurine, certain mucopoly-saccharides and glycolipids, and as sulfate esters in various metabolites. The sulfur present in the amino acids is apparently adequate for formation of the other compounds when the amino acid supply is sufficient. Sulfur enters into taurine along the metabolic pathway of cysteine and into sulfated compounds from inorganic sulfate derived from cysteine; the sulfate is incorporated into 3'phosphoadenosine-5'phosphosulfate which serves as a general agent for esterification of sulfate.

MICROMINERALS (TRACE ELEMENTS)

Table 2.— Microminerals of Interest
(5 mg/day)

1. Iron*	7. Cobalt (-B_{12})†
2. Zinc*	8. Manganese
3. Copper*	9. Molybdenum
4. Iodide*	10. Selenium
5. Fluoride*	11. Vanadium
6. Chromium	

*Human requirement established.
†Cobalt other than that in vitamin B_{12}.

As indicated in Tables 5 and 6, most physicians in this field have made an effort to supply these nutrients in a qualitative way by periodically infusing plasma or blood or by giving parenteral iron. There is only one published report of a trace element formulation which has been used clinically for a prolonged period.[22] The further development of TPN to its full potential necessitates much more information on human requirements for each trace element and their presence as contaminants in parenteral fluids and additives.

Iron

Iron for parenteral purposes is available as an intramuscular and intravenous preparation in the form of iron dextran (Imferon) and for intramuscular use as iron sorbitol (Jectofer). Imferon has been used abroad for a number of years for a single whole dose intravenous administration. Most of the patients in whom this technique has been utilized have been iron-deficient pregnant women. A small and variable number have had reactions. Clay et al noted 13 reactions in 150 women; 7 of these reactions were severe, requiring immediate resuscitative procedures.[42] Others, including Bonnar, noted only 3 serious systemic reactions in 250 patients.[43] The point that impressed me in reading these results, particularly those of Clay et al, was that most of the severe reactions occurred almost immediately after the infusion, despite a slow rate. It may be that patients on TPN may react differently from pregnant women. Nevertheless, if intravenous preparations are to be used, directions are to be followed closely and an emergency tray should be at hand with necessary medications, airway and resuscitation equipment.

Those papers dealing with iron therapy of infants or children receiving parenteral nutrition rarely state the amounts of Imferon given weekly. Other workers give iron in the form of blood transfusions. Preexisting iron deficiency anemia should be corrected immediately. Maintenance iron in growing infants or children should be given perhaps once a week or every two weeks on the basis of 1 mg of iron per day.

Normal adult males and nonmenstruating women have an estimated average daily iron loss of approximately 0.6 to 1.3 mg/day. The menstruating loss contributes an additional and variable 0.1 to 1.4 mg.[44] Any other iron losses should be estimated. Serial determinations of hemoglobin, red cell indices, serum iron, and iron-binding capacity will permit further evaluation of iron requirements. Preexisting deficiency should be corrected. Thereafter, intramuscular or intravenous iron may not be necessary more frequently than once in several months or longer in adults unless iron losses are severe. (Suggestions for routine dosage are indicated in Table 8.)

Table 8.— Trace Elements
(suggested approximate daily intravenous requirements*)

	Infants and young children	Adults
Iron	1 mg/day*	1 mg/day (♂+n-m♀)† +1 mg/day (m♀)
Iodine	5 μg/kg (?)	1-2 μg/kg
Copper	15 μg/kg (?)	1 mg
Fluoride	1 μg/ml	1-2 mg (?)
Zinc	20-40 μg/kg (?)	2-4 mg (?)
Manganese	10-20 μg/kg (?)	1-2 mg (?)
Chromium	0.5 μg/kg (?)	15 μg/day (?)

*To be given daily or weekly; Fe bi-monthly to adults.
†After correction of previous depletion; n-m = nonmenstruating; m = menstruating.

Iodine

Quantitative requirements are not known with certainty. Iodine is efficiently absorbed when taken orally; hence, the parenteral dose is probably fairly close to the oral.[45] The RDA of the National Research Council for iodine are approximately 5μg/kg for infants and young children and approximately 1μg/kg for adults.[13] This ion can be given daily or in intermittent weekly doses (Table 8). There is evidence that ten times this amount has no untoward

effects when given orally and consistently to euthyroid adult individuals.
assume the same holds for intravenous administration.

Copper

This element is not well absorbed in the intestinal tract in most
species, including man. Cartwright and Wintrobe have estimated copper
absorption to be approximately 32%.[46] If one takes the figure of $50\mu g/kg/day$
for infants—suggested in the RDA of the National Research Council—and
estimates that one-third is absorbed, then approximately $15\mu g/kg/day$ should
be adequate for infants. Premature infants with a large copper reserve in the
liver probably will do well with one-third of this amount. For adults, 2 mg/day
appear to be adequate orally, and approximately 1 mg would appear to be
adequate intravenously. I have given a supplement of 1.0 mg of cupric ion from
two to seven times per week for prolonged periods to patients and have found
plasma copper and ceruloplasmin levels to be within normal range.

Zinc

Zinc is another ion which is not efficiently absorbed when given orally.
Spencer et al have found the average absorption of radiozinc to be about
36%.[47] The quantity of zinc excreted in the urine of healthy individuals is small.
It does not vary appreciably with the level of zinc in the diet, nor is it significantly
increased following zinc injections. The major pathway for excretion of zinc
is the feces.[48] Evidence is increasing that zinc is necessary for numerous species,
including man, but evidence of uncomplicated zinc deficiency in man is still
limited. A deficiency syndrome in experimental animals is characterized by
growth retardation, by skin lesions, and by impaired reproductive development and function. Zinc may play a role in wound healing. This ion should be
supplied to patients on prolonged parenteral feeding. Various balance studies
suggest that 6 to 12 mg orally per day are adequate for children or adults; data
on infants are insufficient. Assuming approximately one-third absorption of
this amount, 2 to 4 mg/day given intravenously should be adequate for adults.

Fluoride

The role established for this ion in human nutrition is in conferring
maximal resistance to dental caries by being incorporated in the structure of
teeth. But when the fluoride concentration in drinking water exceeds 1 part
per million (ppm), progressive mottling of the teeth develops as the concentration increases. Above 10 ppm, the dental changes are severe. Abnormalities in bone may occur when fluoride levels reach above 5,000 to 6,000 ppm.
McClure, McCann, and Leone estimate that continuous intake of 8 ppm of
fluoride in the diet for 35 years is necessary before this critical level is
reached.[49] Mixed American diets contain about 0.5 mg of fluoride daily, approximately 80% of which is absorbed.[48] Artificially fluoridated water at 1 ppm contributes another 1 to 2 mg daily. Where there is likely to be prolonged parenteral
nutrition, especially in children, 1 ppm of fluoride appeared to be desirable
in the solution. This does not necessarily mean that the fluoride should be

added to the solutions since this ion may exist as a contaminant in solutions or medications. Information on this aspect is necessary.

Manganese

Manganese deficiency has been demonstrated experimentally in a number of species, but there is no good evidence for manganese deficiency having developed in man. In experimental animals, cardinal manifestations of deficiency are impaired growth, skeletal abnormalities, abnormal reproductive function, and ataxia in the newborn. Experimental data suggest that manganese is poorly absorbed in the intestinal tract, and its absorption is markedly influenced by other ions and materials in the diet. Even when injected, its major pathway of excretion is bile rather than urine. The manganese content of human diets appears to vary from 2 to 9 mg depending on food composition.[48] Assuming 10% absorption of the amount taken orally, approximately 1 mg/day would be adequate intravenously.

Chromium

Since 1959, evidence has been accumulating that trivalent chromium is somehow involved in glucose tolerance and that this ion may be a cofactor with insulin for normal glucose utilization in rats and mice. Indications for a role in human nutrition and the possibility of marginal chromium intakes in individuals living on highly refined carbohydrates have recently appeared. A glucose load leads to a rise in plasma chromium,[50] and much of this chromium may be lost in the urine[51] with the potentiality of depletion of the biologically active chromium stores.[52] If these observations are confirmed clinically, it is possible that the large amounts of glucose infused in TPN will increase chromium requirements. In clinical trials, a portion of patients with diabetes mellitus had significant improvement in glucose tolerance following oral supplementation with chromium as $CrCl_3 \cdot 6H_2O$.[53, 54] The supplementary chromium administered in these diets amounted to 150µg/day, which increased the total intake from about 50 to 200µg/day. With the poor absorption of trivalent chromium ion, it would appear logical to assume at this time that 10 or 15µg of chromium administered intravenously daily would be more than adequate. The amount of chromium present as a contaminant in IV solutions is not certain.

The essentiality for man of other trace elements—vanadium, nickel, selenium, and others—remains to be elucidated through further research.

It is probable that many or all of these trace elements are present in small or significant amounts as contaminants in parenteral solutions and medications. It is essential to have detailed analyses performed on these materials for a large number of trace elements to assure an adequate intake and also to insure against potentially toxic levels.

Finally, it should be emphasized that TPN is given to patients with a variety of diseases. In certain situations there are undoubtedly increased losses of ions. This must be true for the nephrotic syndrome where ions are lost which are closely bound to proteins, such as copper, zinc, and manganese. Large losses of intestinal secretions and lean tissue will also result in deficits that will require replacement. Patients with continued febrile states will have significant increases in the losses of certain materials in sweat.[55-58] I have indicated in Table 9 some approximate mineral losses in sweat. In addition to sodium and potassium, there may be significant losses of iron and zinc.

Table 9.—Minerals in Sweat

Units	Per liter	Reference	Units	Per liter	Reference
Na —meq	50 to 182	55	Fe —mg	0.41 ± 0.13	57
K —meq	6 to 21	55	I —mg	0.009	58
Mg—meq	0.5 ± 3	55	Zn —mg	0.93 ± 0.26	58
Ca —mg	7 ± 2	56	Cu —mg	0.06	58
P —mg	1.1 to 1.6	55	Mn—mg	0.06	58

In conclusion, it is apparent from this brief survey that the nutritional and metabolic implications of minerals are complex and important and that numerous practical aspects are still unanswered.

References

1. Slater JE: Retentions of nitrogen and minerals by babies 1 week old. *Br J Nutr* **15**:83-97, 1961.

2. Filler RM, Eraklis AJ, Rubin VG, Das JB: Long-term total parenteral nutrition in infants. *N Eng J Med* **281**:589-594, 1969.

3. Wilmore DW, Dudrick SJ: Growth and development of an infant receiving all nutrients exclusively by vein. *JAMA* **203**:860-864, 1968.

4. Børresen HC, Coran AG, Knutrud O: Metabolic results of parenteral feeding in neonatal surgery: A balanced parenteral feeding program based on a synthetic L-amino acid solution and a commercial fat emulsion. *Ann Surg* **172**:291-301, 1970.

5. Sherman JO, Egan T, Macalad FV: Parenteral hyperalimentation. A useful surgical adjunct. *Surg Clin North Am* **51**:37-47, 1971.

6. Altman RP, Randolph JG: Application and hazards of total parenteral nutrition in infants. *Ann Surg* **174**:85-90, 1971.

7. Dudrick SJ, Ruberg RL: Principles and practice of parenteral nutrition. *Gastroenterology* **61**:901-910, 1971.

8. Dudrick SJ, Wilmore DW, Vars HM, et al: Can intravenous feeding as the sole means of nutrition support growth in the child and restore weight loss in an adult? An affirmative answer. *Ann Surg* **169**:974-984, 1969.

9. Meng HC, Law DH, Sandstead HH: Some clinical experiences in parenteral nutrition, in Berg G (ed): *Advances in Parenteral Nutrition*. Stuttgart, G. Thieme Verlag, 1970, pp 64-82.

10. Shils ME, Wright WL, Turnbull A, Brescia F: Long-term parenteral nutrition through an external arteriovenous shunt. *N Eng J Med* **283**:341-344, 1970.

11. Jacobson S: Complete parenteral nutrition in man for seven months, in Berg G (ed): *Advances in Parenteral Nutrition.* Stuttgart, G. Thieme Verlag, 1970, pp 6-19.

12. Shils ME: Experimental human magnesium depletion. *Medicine* **48**:61-85, 1969.

13. *National Research Council, Food and Nutrition Board: Recommended Dietary Allowances,* ed 7, publication 1964, Washington DC, National Academy of Sciences, 1968.

14. Shils ME: Magnesium, in Goodhart RS, Shils ME (eds): *Modern Nutrition in Health and Disease,* ed 5. Philadelphia, Lea & Febiger, 1973, pp 287-296.

15. Børresen HC, Coran AG, Knutrud O: Metabolic results of parenteral feeding in neonatal surgery: A balanced parenteral feeding program based on a synthetic L-amino acid solution and a commercial fat emulsion. *Ann Surg* **172**:291-301, 1970.

16. Dickerson JW, Widdowson EM: Chemical changes in skeletal muscle during development. *Biochem J* **74**:247-257, 1960.

17. Jacobson S: Complete parenteral nutrition in man for seven months, in Berg G (ed): *Advances in Parenteral Nutrition:* International Symposium on Parenteral Nutrition, Prague, Sept 3-4, 1969. Stuttgart, Georg Thieme Verlag, 1970, pp 6-19.

18. Moore CA, Bunce GE: Reduction in frequency of renal calculus formation by oral magnesium administration. A preliminary report. *Invest Urol* **2**:7-13, 1964.

19. Whittier FC, Freeman RM: Potentiation of metastatic calcification in vitamin D-treated rats by magnesium. *Am J Physiol* **220**:209-212, 1971.

20. Deitrick JE, Whedon GD, Shorr E: Effects of immobilization upon various metabolic and physiologic functions of normal men. *Am J Med* **4**:3-36, 1948.

21. Hulley SB, Vogel JM, Donaldson CL, et al: The effect of supplemental oral phosphate on the bone mineral changes during prolonged bed rest. *J Clin Invest* **50**:2506-2518, 1971.

22. Shils ME, Wright WL, Turnbull A, et al: Long-term parenteral nutrition through an external arteriovenous shunt. *N Eng J Med* **283**:341-344, 1970.

23. Shackney S, Hasson J: Precipitous fall in serum calcium, hypotension, and acute renal failure after intravenous phosphate therapy for hypercalcemia. Report of two cases. *Ann Intern Med* **66**:906-918, 1967.

24. Goldsmith RS, Ingbar SH: Inorganic phosphate treatment of hypercalcemia of diverse etiologies. *N Eng J Med* **274**:1-7, 1966; Phosphate, sulfate, and hypercalcemia. *Ann Intern Med* **67**:463-464, 1967.

25. Allen TR, Ruberg RL, Dudrick S, et al: Hypophosphatemia occurring in patients receiving total parenteral hyperalimentation. *Fed Proc* **30**:580, 1971.

26. Lotz M, Zisman E, Bartter FC: Evidence for a phosphorus-depletion syndrome in man. *N Eng J Med* **278**:409-415, 1968.

27. Bloom WL, Flinchum D: Osteomalacia with pseudofractures caused by the ingestion of aluminum hydroxide. *JAMA* **174**:1327-1330, 1960.

28. Lotz M, Ney R, Bartter FC: Osteomalacia and debility resulting from phosphorus depletion. *Trans Assoc AM Physicians* **77**:281, 1964.

29. Lichtman MA, Miller DR, Freeman RB: Erythrocyte adenosine triphosphate depletion during hypophosphatemia in a uremic subject. *N Eng J Med* **280:**240-244, 1969.

30. Benesch R, Benesch RE: The effect of organic phosphates from the human erythrocyte on the allosteric properties of hemoglobin. *Biochem Biophys Res Commun* **26:**162-167, 1967.

31. Bunn HF, Ransil BJ, Chao A: The interaction between erythrocyte organic phosphates, magnesium ion, and hemoglobin. *J Biol Chem* **246:**5273-5279, 1971.

32. Lichtman MA, Miller DR, Cohen J, et al: Reduced red cell glycolysis, 2,3-diphosphoglycerate and adenosine triphosphate concentration and increased hemoglobin-oxygen affinity caused by hypophosphatemia. *Ann Intern Med* **74:**562-568, 1971.

33. Travis SF: Alterations of red-cell glycolytic intermediates and oxygen transport as a consequence of hypophosphatemia in patients receiving intravenous hyperalimentation. *N Eng J Med* **285:**763-768, 1971.

34. Jacob HS, Amsden T: Acute hemolytic anemia with rigid red cells in hypophosphatemia. *N Eng J Med* **285:**1446-1449, 1971.

35. Anderson DC, Peters TJ, Stewart WK: Association of hypokalaemia and hypophosphatemia. *Br Med J* **4:**402-403, 1969.

36. Vianna NJ: Severe hypophosphatemia due to hypokalemia. *JAMA* **215:**1497-1498, 1971.

37. Widdowson EM, McCance RA, Harrison GE, et al: Effect of giving phosphate supplements to breast-fed babies on absorption and excretion of calcium, strontium, magnesium, and phosphorus. *Lancet* **2:**1250-1251, 1963.

38. Heaton FW, Hodgkinson A, Rose GA: Observations on the relation between calcium and magnesium metabolism in man. *Clin Sci* **27:**31-40, 1964.

39. Eisenberg E: Effect of intravenous phosphate on serum strontium and calcium. *N Eng J Med* **282:**899-902, 1970.

40. Kahil M, Orman B, Gyorkey F, et al: Hypercalcemia: Experience with phosphate and sulfate therapy. *JAMA* **201:**721-724, 1967.

41. Dudley FJ, Blackburn CR: Extraskeletal calcification complicating oral neutral-phosphate therapy. *Lancet* **2:**628-630, 1970.

42. Clay B, Rosenberg B, Sampson N, et al: Reaction to total dose intravenous infusion of iron dextran (Imferon). *Br Med J* **5246:**29-31, 1965.

43. Bonnar J: Anaemia in obstetrics: An evaluation of treatment by iron-dextran infusion. *Br Med J* **5469:**1030, 1965.

44. Moore CV: Iron. In Goodhart RS, Shils ME (eds): *Modern Nutrition in Health and Disease.* Philadelphia, Lea & Febiger, 1973, p 310.

45. Vought RL: Reliability of estimates of serum inorganic iodine and daily fecal and urinary iodine excretion from single casual specimens. *Metabolism* **23:**1218, 1963.

46. Cartwright GE, Wintrobe MM: Copper metabolism in normal subjects. *Am J Clin Nutr* **12:**224-232, 1964; the question of copper deficiency in man. Ibid **15:**94, 1964.

47. Spencer H, Vankinscott V, Lewin I, et al: Zinc-65 metabolism during low and high calcium intake in man. *J Nutr* **86:**169-177, 1965.

48. Underwood EJ: *Trace Elements in Human and Animal Nutrition.* ed 3, New York, Academic Press, 1971.

49. McClure FJ, McCann HG, Leone NC: Excessive fluoride in water and bone chemistry: Comparison of two cases. *Public Health Rep* **73:**741-746, 1958.

50. Glinsmann WH, Feldman FJ, Mertz W: Plasma chromium after glucose administration. *Science* **152:**1243-1245, 1966.

51. Schroeder HA: The role of chromium in mammalian nutrition. *Am J Clin Nutr* **21:**230-244, 1968.

52. Mertz W: Some aspects of nutritional trace element research. *Fed Proc* **29:**1482-1488, 1970.

53. Glinsmann WH, Mertz W: Effect of trivalent chromium on glucose tolerance. *Metabolism* **15:**510-520, 1966.

54. Levine RA, Streeten DH, Doisy RJ: Effects of oral chromium supplementation on the glucose tolerance of elderly human subjects. *Metabolism* **17:**114, 1968.

55. Consolazio CF, Matoush LO, Nelson RA, et al: Excretion of sodium, potassium, magnesium and iron in human sweat and the relation of each to balance and requirements. *J Nutr* **79:**407-415, 1963.

56. Vellar OD, Askevold R: Studies on sweat losses of nutrients. 3. Calcium, magnesium, and chloride content of whole body cell-free sweat in healthy unacclimatized men under controlled environmental conditions. *Scand J Clin Lab Invest* **22:**65-71, 1968.

57. Vellar OD: Studies on sweat losses of nutrients. 1. iron content of whole body sweat and its association with other sweat constituents, serum iron levels, hematological indices, body surface area, and sweat rate. *Scand J Clin Lab Invest* **21:**157-167, 1968.

58. Altman PL, Dittmer DS (eds): *Metabolism.* FASEB, Bethesda, Md. 1968, p 519.

Vitamins and Minerals

Colloquium

Theodore B. Van Itallie, M.D., chairman and editor
Harold H. Sandstead, M.D. rapporteur

Dr. Van Itallie: We attempted to define desirable combinations of vitamins and minerals for daily administration to patients receiving total parenteral nutrition, hoping to evolve a baseline mixture of nutrients that would be compatible in solution. Tentative estimates were reached for use in initiating TPN until more experimental data are available. Our colloquium protocol progressed through discussions of:

    I. Water-soluble vitamins
       A. Ascorbic acid
       B. B vitamins
          1. Folic acid
          2. Vitamin B_{12}
          3. Riboflavin, thiamin, vitamin B_6
   II. Fat-soluble vitamins
       A. Vitamins A, D, E, and K
  III. Macrominerals
       A. Calcium
       B. Phosphorus
       C. Magnesium
       D. Potassium
       E. Sodium
  IV. Microelements
       A. Iron
       B. Zinc
       C. Iodine
       D. Copper

Dr. Van Itallie: Because parenteral nutrition is unphysiologic, it poses special problems for the physician.

Administration of vitamins (and minerals) via venous catheter may result in excessive losses, particularly of the water-soluble vitamins. These losses may be much greater than those which occur when a similar quantity of the same nutrients is taken by mouth.

Parenteral feeding may involve administration of a nutrient mixture very different from that in the normal diet. Large quantities of carbohydrate are given. Since the need for thiamin seems to be greater when the carbohydrate intake is high, this factor (among many others) must be taken into account.

The patient who is receiving TPN is likely to be quite sick; thus his illness inevitably will have a conditioning effect on his requirements. It is probable also that prior to initiation of TPN the patient was sufficiently ill for a long enough period to warrant institution of this hazardous, albeit lifesaving, procedure. Accordingly, patients on TPN may have reduced reserves of vitamins and other nutrients at the outset of parenteral feeding. While this is not invariably the case, I suspect such a depletion is common.

A recommended formulation of vitamins cannot meet every clinical need and should, accordingly, be considered a baseline preparation to which additional vitamins may be added as clinical circumstances require.

WATER-SOLUBLE VITAMINS

Dr. Hodges: The more we look at vitamins, the more we wonder whether the compound with which we are familiar is really the active vitamin or whether it is the precursor of the active substance. This is true for thiamin. It is true for vitamin B_6, and it may also be true for ascorbic acid.

Ascorbic Acid

Dr. Hodges: Let us look at what can be done when one has a carefully controlled metabolic unit and the expertise of people who know how to use radioisotopes skillfully. If one labels the body pool(s) with ascorbic acid,[1] one can estimate, by use of ^{14}C-labeling, the size of that pool and also, by following the rate of excretion of radioactivity, determine the catabolic rate of the vitamin (see Fig 1).

For ascorbic acid, the body pool size happens to be about 1,500 mg. After the pool is labeled, if a diet free of ascorbic acid is given, the excretory data will permit estimation of the body pool size. In this instance we indicated on the right hand ordinate the rate of catabolism (which averaged 3% of the body pool per day). It can be seen that, at 1,500 mg, the *rate* of utilization of ascorbic acid was 45 mg/day. To put it another way, a person who is ingesting 45 mg/day should maintain a body pool that is full. In contrast, a person who is getting 30 mg/day—as the British and World Health Organization recommend—should maintain a body pool of about 1,000 mg. In experimental deficiency, the body pool size fell to 300 mg at the time manifestations of deficiency became detectable. At this point, the amount of vitamin C catabolized was 9 mg/day, a figure which corresponds to the British estimate of the requirement (ie, approximately 10 mg/day).

Let us try to relate what we know about vitamin C to the problem of parenteral nutrition:

We know that physiologic doses of orally administered vitamin C are absorbed almost completely, but we don't know whether a carrier mechanism is involved.

The renal mechanism for handling ascorbic acid is much like that for glucose. At low plasma concentrations of vitamin C the amount of ascorbate excreted in the urine is small. But, as we increase the plasma concentration of vitamin C, we eventually pass the renal threshold of 1.4 mg/100 ml, and the amount excreted rises rapidly. Once the tubular maximum is reached, renal excretion of ascorbic acid parallels the glomerular filtration rate. Therefore, if we infuse ascorbic acid in parenteral solutions, we should avoid reaching plasma levels in excess of 1.4 mg/100 ml, otherwise we will lose much of the administered ascorbic acid.

Ascorbic acid has other functions apart from prevention of the syndrome we recognize as scurvy. It is involved in the sulfation of some of the ground substances that are necessary for wound healing and for tissue regeneration. In addition, ascorbic acid maintains iron, copper, and probably other metallic ions in the biologically functional reduced state.

We know little about factors that increase the need for ascorbic acid. The concept of it as a stress vitamin is incorrect, with one possible exception: The observation that extreme emotional distress can cause an increase in the rate of catabolism of ascorbate. Presumably the dose of ascorbic acid to give parenterally should not be significantly different from the oral dose recommended by the Food and Nutrition Board, but the rate of administration should be slow to minimize renal losses.

Dr. Butterworth: What is the role of ascorbic acid sulfate in sulfation and excretion of cholesterol?[2]

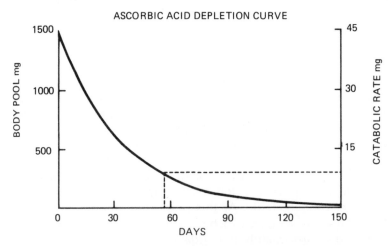

Fig 1. Curve of ascorbate pool derived from data of nine men whose body pool of ascorbate was labeled with ^{14}C L-ascorbic acid.[1] They were then fed a diet devoid of vitamin C. Initially the body pool averaged 1,500 mg. The average daily rate of catabolism was 3% of the existing body pool. Thus, the maximal rate of catabolism approximated 45 mg/day. When the body pool fell below 300 mg total and the catabolic rate below 9 mg/day, signs of scurvy began to appear (about 55 days). From this curve one can estimate the approximate body pool size from the dose. Thus, with a daily intake of 30 mg, the pool size should be about 1,000 mg.

Dr. Hodges: I do not know.

Dr. Shils: You mentioned that you have no evidence for an increased requirement for ascorbic acid in conditions such as trauma or fever. Have you done tracer studies in patients or have your studies been limited to normal subjects?

Dr. Hodges: One individual whose body stores of ascorbate were labeled with ^{14}C fortuitously developed a severe ear infection with regional lymphangitis and lymphadenitis and fever of 103°F.[3] His daily rate of catabolism of the vitamin remained constant.

Dr. Shils: Many surgeons give ascorbic acid in tremendous quantities. Half a gram or a gram a day postoperatively is not unusual. The information you have given would make them reflect about a more appropriate dose. This leads to another question: If you give ascorbate slowly so that it doesn't spill over in the urine, what proportion is metabolized to oxalic acid?

Dr. Hodges: Man metabolizes very little to oxalic acid. The guinea pig converts a higher proportion to oxalate, but the metabolic pathways are different. In our studies, 5% to 10% of the ascorbate was excreted as oxalate.

I would like to comment on use of ascorbic acid in surgical patients. We investigated a report that radioactively labeled ascorbic acid would concentrate in the healing wound margin and asked surgeons to make a full thickness incision on the skin of the thigh of each scorbutic subject. At two weeks and at four weeks, we obtained punch biopsies from the healing wound margins. No concentration of radioactivity was detected in the healing wound margins.

Dr. Van Itallie: King[4] in his review in *Present Knowledge in Nutrition* (1967), cites reports from surgeons who studied patients subjected to major surgery or who had severe burns. The surgeons suggested supplying 150 to 200 mg/day postoperatively to restore normal blood and leukocyte values. Have any of you followed that work?

Dr. Shils: From results of their work the surgeons showed, or claimed to show, that circulating blood levels of ascorbic acid fall with fever or trauma, probably the basis for the suggestion that increased requirements occur under such conditions. Whether changes in blood levels indicate depletion of body stores or whether the vitamin temporarily disappears and returns after the fever or trauma is gone has not been settled.

Dr. Hodges: We have no real evidence to support the widespread practice of administering large doses of vitamin C to surgical patients.

Dr. Van Itallie: Do we really know much about the desirable allowance of ascorbate in total parenteral nutrition? Have the urinary losses been studied adequately when vitamin C is given to patients parenterally? Does any work indicate that parenterally given ascorbate is utilized with sufficient efficiency so that we can reasonably extrapolate from oral administration data? Or should we put a safety factor into our recommendation? Should we increase the parenteral RDA over and above the safety factor that is implicit in the oral RDA of 45 mg, say, to 100 mg/day?

Dr. Hodges: Our ignorance in this area is profound. We don't have anything to go on. Your suggestion is reasonable: we should increase RDA by 50% perhaps, until we learn more about the way the body handles intravenous vitamin C. We should measure the rate of loss in the urine and use ^{14}C-tagging to estimate rates of catabolism under these circumstances.

Dr. Van Itallie: Also, we want to replenish these patients. We have to presume that some of them or many of them are already depleted. In your studies, didn't you find that large doses, up to a certain point, were helpful in replenishing body stores fairly rapidly? When you were treating the subjects in whom scurvy had been induced, you could cure them by giving as little as 10 mg/day, but the rate of improvement was slow, wasn't it?

Dr. Hodges: During the repletion period, the basic diet had about 2.5 mg; in addition we gave a dose of either 4, 8, 16, 32, or 64 mg. Sixty-four was our largest and, for us, a massive dose. The 4 mg dose plus 2.5 mg in the diet cured scurvy slowly.

Dr. Van Itallie: But the operative word is "slowly." We are dealing with sick individuals in whom we want to restore homeostasis as rapidly as possible.

Dr. Hodges: Your suggestion of 100 mg is not unreasonable until we have learned more about it.

Col. Canham: Is there evidence to suggest that 500 mg contained in one vial of Multivitamin Infusion (MVI) would be injurious to a patient?

Dr. Sandstead: The 500 mg of vitamin C in the MVI ampule is not what you worry about. It is the large amounts of the vitamins A and D.

Col. Canham: One of our subjects received 128 mg/day during the repletion period. From oxalate determinations made in our laboratory, we found the rate of excretion of oxalate to be relatively fixed. Derived from the labeled ascorbic acid given prior to depletion and during repletion, it generally represented 10% of the ^{14}C-labeled material in the urine. The 10% figure on normal intakes of ascorbic acid is fairly typical; but in a preliminary study of 5 volunteers given 4 gm/day of ascorbic acid, Briggs et al observed that one subject's daily oxalate excretion rose from 58 mg to 622 mg. The rise for the other four subjects averaged 12 mg/day, as could be expected. Hence the rare individual may develop oxaluria problems in response to pharmacological doses of ascorbic acid. I do not believe that the requirements of the relatively normal adults we have studied are directly translatable to the ill, hospitalized patient. Results of the Ten State Nutrition Survey identified some population groups apparently at risk in their vitamin C status as determined by serum ascorbic acid values.

We surveyed two groups of normal young males. In one group of 196 basic trainees who had been in the Army one week, serum ascorbic acid values ranged from 0 to 0.3 mg/100 ml in approximately 40%. One could attribute these low values to their food consumption prior to entering the service. The second group consisted of 308 men who had been in the service more than a year. They were offered a diet calculated to provide far more than the normal daily requirement of vitamin C. The distribution curve of the serum ascorbic acid values for this second group was almost identical to that of the basic trainees. Presumably the members of this second group had not been eating the food items in their diet that would have provided vitamin C. I am trying to stress that apparently normal subjects may be "at-risk" for vitamin C even before they become ill or are injured.

Animal studies in our laboratory and in others have shown that the form in which ascorbic acid is administered parenterally is important. One form, ascorbic acid 3-sulfate, completely protects against scurvy when administered orally. It is excreted rapidly when given parenterally.

Dr. Van Itallie: Do you think that 100 mg/day is too little as a guide for parenteral alimentation?

Col. Canham: I am inclined to suggest that as a minimum allowance.

Dr. Hodges: I am more conservative than Col. Canham. I would not like the allowance to go to 500 for several reasons. Among the more salient is that antagonisms exist between ascorbic acid and some drug actions. The anticoagulant effects of the coumadin drugs and heparin can be antagonized by large doses of L-ascorbic acid. I am not certain whether 500 mg/day would have a measurable effect, but I think that 2,000 mg might. Unless we can demonstrate a beneficial effect for 500, I would choose a smaller dose.

Dr. Benson: I am unaware that my company has had any problems related to the 500 mg of vitamin C in its multivitamin preparation for parenteral administration.

Dr. Sandstead: MVI comes in a 10 cc ampule; one-third of a 10 cc ampule will provide the daily requirements for vitamins A and D. It has been our practice in parenteral alimentation to give one-third of such an ampule daily. If one administers that quantity, and not a whole ampule, no argument is likely to arise about how much vitamin C is provided in this preparation. Since use of a whole ampule for the patient is general practice, drug companies should be admonished for putting three times the RDA for a given nutrient in one ampule, since use of the whole ampule for the patient is general practice. It would be preferable if the amount in a given ampule never exceeded the amount intended for administration over one 24-hour period.

Dr. Van Itallie: Dr. Benson, would you give us reasons for the 500 mg dose?

Dr. Benson: I don't know the answer. Recently, my company introduced a concentrated vial of the vitamin mixture so that aliquots may be taken out and used. This should assist the physician who will be making up these infusions. He can select the amount he needs.

Dr. Hodges: I would much prefer to see amounts in one vial that are in accord with recommendations of the Food and Nutrition Board, as Dr. Sandstead suggested.

Dr. Benson: I understand that the new package is a rubber-stoppered vial, not just a sealed glass vial. Thus, multiple units are obtainable from it.

Mr. Klotz: I am a pharmacist from Children's Memorial Hospital affiliated with Northwestern University and we use MVI. One reason was ease of handling with less chance of contamination. Contamination with *Candida* has been one of the major problems in total parenteral nutrition. But this rubber-stoppered vial is not meant to be used as a multiple dose vial. It should not be reentered; every such reuse increases the risk of contamination. If the whole unit is not used at once, I would suggest destroying it. That is one reason pharmacists in our hospital monitor each patient. No nurse or resident physician is allowed to add anything to the system. Every ingredient is added under the laminar air-flow hood. In this way, we minimize that type of problem.

Dr. Shils: The formulation of intravenous vitamin preparations for various purposes is a basic problem. One of the good things that should come out of this meeting is a recommendation that dosage of therapeutic vitamins be carefully reexamined and a new set of standards established.

Dr. Van Itallie: I agree. The Food and Nutrition Board is interested in developing standards for nutritional management of persons who are sick as well as for healthy individuals. Obviously such standards will have to be flexible. Perhaps they will be expressed as principles rather than as absolute values.

B Vitamins

Dr. Butterworth: Vitamin B_{12} is a water-soluble vitamin, but folic acid is only sparingly soluble. Yet it is in the water-soluble category.

Folic acid

Dr. Butterworth: Functions of folic acid are primarily those of transport of single carbon fragments. Conversion of the pteridine part of the folic acid molecule into biopterin has been conjectured, but there is evidence that this does not occur in man. The reactions involving carbon transport are concerned primarily with cell division, also DNA synthesis; therefore, deficiency of folic acid is manifested readily in the most rapidly dividing tissues. One first sees the effects of deficiency in the epithelial surfaces of the intestine and in the blood forming lines in the bone marrow.

After an oral dose of 5 mg folic acid is given, the urine in 24 hours will contain an average of about 25% to 45% of the administered dose. If one gives the same amount IV, the urine will contain 30% to 60% of it. We are talking about PGA, the synthetic precursor. We are not talking about the biologically active form. This fact must be emphasized. We have little information about the renal excretion of the predominant form that is in plasma, that is the 5-methyltetrahydrofolate. Folate binding proteins are in plasma, apparently.

Oral absorption of the monoglutamate and polyglutamate forms of the vitamin differ. We have looked at the excretion as a reflection of the absorption of folic acid variants containing 1, 2, 3, 4, 5, 6, or 7 glutamic acid residues on the chain. Following administration of the monoglutamate, less than 10% of the amount given—say 2% to 5%—will be found in the feces, while the urine will contain about 50%. When the dosage includes long-chain lengths, the urine will contain, in 24 hours, less than 5% to 10% of the administered dose, the feces as much as 40% to 50%. Hence, the absorption and excretion of folic acid are directly related to the chain length of the orally administered compound. Folic acid absorbed from the intestine goes through the liver first. When given parenterally, it may not experience the transformations it is exposed to when absorbed orally; hence, the renal losses are greater.

The daily requirement is still a controversial subject.[5] When Herbert put himself on a low folate diet,[6] it took him approximately four months to become depleted; subsequently, when he and his two technicians studied the effectiveness of graded levels to prevent the onset of a low plasma folate, they found that 35 to 50 μg of PGA prevented such depletion.

An unknown factor in Herbert's studies was the amount of polyglutamate that may have remained in the diet he consumed. The experimental subjects were on folate-low diets for prolonged periods. One may still question how much additional folic acid as polyglutamate they were receiving.

Sheehy[7] was first to report microgram amounts of folate as being effective in sprue in Puerto Rico. However, the subjects who responded to doses of 25 μg were exceptional cases and were not representative. Some patients did not respond to 200 μg of PGA in addition to the diet. Clearly more work is needed to establish the requirement for folic acid among normal subjects, also for patients with sprue and other disorders associated with folate deficiency.

The monoglutamate has the disadvantage of being lost in the urine while the polyglutamate has the disadvantage of not being readily or rapidly absorbed. This may mean that the gut cells absorb it and hold it temporarily, as they do iron. We don't know. What matters is that about half of what is eaten is absorbed and retained. If 200 μg/day are required, 400 μg must be consumed. This seems to be a reasonable figure for adults and is, I recall, the figure that is given in the last report from the World Health Organization. In pregnancy, the allowance is 800 μg/day; for very young infants, about 200 μg/day.

In parenteral nutrition, there is a margin of safety in the products that are available, allowing for renal excretion of 50% or 60% of the administered dosage. As I recall, Folbesyn® (Vitamins B with C) containing 3 mg of folic acid is the one used most often. I believe Dr. Shils' regimen calls for using this twice a week, is that right?

Dr. Shils: Once a week.

Dr. Butterworth: If only 1.5 mg of the 3 mg administered are lost in the urine, this still leaves a modest excess. As far as I know, there are no harmful effects associated with any excess of folic acid in this range. A small group of subjects took 45 mg/day orally for several weeks, as I recall, and became irritable, confused, fussy. They didn't like the side effects and quit. That is the only report of overdosage I know of.

Dr. Hodges: What about the reported antagonism between folic acid and the anticonvulsant drugs, particularly dilantin?

Dr. Butterworth: All the answers are not in. Everyone agrees that a megaloblastic anemia can occur in patients taking dilantin, and that it responds to folic acid. One can continue the anticonvulsant with added amounts of folic acid, increasing the convulsive tendency in people who previously were deficient. But these effects are not clearly established. Nor is the mechanism established. Some investigators report that dilantin interferes with absorption of polyglutamate. Preliminary evidence suggests that dilantin may interfere with the glucose-dependent pathway for the absorption of folic acid.

Dr. Van Itallie: Is there any advantage in giving one form of folic acid over others as the parenteral substance?

Dr. Butterworth: The main form available is synthetic PGA. The citrovorum factor (Leucovorin) is also available but is not widely used. I suppose people who have had dihydrofolic reductase blocked by aminopterin or such drugs might benefit from the use of the citrovorum factor. For routine purposes, I don't know of any advantage.

As for increased needs, have we mentioned, or should we mention, the problems of hemolysis, diarrhea, burns, and pregnancy?

Dr. Van Itallie: One more question! You mentioned the practice of giving folate once a week. From the standpoint of practicality, does it make sense? Would it be better to include folate as part of an IV package to be given every day, rather than once a week, with an appropriate adjustment of dosage, of course.

Dr. Shils: Our present practice stems from the unbalanced vitamin forms available for parenteral use. I use Folbesyn because it is available. I am concerned about periodic high doses, too. I would prefer that there be one single good IV parenteral vitamin preparation for daily use.

This raises another point which should be considered, however. I have read somewhere that, when one induces high blood levels, the tissue uptake of both water-soluble and fat-soluble vitamins is significantly greater than when relatively low levels obtain. If this is so, giving these nutrients less frequently in higher dosages, then falling off, might saturate tissues more efficiently. Does anyone have any information concerning that possibility?

Dr. Van Itallie: We are trying to get as close to the ideal combination of parenteral nutrients as possible but will leave the technique of formulating such a preparation to the drug industry. We should not, however, accept any product that is short of convenient. We would like to have in one preparation all of the ingredients to be added to an appropriate parenteral solution. We could then decide on daily recommendations under ideal circumstances of administration.

Mr. Klotz: Is Folbesyn a sodium salt? Because most of the time that will solubilize the folic acid. The pH of the hyperalimentation solution is usually well below the pH where it will go back to folic acid, and folic acid is soluble at 1.4 mg/liter. We figure that 1 mg/liter can be added to prevent precipitation. A precipitate wouldn't do any harm because it would be collected by a Millipore filter; but why create a precipitate if you don't have to?

Dr. Shils: We have examined our Millipore filters. I have not noticed any yellow precipitate.

Dr. Van Itallie: Can we give a tentative recommendation? Can we say something about the desirable folic acid activity we would like to see per day in a parenteral solution, taking into account urinary losses, the need for a substantial margin of safety, and the increased need associated with the repair of damaged tissue?

Dr. Butterworth: To answer your question specifically, and maybe precipitate discussion, I would say $1,000\mu g$/day would be a reasonable starting point.

Dr. Shils: May I ask why you go so high as 1 mg/day?

Dr. Butterworth: Because I would assume that $500\mu g$ are lost in the urine; $500\mu g$ are available for tissue repletion and utilization. This is a perfectly reasonable and nontoxic level. Some diets, although they might be consumed only occasionally, can provide up to 2,300 or $2,500\mu g$/day; hence, $500\mu g$/day is a reasonable allowance. But I can see that this amount could be higher in a patient who has hemolysis or a burn or is pregnant.

Vitamin B_{12}

Dr. Butterworth: Vitamin B_{12} does many of the things that folic acid does. It has a host of substituents. Methyl is one of more universal consequence; but cobalamin can also be substituted with the cyanide group, hydroxy group, nitro groups, and perhaps other larger fragments, the case apparently in methylmalonyl coenzyme A isomerization, in which, in essence, a glycine unit is replaced or relocated.

Hydroxycobalamin is better retained, the glomerular filtration of hydroxycobalamin being less than that of cyanocobalamin. Cyanocobalamin is excreted quantitatively by the glomerulus; hence it is used as a test for kidney function. Thus, the cyanocobalamin that is presented to the kidney is likely to be excreted. If, in the meanwhile, the cyano group has been replaced with something else, and the cobalamin can be utilized in tissue, this opportunity for urinary loss does not occur as readily. Cyanocobalamin is the form we usually obtain, although there are hydroxycobalamin preparations on the market. Neo-Betalin 12® (hydroxycobalamin, injection) is one of these and may be somewhat more physiological. It is an inexpensive water-soluble vitamin and is readily available in dosages of $100\mu g$/ml to $1,000\mu g$/ml.

The need for vitamin B_{12} is increased in patients who have had ileal resection or large portions of the stomach removed. Such procedures interfere with recycling of B_{12} which is excreted in the bile and normally reabsorbed in the terminal ileum.

The requirements for vitamin B_{12} have been estimated to range from 3 to $6\mu g$/day. Results of animal experiments indicate that high protein diets increase the requirement for vitamin B_{12}.[8] This is particularly true if the protein contains amino acids that lead to large amounts of branched-chain amino acids and to methylmalonate formation.

Dr. Van Itallie: What is your estimate of a likely daily dose?

Dr. Butterworth: I would say 10μg/day.

Dr. Shils: One of our patients was given Folbesyn once a week for over a year. Folbesyn contains 3 mg of folate and 15μg of vitamin B_{12} per dose. In our patient, the folic acid and B_{12} levels remained within normal ranges throughout. Thus, with as little as 15μg of vitamin B_{12} and 3 mg of folic acid given once a week, this patient, with normal renal function, was able to maintain her serum levels.

Dr. Butterworth: At 15μg/week of B_{12}, that would be about 60μg/month, which calculates to around 2μg/day. Some estimates are 3 to 5μg/day, depending on size. Was your patient a small person?

Dr. Shils: No, she was rather large. Is it true that 1μg/day intramuscularly will cure pernicious anemia?

Dr. Butterworth: It is said to be adequate. The statement that 1μg is equivalent to one unit of refined liver extract was questioned, and the amount people recycle varies.

Dr. Van Itallie: What about urinary losses of B_{12}? This is normally given intramuscularly, isn't it? If it were given in an intravenous solution, would that make a difference? Would this affect the loss?

Dr. Butterworth: With large doses—1,000μg of cyanocobalamin—the urinary loss is 90% + with an intramuscular dose. I assume that one might lose at least this much, if not more, through the intravenous route. Hydroxycobalamin is more slowly excreted, of course. I don't know the amounts of vitamin B_{12} present in the urine of a normal person. Do you know, Dr. Sandstead?

Dr. Sandstead: I don't; but vitamins given to patients during parenteral alimentation should be included in the IV, primarily because one does not like to stick needles into patients unnecessarily. Also, if the mixture is included in the IV, in whatever dosage pattern we finally recommend, one can be certain that the patient will get it. With a number of different persons involved in the care of the patient, administration of a single injection of certain vitamins once a week may be overlooked.

Dr. Van Itallie: Would you suggest a range for vitamin B_{12}? I assume that 10μg/day is a safe dose. Would you settle for 5 to 10μg/day?

Dr. Butterworth: Five would be a safe and reasonable lower limit of a range. As Dr. Shils has already pointed out, one can get by with even less. For parenteral nutrition, 5 to 10μg/day would be reasonable.

Riboflavin, Thiamin, Vitamin B_6

Col. Canham: Our studies, designed to evaluate the requirement for many of the water-soluble vitamins, were conducted with normal healthy adult males. The limited data available relating to the water-soluble vitamins in TPN were covered by Dr. Greene (see p 241).

Since many of the patients who will be placed on TPN will have been partially or completely starved prior to hospitalization, their vitamin pools will be depleted. Refeeding, even by TPN, may further deplete their stores and bring out biochemical or clinical evidence of deficiency. Symptoms of thiamin deficiency have been observed as early as seven days on a calorically adequate but thiamin-deficient diet. Biochemical evidence of vitamin B_6 deficiency can be produced in seven days, particularly if the intake of protein is high. Clinical evidence of riboflavin deficiency takes longer to develop. Horwitt reported that a high intake of protein will increase the need for riboflavin. Other investigators have not found this to be true.

While the definitive studies to identify the requirement for water-soluble vitamins during TPN have not been done, consideration should be given to use of two separate vitamin preparations. The oil-soluble vitamins should be separate from the water-soluble vitamins. We have not encountered clinical evidence of toxicity during studies involving prolonged administration of 300 mg/day of vitamin B_6 or 3 gm/day of ascorbic acid to normal male adults.

Dr. Van Itallie: Little information is available concerning the need for an appropriate dose level of parenterally or intravenously administered vitamins in sick individuals, and how this route of administration changes the amount we should give. No two patients are alike and we don't know what the range of change in requirements might be as influenced by the patient's illness. I propose, when we are giving parenteral vitamins, that we provide adequate nutritional insurance without harming the patient. Although it sounds sensible, this statement may not be correct, because we do not know how various disorders may affect the metabolism and excretion of vitamins.

Dr. Greene: The dose usually considered adequate for oral administration of a water-soluble vitamin should be increased if it is to be given intravenously. This statement is based on work with two patients and refers to the renal excretion of vitamins B_2 and B_6. Our results should not be construed to represent all subjects and all water-soluble vitamins, but the data suggest that renal losses increase when the parenteral route is used.

Dr. Van Itallie: By a factor of what?

Dr. Greene: From the data we have on two patients (and these were individuals at bed rest, not in a hypercatabolic state), the increase would be about 35% to 50%.

Dr. Shils: Would you elaborate on the study? Was it a rapid injection, or was it given slowly?

Dr. Greene: This was a constant intravenous infusion. When given orally, the vitamins were in tablet form and given at eight-hour intervals.

Dr. Shils: Over how many hours was the intravenous administration maintained?

Dr. Greene: The vitamins were mixed with the TPN solution and given continuously. Both subjects received total parenteral nutrition in amounts to meet calorie and protein requirements. One was given oral vitamins. The other received the vitamins intravenously. Clearly, the requirements for these and other vitamins are modified by catabolic state. The requirements for B_6 vary, depending on the amount of protein that is being utilized. The need for thiamin is modified by the concurrent intake of carbohydrate. Other vitamins are affected similarly by the nutritional and metabolic climate obtaining at the time.

One question concerns the precise effect of carbohydrate on thiamin requirements. Col. Canham can answer that better than I.

Col. Canham: Unfortunately the studies conducted by Sauberlich et al in our laboratory did not include comparison of the influence of the oral versus the parenteral route of carbohydrate administration. The effect of varying levels of carbohydrate intake upon the thiamin requirements was compared. Results indicated that the level of 0.33 mg of thiamin/1,000 kcal (recognized by a joint FAO/WHO Expert Group as the requirement) was correct. The RDA include the recommendation of 0.5 mg/1,000 kcal.

Dr. Sandstead: The RDA refer to the calorie level in the diet. What is the relationship between thiamin requirement and the metabolic rate of the patient? That is the more critical concern in the kind of patient we are talking about.

Dr. Van Itallie: I believe this is tied to the patient's overall energy needs, not to his resting metabolic rate only.

Dr. Sandstead: How about the patient with burns, the person who is a supermetabolizer due to stress? What happens to his thiamin?

Dr. Hodges: I don't know. May I comment on one other item? In addition to the factors we have discussed, we also should consider the potential pharmacologic effect of truly massive doses for each nutrient, because undoubtedly there will be instances where massive doses are used. Intravenous infusion of riboflavin has been reported to induce cardiac arrhythmias, even death, when given in large amounts.

Dr. Shils: We know that riboflavin and B_6 requirements are directly related to the level of protein. The question is whether just protein in general is responsible, or whether the amino acid pattern is critical. Certain amino acids may affect the requirement of one vitamin more than another.

Dr. Van Itallie: What emerges from this discussion is a great array of variables. We cannot rely on the RDA in all cases. We are not dealing with a standard intake of calories or protein. The only fact we can be sure of is that the patient is lying in bed or sitting in a chair. But we can't be certain that his disease is not creating a substantial increase in his energy needs and in his protein needs. Thus, if we are trying to formulate a mixture of vitamins to be given parenterally and if we accept the fact that these are relatively safe materials (aside from the fact that allergic reactions may occur), all that we can reasonably do is develop a policy statement on what level of intake might be appropriate for various individuals: Those who are exhibiting urinary losses of vitamins that are given intravenously; those who may develop diuresis as a result of glucose overload; and those whose nutritional requirements may be increased by disease and stress.

We should avoid giving too low a vitamin dose on the one hand, and avoid giving too high a dose on the other. Should we be setting upper limits on the vitamins that we recommend? Should we also indicate levels below which we would encounter a significant number of patients who are not getting enough?

Dr. Hodges: I suggest that we agree on a few simple points:

We do not know the desirable levels of intravenously administered vitamins.

In all probability there is a greater than normal rate of loss or wastage of a given vitamin, either because of increased urinary excretion, or because it is not bound to its appropriate carrier vehicle.

Any toxicity that may be inherent in a given nutrient might be exaggerated by giving it parenterally.

We should strive to select an arbitrary coefficient that is reasonable both in terms of effectiveness and safety. Two-fold has been suggested. That probably is a good number, realizing that we need definitive investigations to determine true requirements and rates of loss under this entirely artificial situation.

Dr. Sandstead: We have had to approach this problem empirically. I don't recall the levels of the water-soluble B vitamins in MVI, but utilizing their preparation, with one-third of an ampule to take care of the need for vitamins A and D, we did not observe clinical deficiency in patients to whom total parenteral alimentation was administered for several months. We have measured transketolase activity in a few of these individuals, and it was perfectly normal. I would think that quite empirically we should pick a level that is safe until more research has been done.

Dr. Van Itallie: Your approach is a good one. The point you make, as I understand it, is that we ought to consider what preparations have been given and how these have worked out. If deficiencies have not occurred at these levels, we can make the preliminary judgment that such levels are adequate. Then, maybe what we need to do is to work down from these levels if they seem to be unreasonably high. At least we know that we probably don't have to go much higher. From what you say, one-third of the ampule of USV parenteral preparation—which was so divided in order to avoid toxic quantities of vitamin A and D—seems to have been adequate in your hands. Perhaps Dr. Shils and others can tell us whether their experience has been similar.

Dr. Shils: Yes, our experience is similar. We have not noticed any evidence of deficiency in the water-soluble vitamins, but we are giving large doses. We should encourage drug companies to cooperate in making an experimental formulation based on the recommendations of this conference.

The preparation should be given to investigators who are willing to follow blood and urine levels and provide other appropriate information.

You said earlier that the Food and Nutrition Board is interested in this problem, but without more basic data we are right back to the earlier recommendations which were not generally acceptable.

Dr. Van Itallie: You are right. All the Food and Nutrition Board can do at the present time is what we are doing also—that is, to enunciate some principles and bemoan the fact that we lack hard data. Dr. Benson, do you have the formulation of the USV preparation with you so that we can refresh our memories about this?

Dr. Benson: USV's first preparation was introduced many years ago at a time of great need for multivitamin preparations of high dosage in treatment of deficiency states. I would like to be assured that you are dealing with therapeutic needs.

Dr. Van Itallie: We are not concerned at this point with conventional therapy of pellagra, beriberi, and other deficiency diseases. We are dealing with the maintenance of people who cannot take food by mouth, in awareness that there are special circumstances of the concomitant illness and the route of administration. This is not the same as therapy, as we understand it.

What we need is information concerning the precise composition of this parenteral vitamin formulation.

Contents of this multiple vitamin preparation* are as follows:

Ascorbic acid, 500 mg. If we divide that by 3, we have 167 mg, certainly within the range we were discussing.
Thiamin, 50 mg. One-third of that would be roughly 15 mg.
Riboflavin, 10 mg. We would be talking about 3 mg roughly.
Niacinamide, 100 mg. We are talking about 33 mg.
Pyridoxine, 15 mg. We are concerned with about 5 mg.
Dexpanthenol, 25 mg. Let's say, 8 mg.
Folic acid is not listed.
Vitamin B_{12} is not listed.
Vitamin A, 10,000 USP units.
Vitamin D, 1,000 USP units.
Vitamin E, 5 IU.

Dr. Sandstead: That is about what we used. Dr. Shils, are you aware of any deficiencies occurring with doses of this sort?

Dr. Shils: No. I give MVI only twice a week, and I would give even less except that I want to provide more vitamin E.

Dr. Van Itallie: If you give it twice a week, you are doing essentially what Dr. Sandstead is doing.

*According to *AMA Drug Evaluations* (ed 2, 1973), the contents of each 10 ml of solution or 5 ml of concentrate of this multiple vitamin preparation are: Ascorbic acid, 500 mg; Thiamin hydrochloride, 50 mg; Riboflavin, 10 mg; Niacinamide, 100 mg; Pyridoxine hydrochloride, 15 mg; Dexpanthenol, 25 mg; Vitamin A, 10,000 units; ergocalciferol, 1,000 units; d-α-tocopheryl acetate, 5 IU.

Dr. Shils: That is right.

May I raise a point concerning Dr. Greene's statement on increased excretion? Water-soluble vitamins—like minerals—are going to build up until they exceed the renal threshold. Even provision of relatively small amounts of vitamins will gradually increase the blood level and the tissues will remove them until they become repleted. Then, the vitamins will increasingly spill as the blood level rises. We should look at such spillage as reflecting the fact that the renal threshold has now been reached and exceeded. The tissues probably are well stocked at this point, even though spillage is going on. Such spillage does *not* imply an *increased* requirement.

Dr. Van Itallie: If I understand you, the only problem with this argument is that vitamins are consumed by mouth normally, so that nature's way of dealing with the renal threshold involves spillage after the vitamin has traveled a certain route. We can't assume that nutrients added directly to the systemic circulation are necessarily going to be handled in an appropriate way. Thus, there would be some difficulty in interpreting the spillage of a given vitamin into the parenteral circulation.

Dr. Shils: I am not saying that we do know. I wanted to call attention to the vitamin thresholds and point out that we don't know what their significance is for intravenous feeding.

Col. Canham: One must distinguish between excretion of metabolites of the vitamin and excretion of the vitamin. The amount of metabolite excreted in the face of a deficient intake appears to be proportional to the rate of utilization of the body stores; but the amount of vitamin in the urine appears to be proportional to the intake. Consider a man on a vitamin C-deficient diet. Reduced ascorbic acid will disappear from the urine early during the deficiency, while the decrease in metabolites occurs in an exponential fashion. Blood or plasma ascorbic acid level will still be normal after cessation of the urinary excretion of reduced ascorbic acid and the blood values may remain in what is considered the normal range until his ascorbate body pool has been sufficiently reduced. In vitamin A deficiency, a similar picture is observed. The level of excretion of the urinary metabolites drops faster than the plasma levels of the vitamin. A conservation mechanism appears to exist.

Dr. Van Itallie: To summarize:

Information is sparse as to desirable quantities of water-soluble vitamins in parenteral solutions.

The most reliable information we have is derived from the experience of those who have administered USV parenteral preparations for various periods of time. Apparently no reports are available on toxicity or deficiency resulting from such treatment. With this and additional information based on studies of normal individuals, we are left with figures that are purely empirical.

We agree that a mixture should be available to be added to parenteral solutions on a daily basis. We would start empirically using as a point of departure about one-third of the quantity of water-soluble vitamins present in the current USV parenteral preparation (see p 290).

Any recommendations we might make beyond this point would be based on experimental data. Such data should be developed from studies of nutrient blood and tissue levels and excretion rates in patients with a variety of medical problems who are carefully followed during total parenteral nutrition.

FAT-SOLUBLE VITAMINS

Vitamin A

Dr. Van Itallie: Should fat-soluble vitamins be in these parenteral mixtures? Should retinol be included, or should it be retinoic acid, or what? Do we need it at all, considering how long it takes to develop vitamin A deficiency?

Dr. Hodges: It takes between one and two years of sustained deprivation for vitamin A deficiency to develop in normal middle-aged men who were well fed initially. We know from the work done in Canada[9] and confirmed in this country[10] that evaluation of liver samples from routine autopsies in our city hospitals shows between 15% and 35% incidence of deficiency. By that, we mean that the liver tissue contained fewer than $40\mu g$ of retinol per gram of liver tissue. If such a person who had $10\mu g$—and that is not uncommon—were to have some disaster or illness that necessitated total parenteral nutrition, he might become vitamin A-deficient within a month or two.

You ask if we should provide vitamin A in parenteral solutions. The answer is yes, we should. Vitamin A does many things, some of which we don't understand. It functions in growth and possibly in wound healing and tissue repair. It has a series of functions in maintenance of epithelial integrity. Most membranes depend upon some of the functions of vitamin A for their preservation and function. Therefore, vitamin A must be considered an essential in total parenteral nutrition.

What is the best way to give it? Shall we use water-miscible preparations? Shall we use retinoic acid? Shall we give vitamin A intramuscularly? How shall we give it?

One of our experiences may bear on this. When we were preparing to induce vitamin A deficiency in a group of volunteers, we drew a sample of their blood, separated the plasma, and mixed it with retinol acetate, which was ^{14}C-tagged. We then homogenized it, reinfused it intravenously, and followed CO_2 excretion in expired air. Within 48 hours they had lost between 40% and 60% of the administered dose.

The intravenous route is not physiologic. We gave the same type of dose to a man orally. He absorbed it and catabolized less than half as much. The gut is smarter than we are in moving nutrients from the outside into the circulating blood.

I wonder how many patients who need total parenteral nutrition still have enough gastrointestinal function so that we could put in a few milliliters of an oily or an aqueous solution containing essential nutrients? This might not work, but the concept has possibilities.

Question: How much vitamin A?

Dr. Hodges: Assuming that the 5,000 IU figure represents a target, I would oppose doubling this because of potential toxicity.

Dr. Van Itallie: You suggested, though, that, if given parenterally, up to 60% of the administered dose might be lost.

Dr. Hodges: Intravenously, this is true, yes.

Dr. Van Itallie: Are you prepared to accept 2,000 IU per day as adequate?

Dr. Hodges: No. We could afford to go a bit higher, but we don't have enough data on which to base a firm decision.

We found that people who were deficient experimentally had different tissue levels of requirement. We could reverse dark adaptation with $75\mu g$/day. We found that $150\mu g$ were necessary to correct the electronystagmogram. Advancing to cutaneous changes, we needed in excess of 1,200 mg. This evidence suggests that each different function of the vitamin requires a different amount; thus, when dealing with what amounts to tissue maintenance and repair, we may need substantial amounts. Therefore, I would not object—if we are going to give it as an emulsion intravenously—to providing vitamin A in somewhat higher amounts. (For convenience, conversion of micrograms to IU can be approximated by multiplying by three.)

Dr. Van Itallie: Seven or eight thousand IU equivalents of vitamin A, as retinol?

Vitamin D

Dr. Hodges: That is reasonable. Let us progress to another nutrient, vitamin D. According to some investigators vitamin D is an essential in adults. The active form is considered to be a hormone, 1,25-dihydroxycholecalciferol. Its main function is to enhance calcium absorption. One wonders what the function is in one whose gastrointestinal tract is temporarily nil. I don't know.

Also, it has been many years since the ergosterol mechanism was demonstrated. What would happen if we used an ultraviolet light to give people a brief sun treatment each day? Would they make enough vitamin D to cover their needs?

Comment: We tried that.

Dr. Hodges: Did you? Did it work?

Comment: We had no way of measuring.

Dr. Van Itallie: Maybe Haddad will work that out using his special assay procedure.[11]

Vitamin E

Dr. Hodges: There is still another consideration: vitamin E, or the tocopherols. If we are giving fat emulsions, especially if we are using the poly-unsaturated fats such as soybean oil or cottonseed oil, we will probably increase the need for tocopherols. Again we are dealing with a lipid-soluble substance. How are we going to administer it? Are we going to emulsify it? If we are going to administer fat emulsions, it may be wise to incorporate the tocopherols in them. Or it may be that during processing the natural toco-pherols already present in these vegetable oils will not have been destroyed. I would propose using 50 mg of vitamin E.

Dr. Sandstead: A water-soluble vitamin E may be added to our solu-tions, but we do not know whether it is metabolized properly.

Vitamin K

Dr. Hodges: We must also consider vitamin K. Many of these patients have hepatic disease, or at least hepatic dysfunctions. If they have superim-posed upon this a lack of vitamin K, their prothrombin time may be prolonged, and they may have a bleeding problem.

We do not know the best way to give vitamin K, but we have water-soluble substances available, some of the quinone derivatives.

Dr. Van Itallie: Vitamin K_1 is the best by far; I propose 3 to 5 mg/day. How do you want to give vitamin A? As retinol?

Dr. Hodges: Retinol equivalent, at least.

Dr. Van Itallie: That would be 7,000 to 8,000 IU of vitamin A.

Dr. Hodges: Yes.

Dr. Van Itallie: Vitamin E, 50 mg?

Dr. Hodges: That is generous.

Dr. Van Itallie: Vitamin K_1, 3 to 5 mg/day?

Dr. Hodges: That would be plenty.

Dr. Van Itallie: Vitamin D?

Dr. Hodges: Question mark.

Dr. Van Itallie: That is, an active form like 1,25-dihydroxycholecalciferol when it becomes available.

MACROMINERALS

Calcium

Dr. Shils: Administration—by four different groups—of calcium, phos-phorus, and magnesium to adults is illustrated in Table 6 (see p 260). Most TPN regimes provide an amount of calcium ranging usually between 200 and 400 mg/day.

One of the characteristics of parenteral formulas is that their origina-tors do not disclose the thought processes that led them to a given formula. It would be an interesting intellectual exercise to have these people put their rationales on paper. If one assumes that an adult needs about 800 mg of calcium per day (in accord with the RDA) and that approximately one-fourth of this amount is absorbed, one could expect an adult to absorb about 200 mg/day. But individuals getting fewer than 800 mg/day do well as far as calcium balance is concerned. The evidence is clear that the absorption of calcium bears some relationship to the previous level of calcium intake and the calcium needs of the individual. Hence, I don't believe there is an absolute requirement for calcium.

If one has patients who are mainly or totally at bed rest, is there danger in giving intravenous calcium when they probably are going to resorb calcium from bone? In such bedridden patients, might additional calcium not increase the risk of calcium deposition in soft tissues? Kinetic studies with calcium would provide information that would help us make decisions about the problem.

For an individual who is active and out of bed, 200 mg presumably would be a reasonable amount to give.

Phosphorus

Dr. Shils: No question remains about the need to maintain serum inorganic phosphate levels. Various workers, including ourselves, suggest that approximately 300 to 350 mg/day are adequate to maintain normal serum levels. (See Table 3, p 258.) More is necessary when TPN is instituted in pre-viously debilitated patients since the phosphorus level often falls markedly.

Magnesium

Dr. Shils: The range for magnesium supplied by various research groups is tremendous, from 4 to 25 mEq/day. (See Table 6, p 260.) The available data are inadequately supported by balance data. Between 8 and 10 mEq/day for an individual without tubular defect or gastrointestinal losses should be sufficient.

Dr. Friend: I have a question about your reference to phosphorus. This is the elemental phosphorus, not the phosphate ion, right? Have you made the conversions from the reports and the literature to the elemental phosphorus in your slides?

Dr. Shils: A good point. We are in a period when milliequivalents and millimols are fashionable. In a discussion of phosphorus one has to be careful, because the form of phosphorus in which we are principally interested is orthophosphate, $HPO_4^=$ and $H_2PO_4^-$. The ratio of $H_2PO_4^-$ to $HPO_4^=$ depends on pH. In blood at pH 7.4 there is a ratio of 4 to 1 of the divalent to monovalent ion. But in urine, with a pH about 5, you are dealing with a ratio which is altered to 4 to 100. For this reason, use of milliequivalents of phosphate is confusing.

We should express the data as millimols or milligrams of phosphorus; one millimol equals 31 milligrams of phosphorus. I have expressed my data as milligrams of phosphorus in the form of inorganic phosphate.

Dr. Sandstead: In the past we had not thought it necessary to add calcium or phosphorus to intravenous solutions for adults, particularly during relatively short periods of TPN. We had not recognized difficulties in adults that could be attributed to lack of calcium and phosphorus. But if TPN is provided for long intervals, we believe both calcium and phosphorus should be added. Perhaps we have been wrong not to add calcium and phosphorus to all solutions.

We have had some experiences with magnesium which suggest to us that giving fewer than 15 to 20 mEq/day of magnesium may not be wise if the patient is highly anabolic. We observed a syndrome consisting of quadriplegia, hysteria, hyperventilation and other emotional abnormalities that occurred in a patient who was retaining approximately 12 mEq/day of magnesium. His abnormalities appeared to be relieved soon after extra magnesium was administered. He was receiving 2,700 kilocalories and 85 grams of protein as amino acids, using the FreAmine preparation. He also was receiving between 150 and 200 mEq/day of potassium. As a consequence of regional enteritis with chronic diarrhea, he had been magnesium-depleted. He was putting on weight at a rapid rate. He did well for about four weeks, then he began to experience the syndrome described above.

By trying a variety of treatments, we found that magnesium dramatically relieved his quadriplegia, his abnormal behavior, and other problems on the first day given. Twenty-five mEq/day in the intravenous infusion had apparently not been adequate to meet his requirements. Unfortunately the seriousness of his illness did not allow repeated study of the syndrome, so our observations must be considered only tentative. In addition, at the time we saw the patient we were not aware of syndromes caused by phosphorus depletion. I cannot tell you, therefore, whether he was also phosphate-depleted, or whether he would have responded to phosphate.

Potassium

Dr. Sandstead: One factor that may have contributed to his problem was the large amount of potassium we were giving him. Investigators at the USDA Soils and Nutrition Laboratory in Ithaca, New York, have found that grass tetany, or acute tetany in nursing cows on fresh grass, is due, at least in part, to change in the ratio of potassium to magnesium intake. When cows eat the young spring grass, which is high in potassium, they may become tetanic, without any change in their magnesium intake, and are responsive to therapy with extra magnesium. This effect of potassium on magnesium metabolism is in contradistinction to potassium wastage induced by magnesium deficiency described by Dr. Shils and others.

Potassium requirements in parenteral alimentation are related to patient's previous experience. If the patient has had prolonged protein-calorie depletion, as has been the case in patients we have seen, one can assume that the total body potassium is depressed. Providing TPN with a high carbohydrate load will precipitate a drop in serum potassium also. If the patient is on digitalis, digitalis toxicity and other complications are likely to ensue. Thus, consideration of the amount of potassium added to the mixture is critical.

Dr. Dudrick reported that a patient receiving TPN required 300 mEq/day of potassium to maintain a normal serum potassium. We have seen patients who required 200 mEq/day. This may have been related to their previous state of depletion and because they were receiving 2,700 or 3,000 kilocalories as glucose. As the patient becomes anabolic, potassium moves into the cell. It is the primary intracellular cation. Potassium requirements are variable and require close monitoring. The need for potassium is hard to predict. We usually start with about 120 mEq/day and increase the amount as indicated. One useful and convenient way of monitoring is to measure the 24-hour urinary potassium excretion.

Sodium

Dr. Sandstead: For the elderly TPN patient, 100 mEq/day of sodium may be a high intake. Initially I recommend 40 mEq/day, increasing further from that initial level if necessary. If one finds biochemical evidence that the patient needs more, sodium is easily provided.

Dr. Weston: We started total parenteral nutrition about 10 or 12 years ago and were successful as a consequence of developing a 50% dextrose solution with 1 mg of hydrocortone (Melodex). This preparation permitted us to give a 50% dextrose solution into a peripheral vein as long as we infused it for no more than 17 to 20 hours.

We went from arm to arm each day and were able to provide TPN with remarkable results. We used a 10% protein hydrolysate which included a 5% alcohol solution. When we piggybacked this into the 50% dextrose solution, we were able to give 3,400 to 4,000 kilocalories a day.

The reason we were successful—and the reason Dr. Dudrick was successful—in demonstrating that total parenteral nutrition is feasible was the fact that from the beginning we recognized the need for potassium. We also recognized the need for magnesium, and we recognized the need for phosphorus.

In review, remember that, although the principal intracellular cation is potassium, magnesium comprises one-quarter of total intracellular cations. For each gram of nitrogen that is deposited during tissue anabolism, approximately 2.7 to 3 mEq of potassium are needed. If a patient develops a 10-gm positive nitrogen balance—as some of these people will early in nutritional rehabilitation—that process requires a minimum of 30 mEq of potassium. At the same time, one quarter as much magnesium is needed just for the newly laid down tissue. In addition there is a much more important consideration: Most of these patients are, or have been, desperately sick, and many of them develop what Elkington called the "sick cell syndrome."

Characteristic of the sick cell syndrome is an inability of the cells, by virtue of their metabolic disorder, to maintain a normal intracellular cation concentration. To maintain high potassium intracellular concentration versus low extracellular concentration means that the sodium pump has to be working efficiently. Thus, intracellular potassium and intracellular magnesium may be low in the sick patient. This is why, when you provide such patients with total parenteral nutrition and follow their balances or do exchangeable potassiums on them, you find that for 10, 15, or 20 days they can have a positive potassium balance of anywhere from 30 to 50 or 70 mEq/day; and these patients generally need about one quarter as much magnesium. This is to replete their depleted stores as well as to cover their anabolic needs.

Initially, when we started our studies, we added 1 gm of magnesium sulfate to each liter that we gave, roughly 16 mEq. We were providing as much as 50 mEq/day of magnesium, never finding any difficulty with elevated serum magnesium levels. This was in patients with good renal function. We gave large amounts of phosphorus, too. We gave as much as 80 mEq/day of phosphorus. We measured our phosphorus in milliequivalents because a solution was prepared for us as potassium phosphate. We gave a good deal of our potassium as potassium phosphate, and the potassium phosphate solution was buffered to 7.4, so that the average valence was 1.8, the classical picture. Thus, we knew exactly what we were giving.

As a consequence of giving 200 to 300 mEq/day of potassium, 80 to 90 mEq/day of phosphorus, and this amount of magnesium, we promoted a much more positive nitrogen balance. This is what you will find. Others are discovering the same thing when they measure nitrogen balances.

Question: How high was the magnesium?

Dr. Weston: We went to 50 mEq but soon decided we did not need that. What we recommend is to stay between 25 and 40 mEq/day of magnesium.

Question: You gave how many grams?

Dr. Weston: We gave 3 gm of magnesium sulfate.

Question: Isn't it about 8?

Dr. Weston: No. If you calculate it out, it is not. The ampule says 8¼ mEq, but it is not. It is 8¼ millimols.

Dr. Shils: One should not forget that magnesium sulfate comes as the heptahydrate, that is, with 7 molecules of water, and this must be considered in calculating magnesium content.

Dr. Weston: May I stress again the importance of phosphorus. For each gram of nitrogen laid down in tissue, 65 mg of phosphorus is required. Therefore, if you are going to a positive nitrogen balance of 10 gm, you also need 650 mg of phosphorus. This applies to the sulfate also. An equivalent amount of sulfate is needed.

My plea is that we provide the very sick patient with all the nutrients he needs in slight excess initially. Dr. Sandstead made an equally important point about dealing with a glycogen-depleted liver in the early days of total parenteral nutrition. For each gram of glycogen that is deposited, approximately 0.34 mEq of potassium and an equivalent amount of phosphate must be put down. Thus, the equivalent of 50 mEq of potassium is needed merely to replete liver glycogen and quite a large amount of phosphorus in those first few days to replete liver phosphate as glycogen phosphate.

I suggest that all of you, when you return to your investigations, increase magnesium, potassium, and phosphorus. You should note an increased retention of magnesium, phosphorus, and potassium, also an improvement in nitrogen balance.

As for sodium, I agree with Dr. Sandstead. There is no blanket recommendation for sodium administration. The amount of sodium one provides has to be dictated by the needs of the patient; starting with a relatively small amount of sodium, one can always add sodium. Why be burdened with the problem of extracting sodium from a patient who may be a salt retainer?

But, let me also caution you that sodium depletion can develop if you do not pay attention to the sodium requirements. You simply have to rely on titration. Fortunately you can easily measure sodium and potassium output in the urine, as has been indicated, and you can very easily monitor serum, sodium, and potassium.

In conclusion, I recommend from 150 to 200 or 250 mEq of potassium for very sick patients; small amounts of sodium, 25 to 40 mEq/day for such patients, and as much as 150 or 200 mEq for individuals who are losing larger amounts of sodium; and somewhere between 20 and 40 mEq of magnesium. I suggest about 600 mg/day of phosphorus initially. It can always be reduced.

Dr. Van Itallie: Should these macronutrients be given together? How much should be given? Opinions on these questions vary with the experience and preconceptions of the physician taking care of the patient, also with respect to the patient's nutritional status. Thus, I question whether we could ever formulate a standard solution containing a suitable mixture of these substances or whether we should provide these individually, according to principles we might establish through research.

When we add potassium to a parenteral solution, we usually add it separately. Wouldn't the same apply to magnesium, calcium, and phosphorus?

Dr. Shils: Unlike vitamins—certainly unlike the water-soluble vitamins, which I would like to see in one daily dose formulation—I would prefer to have each of the macrominerals given in a separate solution according to the patient's needs. I am not convinced that calcium is safe in all instances. I would want to be able to handle magnesium in the amounts required by the patient, and the same applies to potassium and sodium. On the basis of information that is coming through, I believe that phosphorus is absolutely essential, but again it will vary from patient to patient. Thus, I agree that the minerals ought to be given on an individual basis.

Dr. Van Itallie: All we can do in our consideration of these macrominerals is to set ranges which have been found useful and which seem to make sense nutritionally, but with the admonition that they be used on an individual basis by physicians according to their best judgment.

Dr. Ruberg: I was interested in Dr. Sandstead's remarks on the use of calcium and phosphorus in solutions for adults. Since you have seen no significant difficulties, what solutions were you using?

Dr. Sandstead: FreAmine.

Dr. Ruberg: We looked into the incidence of hypophosphatemia in a series of patients.[12]

Dr. Weston: That is a different matter. Hypophosphatemia is precisely what one would predict if phosphorus is not given. If you wait long enough, you will get the symptoms that go with it.

Dr. Ruberg: Essentially Dr. Weston is correct. Monitoring serum levels in a series of 20 consecutive patients receiving solutions without phosphorus, we found 100% incidence of hypophosphatemia. The incidence of what you might call significant hypophosphatemia (ie, patients with symptoms) was on the order of 1 to 2 out of 20, but this depends on the level to which you drive the serum phosphorus. Significant symptoms were observed in patients with serum phosphorus levels below 1 mg/100 ml. This does not occur, of course, in the great majority of patients. This is why, perhaps, in our earlier series—using fibrin hydrolysate, which did not have calcium and phosphorus, and using amino acid solutions for a while—we did not recognize this problem, because the incidence of obvious complications from hypophosphatemia is low. The incidence of measurable hypophosphatemia, however, will be 100%. For this reason, the addition of phosphorus to solutions is indicated. We can't predict which patient with hypophosphatemia is going to develop the syndrome described by Dr. Shils. We have seen this picture in 8 or 10 patients receiving a variety of solutions.

I suggest that the amount of phosphorus required to prevent hypophosphatemia is proportional to the amount of parenteral solution given and is not necessarily a matter of absolute daily requirement. Thus, the more solution given, the greater the phosphorus requirement.

Dr. Van Itallie: Do you want to estimate the range of phosphorus needed under such circumstances?

Dr. Ruberg: Dr. Shils may criticize me for using milliequivalents, but the solutions our pharmacy uses for adding phosphorus to our parenteral nutrition solutions are labeled in milliequivalents per milliliter. Perhaps criticism concerning terminology of units should be directed to the companies preparing solutions. Because there is no uniform system for labeling, different groups of investigators list their recommendations in different types of measurements. We are recommending between 6 and 20 mEq/liter of phosphorus per liter of solution to prevent hypophosphatemia.

We have seen a case of magnesium deficiency similar to the one Dr. Sandstead described. This patient was receiving from 8 to 16 mEq/day in an anabolic state. He gained approximately 20 pounds in 30 days. Despite magnesium replacement at the level we indicated earlier, the patient developed a neurologic syndrome with dysarthria and some paresthesias, which was corrected by adjusting the levels of magnesium.

Dr. Van Itallie: Can you describe the syndrome you have seen with phosphate deficiency?

Dr. Ruberg: Yes, although Dr. Shils pointed out most of its features. We observed circumoral tingling, fingertip and extremity paresthesia. Often a dysarthric speech occurs, together with some mental confusion and an abnormal respiratory pattern, not exactly hyperventilation. We have seen this in a number of cases of hypophosphatemia, usually in patients exhibiting phosphorus levels of 0.4 to 0.6 mg/100 ml. The syndrome was reversed with the addition of phosphorus, but on a delayed basis. Some of the specific metabolic abnormalities (eg, decreased levels of ATP and 2,3-DPG) are fairly rapidly reversed. Improvement of the overall syndrome of hypophosphatemia may require two to three weeks despite a return of the serum phosphorus level to normal. This raises the question: what is the tissue phosphorus level at that time?

Dr. Van Itallie: How long does it take for this syndrome to develop during total parenteral feeding?

Dr. Ruberg: We have seen it appear in one to two weeks or occasionally even longer. It varies, reflecting, perhaps, the prior state of the patient in terms of phosphorus balance when TPN is started. We have seen it appear within one to two weeks on solutions containing no phosphorus.

Dr. Shils: Would you tell us about the development of hypocalcemia which is reported as occurring when you gave phosphate to some patients?

Dr. Ruberg: I have never produced this type of hypocalcemia, because I have always followed the recommendations of Dr. Dudrick not to give phosphorus alone. These situations arose in patients who were hypophosphatemic initially. Infusion of solutions containing approximately 10 mEq/liter of phosphorus over a period of 6 to 8 hours in hypophosphatemic patients in an attempt to raise the serum phosphorus level rapidly resulted in a significant hypocalcemia.

Dr. Shils: Significant to the point of symptoms?

Dr. Ruberg: Symptoms of hypocalcemia were precipitated in hypophosphatemic patients. As I said, I have never done this, because I have always given calcium during phosphorus infusion. This is the reason we recommend the addition of both calcium and phosphorus to IV nutritional solutions. In all of the patients we studied who became hypophosphatemic without calcium and while receiving phosphorus, the serum calcium remained normal. In general, the serum magnesium also remains fairly stable with replacement in the lower range that we have discussed today. The calcium remains normal despite the fact that the phosphorus decreases. We tried to discover where the phosphorus goes. We have seen—paralleling the serum phosphorus decrease—a similar decrease in urinary phosphorus. In some patients excretion levels may start in the range of 300 to 1,000 mg/day, then diminish to 5 to 10 mg/day, a significant reduction. Presumably, as Dr. Weston suggested, this is because of intracellular use of the phosphorus.

Dr. Van Itallie: Are you saying that when we administer phosphorus, we should always give calcium as well?

Dr. Ruberg: We are saying that we have to give phosphorus, and we must give it in a safe way. In our experience, at least, that means a concurrent administration of calcium. This might not be necessary in every case, but we have not had any problems with such an approach.

Dr. Van Itallie: Since a significant number of people who develop hypophosphatemia are on total parenteral nutrition for more than a week, your notion is to prevent it rather than to have to treat it. Is that right?

Dr. Ruberg: Yes sir.

Dr. Weston: I don't understand why this problem exists. Data in the literature establish the facts that we alluded to before. All one has to do is pick up Albright's text, look in the appendix on how to run a metabolic ward, and read his suggestions on analyzing metabolic data. The facts are clear enough. One does not have to worry about the necessity for giving calcium with phosphate, as long as one starts out with the correct assumption that, when a patient goes into positive nitrogen balance, he lays down phosphate, magnesium, and potassium with the protein. In such a situation, phosphate, magnesium, and potassium should be given in significant amounts.

We have established a need for phosphorus, but I want to go further. I want to make the point that the worst index of how much phosphorus to give is necessarily the serum phosphorus level. You are measuring serum phosphorus levels in individuals in whom you are infusing a phosphorus solution. Thus, a normal phosphorus level does not tell you much. Your observation was better. As you measure the urine for phosphorus content, the amount of phosphorus you give intravenously should be a function of what you find in the urine. You continue to increase the phosphate in your infusion, Dr. Ruberg, without getting to a ridiculously high level. You try to do it until you cover the positive balance in the patient. Fortunately these patients don't put out stools.

You are giving an infusion that you prepare. You know what the intake is. It is easy to do a metabolic study. You measure the phosphorus in the urine, the potassium in the urine, magnesium in the urine, and you know what you are infusing. You give enough magnesium, enough potassium, and enough phosphorus to more than supply what you need for positive balance. You described patients in whom the 24-hour urinary phosphorus went down to 5 mg during TPN. I have seen patients whose urine contained no phosphorus; on concentrating the urine, there was still no phosphorus, if phosphorus was not being infused.

Manufacturers are seeking a single electrolyte preparation that can be given to every patient. We agree that this shotgun approach is not feasible. To the contrary, you have to rely on titration. Broad ground rules can be set up for electrolytes to be given, but to prepare a single electrolyte additive for the general practitioner to use with ease is an unwise step.

Dr. Friend: I have two questions. The first is simple, perhaps trite, to Dr. Weston. In the calculations of the additions of electrolytes, are those electrolytes already present within the products taken into account? If they are not, you are giving more than you have claimed.

Dr. Weston: We always calculate that.

Dr. Friend: We have listed four cations. What about the anions? What are we going to do about them? Are you going to add magnesium sulfate?

What about the sulfate? Are you going to add calcium gluconate? What about the gluconate ion? With potassium chloride, you are adding chloride, and with sodium, you can add sodium chloride, but there again you are imposing a chloride load. My question arises from a conviction that discussion of macroions or elements should include the total additive, not just the single cation.

Dr. Weston: This is a good question, and we should devote time to it. I use calcium gluconate, a useful form of calcium. I generally give 200 mg/day of calcium, roughly 2 gm of calcium gluconate put in the first liter for each day so that it does not interfere with the phosphate.

To provide the phosphate and also to neutralize the excess chloride in those preparations which we will use until the newer amino acid solutions come out—in these the anion is going to be acetate, which is metabolized—I give potassium in three forms: potassium chloride, potassium phosphate as my principal source, and potassium acetate for additional potassium in a form which provides bicarbonate precursor.

The same applies to sodium. I use sodium as a concentrate, 3 or 4 mEq/ml, and either sodium chloride or sodium acetate. The acetate is used instead of bicarbonate, particularly in the calcium solutions to avoid precipitating the calcium.

Then there is the problem of the metabolic acidosis that develops to a greater degree when you use the free amino acid solutions than when you use the protein hydrolysates. This may be due to the nature of the amino acids contained in the mixture, also to the excess chloride.

Recognizing that there is a potential for metabolic acidosis with hyperchloremia, you try to correct for this by using more acetate forms. You use some sodium acetate, some potassium acetate, and end up with a solution designed to correct acidosis for the individual patient, if it is going to develop. By use of such additives, one is able to devise a proper solution.

I suggest metabolic studies on the effects of nitrogen balance of increasing magnesium and phosphorus, also potassium intake.

Dr. Ruberg: Dr. Weston said he thought that measuring serum levels of various ions (eg, serum phosphorus levels) was of little value in determining the effectiveness of the therapy, and that measuring urinary values was of more significance. What is the opinion on this? Measurement of urinary levels appears to be of little value, particularly in the case of phosphorus.

Dr. Van Itallie: I understood Dr. Weston to mean that levels obtained while infusing a substance don't reflect the individual's nutritional status, just as when you give glucose intravenously, the blood glucose concentration does not have too much meaning during the infusion period.

Dr. Shils: If you are infusing, say, 300 mg in a liter, this should not change the serum level, particularly if the phosphorus is given slowly. One *can* use serum phosphorus levels if it is a slow infusion.

Dr. Ruberg: That is 30 mg/100 ml.

Dr. Shils: Yes. If it is going in slowly, and if you take samples from the opposite arm, it doesn't make that much difference.

Dr. Ruberg: That is the circulating level of the phosphorus?

Dr. Shils: I think the tissues are going to take it out. In studies in which we infused high amounts of potassium and took blood samples out of the opposite arm, we discerned very little influence on the serum level. I assume the same thing happens with phosphorus.

Dr. Ruberg: That is my point. Dr. Munro has mentioned the validity of measuring serum levels of amino acids despite the fact that this was during constant infusion. I believe there is a great deal of significance in measuring levels of the elements we are talking about.

Dr. Sandstead: One more comment! We have suggested ranges of minerals that can be added to parenteral fluids. From the pharmacist's point of view, it is desirable to have a baseline electrolyte solution as a point of departure. This is the initial solution on which patients can be started as far as electrolytes are concerned. The availability of such a solution will allow the house officer to begin parenteral alimentation prior to receiving complete chemistries on the patient. Thus if he wishes to begin TPN in the evening and the laboratory operates only in the morning, he will be able to order a standard mixture, which is conservative. It should contain electrolytes sufficient to cover most contingencies. The data which describe the true electrolyte status of the patient will be available subsequently and the electrolyte orders can be modified to meet the patient's needs.

Of course it is necessary to know the BUN before deciding that 80 mEq of potassium and 10 mEq of magnesium can be administered with safety.

Dr. Van Itallie: Perhaps the chairman and rapporteur can work out a suggested baseline solution.

Mr. Klotz: If we have a baseline to go from we can calculate what must be added to amounts of minerals already present in certain solutions, such as amino acid preparations. We develop such a baseline and use it to make a standard formula. When a particular patient deviates in his needs, we can modify it at that time. But at least we have a baseline solution available for quality control and for discussion between physician and pharmacist.

Dr. Van Itallie: These points are well taken. We know that when parenteral feeding begins, conditions are not always optimal to calculate the most desirable quantities of each of these electrolytes or macrominerals. It makes sense to have the kind of basic mixture Dr. Sandstead is talking about. This could provide some nutritional insurance until more enlightened calculations can be made, based on subsequent laboratory data.

As I recall, the basic mixture suggested included the following ranges of macrominerals:

Calcium	100 to 300 mg/day
Phosphorus	100 to 300 mg/day
Magnesium	4 to 50 mEq/day
Potassium	80 to 200 mEq/day
Sodium	20 to 80 mEq/day

MICROELEMENTS

Dr. Sandstead: We don't know much about trace elements. The trace elements essential for man are the transition elements, probably all of them, in addition to elements on the right hand side of the periodic table near iodine.

What these elements do is in some cases not known, but it is our reasoning teleologically that if they are required by any form of life, they are probably required by all higher forms of life; this is because we originate from the sea, and simple organisms clearly require these substances.

Iron

Dr. Sandstead: We should be concerned about iron in patients who are receiving parenteral alimentation for long periods of time. I do not recommend adding iron to intravenous solutions. If one is unable to give oral iron to a patient, one can restore iron by careful administration of intramuscular iron. But one should realize that intramuscular iron is not without risk. Anaphylaxis may occur and is even more likely with intravenous administration. Thus, it should only be given by a physician.

Dr. Hodges: What is your opinion on administration of packed red cells as a source of iron in these patients?

Dr. Sandstead: Unnecessary transfusions are not wise because of the high incidence of hepatitis. In some centers, one of every 200 transfusions is said to be associated with hepatitis. Transfusions should be avoided unless indicated for bleeding or other cause of rapid erythrocyte loss. Under usual circumstances patients will regenerate their erythrocytes if adequately nourished and given iron.

Because viral hepatitis can be transmitted in plasma, it is not wise to give plasma to patients as a source of trace elements. We have avoided this approach. Others have given plasma for this purpose, but I don't know of any data to indicate that such treatment is beneficial. Our first duty to the patient is to do him no harm.

Zinc

The only other transition element we have given intravenously intentionally is zinc.[13] We have empirically added zinc sulfate to our preparation, giving from 5 to 10 mg of zinc sulfate daily. The reasons for giving zinc are based on experimental observations that zinc is required for protein synthesis, for nucleic acid synthesis, and is involved therefore in wound healing.[14] One can demonstrate this readily in the experimental animal, and it has been shown in patients in studies having variable degrees of control.

On this basis we have added zinc. We have no unequivocal evidence that we have done any good. We have observed granulation tissue appear. But when you improve a patient's nutrition, wound healing probably will accelerate. At present, zinc is the only trace element for which I have sufficient evidence to justify its addition to an intravenous solution.

It is difficult to produce zinc deficiency or, indeed, any trace element deficiency in animals. You have to have special conditions. I suspect that one is only liable to get into trouble when the requirements of the particular transition element are high. Zinc may be a case in point.

The NRC allowance for zinc of 15 mg/day may be conservative. We need to test our hypothesis, though under controlled conditions. The serum zinc level will be low in the malnourished patient with large wounds. Zinc should be given to these patients.

Dr. Van Itallie: May I point out that some of these substances given parenterally have not been approved as drugs by the Food and Drug Administration. Zinc and certain sugars (eg, maltose) are not approved.

Dr. Forbes: Zinc is approved as a dietary supplement, but not as a drug.

Dr. Van Itallie: If this is the case, would the company need to go to FDA and ask for an IND number? (See pp 398, 450.)

Dr. Forbes: Any change in their basic standards for parenteral use is unlikely, and they will remain drugs.

Dr. Van Itallie: The parenteral nutrient is considered to be a drug. Is that right?

Dr. Forbes: Yes.

Dr. Greene: At the dose we were giving, the serum levels for zinc were normal. We are giving the adult about 1 mg/1,500 ml of intravenous fluid in the form of zinc sulfate. This would appear to be slightly more than the requirement, because the hair levels are quite high after approximately 30 days on this regimen.

Dr. Van Itallie: Dr. Sandstead, the zinc level you cited was considerably higher than 1 mg/1,500 ml. Do you worry about giving too much?

Dr. Sandstead: The reason we chose a higher dose than 1 mg/day of zinc sulfate is the reported daily intake in our diet. With a good diet, it is between 12 and 15 mg of zinc per day. Evidence from balance studies indicates that as much as 50% of the dietary zinc may be absorbed by some individuals, with more usual levels between 20% and 40%. Ten mg of zinc sulfate is roughly equivalent to 3 mg of zinc. This is below the amount apparently absorbed daily from the GI tract. Therefore, we have added 5 to 10 mg of zinc sulfate to our parenteral solution each day.

A 150-gm rat, given 1 mg of zinc intraperitoneally, tolerates it well. Hence, 3 mg of zinc were suggested in human studies as a dosage for the adult.

Iodine

Dr. Sandstead: I know of no one who is adding iodine to intravenous fluids, nor do I know any clear clinical indication for adding iodine. I would like to learn of any evidence that we should.

Dr. Shils: I add small amounts of sodium iodide.

Dr. Van Itallie: How about fluoride?

Dr. Sandstead: I know of no indication for giving fluoride.

Dr. Van Itallie: Manganese?

Dr. Sandstead: No data.

Question: How about cobalt?

Dr. Sandstead: It is my impression that the requirement of cobalt for man is available from vitamin B_{12}.

Copper

Question: How about copper?

Dr. Sandstead: Copper deficiency is exquisitely difficult to produce.

Dr. Van Itallie: We have not discussed copper deficiency, except to say that it is rare. Dr. Sandstead, would it be helpful to follow copper during parenteral alimentation? Is this a feasible procedure?

Dr. Sandstead: These are research questions. That's the problem. We don't know enough about the subject to make a recommendation.

Dr. Hodges: I would go along with the concept of giving small quantities of iron—which almost certainly would be contaminated with copper—and this might be one way of providing copper. Would 1 mg/day of elemental iron (approximately the amount that is converted into red cells per day) carry a significant hazard? Even this amount might preserve iron stores.

Dr. Sandstead: That would be reasonable, but I don't know about the hazard.

Dr. Greene: In two subjects we studied—one for approximately three months and another for a total of about two months—the copper content at the scalp level is lowest, whereas out at the tip it is highest. We know also that people tend to accumulate copper toward the ends of the hair. I don't know if this decrease in serum copper will be clinically significant. But a recent report[15] in the *Journal of Pediatrics* concerns one patient who had documented copper deficiency during parenteral alimentation and associated clinical symptoms which responded to copper treatment.

We have measured, or Hambidge[16] (at the University of Colorado) has measured, trace elements in many of the solutions that we give parenterally: FreAmine, Aminosol, two of the casein hydrolysates, and the electrolyte solutions we put into these units, including MVIs as sources of vitamins. Copper appears to be deficient in many of these final mixtures. Chromium is also low.

Dr. Van Itallie: Analysis of the hair for trace elements might be done in patients who are receiving parenteral alimentation. Part of our recommendation as a group would be encouragement of clinical investigation to find solutions to the questions we are unable to answer.

We could summarize by saying that of all the trace elements, iron is most needed, but should not be given intravenously because of the high risk

308

of anaphylaxis. If it is really necessary, it should be given *by* a physician and *only* by a physician, preferably intramuscularly.

It also seems clear that the evidence is growing that it would be useful to have zinc available for IV administration, particularly in individuals in whom the problem of wound healing exists.

References

1. Hodges RE, Baker EM: Ascorbic acid, in Goodhart RS, Shils ME (eds): *Modern Nutrition in Health and Disease.* Philadelphia, Lea & Febiger, 1973, chap 5, section K.

2. Mumma RO, Verlangieri AJ: *In vivo* sulfation of cholesterol by ascorbic acid 3-sulfate as a possible explanation for the hypocholestemic effects of ascorbic acid, abstracted. *Fed Proc* **30**:370 (abstract #991), 1971.

3. Hodges RE, Baker EM, Hood J, et al: Experimental scurvy in man. *Am J Clin Nutr* **22**:535-548, 1969.

4. King CG: Present knowledge of ascorbic acid (vitamin C), in *Present Knowledge in Nutrition, ed 3.* New York, The Nutrition Foundation, Inc., pp 76-79.

5. Hunter R, Barnes J, Oakeley HF, Matthews DM: Toxicity of folic acid given in pharmacological doses to healthy volunteers. *Lancet* **1**:61-63, 1970.

6. Herbert V: Experimental nutritional folate deficiency in Man. *Trans Assoc Am Physicians* **75**:307-320, 1962.

7. Sheehy TW, Rubin ME, Perez-Santiago E, et al: The effect of "minute" and "titrated" amounts of folic acid on the megaloblastic anemia of tropical sprue. *Blood* **18**:623-636, 1961.

8. Dryden LP, Hartman AM: Vitamin B_{12} deficiency in the rat fed high protein rations. *J Nutr* **101**:579-587, 1971.

9. Hoppner K, Phillips WEK, Erdody P, et al: Vitamin A reserves of Canadians. *Can Med Assoc J* **101**:84-86, 1969.

10. Underwood BA, Siegel H, Yeiweisell RC, et al: Liver stores of vitamin A in a normal population dying suddenly and rapidly from unnatural causes in New York City. *Am J Clin Nutr* **23**:1037-1042, 1970.

11. Haddad JG: Competitive protein-binding radioassay for 25-hydroxycholecalciferol. *J Clin Endocrin Metabolism* **33**:992-995, 1971.

12. Ruberg RL, Allen TR, Goodman MJ, et al: Hypophosphatemia with hypophosphaturia in hyperalimentation. *Surg Forum* **22**:87-88, 1971.

13. Sandstead HH: Zinc nutrition in the United States. *Am J Clin Nutr* **26**:1251-1260, 1973.

14. Sandstead HH, Lanier VC Jr, Shephard GH, Gillespie DD: Zinc and wound healing. Effects of zinc deficiency and zinc supplementation. *Am J Clin Nutr* **23**:514-519, 1970.

15. Karpel JT, Peden VH: Copper deficiency in long-term parenteral nutrition. *J Pediatr* **80**:32-36, 1972.

16. Hambidge KM: Use of static argon atmosphere in emission spectrochemical determination of chromium in biological materials. *Anal Chem* **43:**103-107, 1971.

Digest of Colloquium

Owing to lack of relevant experimental data, desirable quantities of vitamins and minerals for daily administration to patients receiving total parenteral nutrition have not been defined. But every nutrient which might be essential for man probably should be administered during prolonged parenteral nutrition, provided no contraindication exists.

Patients requiring TPN may be seriously ill. They may need extra vitamins to repair prior depletion, to meet increased metabolic requirements associated with fever, infection, and other stresses, and to fulfill the needs of anabolic processes. Also, the underlying disease process may cause an accelerated catabolism of one or more vitamins.

Administration of vitamins via the venous catheter is unphysiologic and may result in excessive urinary losses, particularly of water-soluble vitamins. When the blood concentration of ascorbic acid is higher than 1.4 ml/100 ml, the renal threshold for this vitamin is exceeded, and large quantities are lost. Sixty percent of a modest dose of folic acid or of vitamin A given intravenously may be excreted. Over 60% of intravenously given pyridoxine may be lost in the urine in unbound form. Riboflavin is similarly wasted, although not in as dramatic a fashion.

Since little reliable information is available concerning the physiology of intravenously administered vitamins, determination of desirable dosage must be made empirically. The quantities of water-soluble vitamins recommended are, in general, one and one-half times the Recommended Dietary Allowances (RDA). A higher figure for thiamin is recommended because of extra need for the vitamin when dietary calories are derived principally from carbohydrate (glucose). Requirements for vitamin B_{12}, vitamin B_6, and possibly riboflavin are influenced similarly by protein intake.

Since no recommended formulation can meet every clinical need, we attempted to develop a baseline preparation to which additional vitamins may be added as clinical circumstances require. It was agreed that a mixture should be available for addition to parenteral solutions on a daily basis, using as a point of departure about one-third the quantity of water-soluble vitamins present in a USV parenteral preparation (see p 290). This modification avoids administration of potentially unsafe quantities of vitamins A and D.

Vitamin A is needed because patients may come to parenteral alimentation with a vitamin A deficiency. Vitamin K is desirable. The question of vitamin E was not resolved. Addition of vitamin D to the formulation was not thought to be necessary for most adults. Although it was suggested that an essential fatty acid (EFA) deficiency might develop in the patient on TPN, no agreement was reached on the need for essential fatty acids for the adult.

Ranges of macrominerals suggested for addition to parenteral fluids included the following:

Calcium	100 to 300 mg/day
Phosphorus	100 to 300 mg/day
Magnesium	4 to 50 mEq/day
Potassium	80 to 200 mEq/day
Sodium	20 to 80 mEq/day

For the pharmacist, a baseline electrolyte solution of this kind serves as a point of departure, a solution that might be used to initiate total parenteral alimentation. It contains electrolytes to cover most contingencies. Later—when data concerning the patient's electrolyte status become available—the electrolyte orders can be modified in terms of patient needs.

Of the trace elements, iron is most needed but should not be given intravenously because of anaphylaxis. If it is required for the patient, it should be given only by a physician, preferably intramuscularly. Evidence has accumulated for the use of zinc in IV administration, particularly in individuals in whom the problem of wound healing exists.

Recommendations beyond those made during the colloquium discussion should develop from studies of blood and tissue levels and excretion rates in patients with a variety of medical problems who are carefully followed with parenteral nutrition.

The task of formulating recommendations for vitamin and mineral components of parenteral fluids is fraught with difficulties. Much of the available information is anecdotal or has been obtained from studies with normal subjects. The Nutrition Advisory Group on TPN of AMA's Department of Foods and Nutrition has prepared recommendations based in part on this discussion (see p 458).

PART THREE

Section One

A. Microbiological Safety

8 Problems in Preparation and Handling of Solutions
  William F. Schaffner, M.D.
9 The Problem of Sepsis
  Donald A. Goldmann, M.D., and Dennis G. Maki, M.D.
10 Preparation and Guidelines to Utilization of Solutions
  W. Arthur Burke, Pharm.D.
11 Hospital Practice of Total Parenteral Nutrition
  Robert L. Ruberg, M.D.

  Colloquium: Safety
  Digest of Colloquium
  P. William Curreri, M.D., and Robert H. Henry, M.S.

SAFETY AND DELIVERY OF SOLUTIONS

Chapter 8

Problems in Preparation and Handling of Solutions

William F. Schaffner, M.D.

Contamination in preparation and handling of fluids for intravenous use is an ever-present problem. The problem areas— preparation of the fluids in the hospital, manufacture of the fluids by industry, actual delivery to the patient—are pinpointed and possible solutions are offered.

A review of the literature reveals that bloodstream infection is recognized, with but rare exceptions, as the major complication of total parenteral nutrition.[1-5] Infection may arise in three areas related to TPN:

Preparation of TPN solutions in the hospital;
Manufacture of the solutions by industry;
Delivery of the solutions to the patient.

Infection surveillance within the hospital and nationwide is an essential feature of appropriate measures of control.

PREPARATION OF FLUIDS

If solutions for hyperosmolar alimentation (HA) are to be produced in the hospital (as most are), an integrated approach encompassing clinicians and pharmacists is necessary. This systematic approach has advantages for both patient safety and patient nutrition. It is vastly superior to bottle-by-bottle uncoordinated procedures.

Solutions for hyperosmolar alimentation should be prepared according to a written protocol which has been approved by the appropriate standing committees of the institution, such as the Pharmacy and Infection Control Committees. An ad hoc combined subcommittee might be designated to work with the director of pharmacy to facilitate the design of an appropriate process. Such formal approval has two purposes. It allows for those not working directly with the project to introduce additional safety factors (eg, an infectious disease consultant might have special concern for the type of microbiological sampling which is done). It also provides some medicolegal insurance for the participants and for the hospital.

The hospital must have the proper facilities for preparing the solutions. The ward does not qualify as a proper facility. These fluids should be prepared in the pharmacy under a laminar air-flow hood. In our hospital, the pharmacists employ sterile pyrogen-free chemicals and triple-distilled sterile water. During the manufacturing process, samples are taken at the beginning, in the middle, and at the end of the procedure for sterility and pyrogen testing. When single bottles of an unusual mixture are compounded, these are mixed under the laminar flow hood, but are not sampled for bacteriologic testing. Perhaps they ought to be. The fluids are prepared no more than 24 hours before administration, are dated, and are then refrigerated until delivered to the ward. Ward personnel are not permitted to add medicaments or other additives to TPN solutions.

MANUFACTURE OF HYPEROSMOLAR ALIMENTATION FLUIDS

With the large-scale manufacturing methods now in use and with coast-to-coast distribution patterns of final products, contaminated intravenous fluids can evoke a national (even international) outbreak of nosocomial sepsis. Such hospital-acquired illness strikes the most debilitated patients. This is even more true for those patients receiving total parenteral nutrition. An extraordinary propensity to bloodstream infection among these patients is amply documented. [2-5]

The nationwide outbreak of gram-negative sepsis caused by contamination of the closure systems of intravenous fluid bottles produced by a leading manufacturer [6, 7] provoked a careful reappraisal of the safety factors currently employed to guard against microbial contamination of the final product. I do not believe we have as yet developed a mechanism which affords us maximum security.

We realize that "sterility" is *not* an absolute concept. Sterility is a statistical phenomenon defined operationally in terms of the nature of the product, its microbial contamination (qualitatively and quantitatively), the sterilization process employed, the duration of its application to the product, and the sampling methods used to detect covert contamination. What we are left with is some measure of the *probability* that a given batch of intravenous fluid is free of microorganisms.

I suggest that we revise our labeling methods. "Sterile" has implications of an absolute state. The term should be discarded in favor of a grading system that will take the various factors into account.

Traditionally, industry has relied on sampling the final product in an attempt to detect microbial contamination. The current ground rules for terminal sampling are inadequate as the major screen for sterility. They are statistically inappropriate. First, the number of items sampled is small. Let us calculate, therefore, how often a contamination lot is passed using such a small sample: If one assumes 1% contamination of the items in a lot—a very high figure, I hope—80% of the time the lot will be passed as sterile if only 20 items are tested. Furthermore, if some contamination is discovered, the manufacturer is permitted to draw another sample of 20, and, if these are sterile (at the same probabilities), the lot will pass.

Not only are the statistical assurances of sterility weak, the qualitative bacteriology is equally inadequate. Only the simplest of anaerobic bacteriology tests are performed (thioglycolate broth), and the isolates obtained are not further speciated. A single colony of *Pseudomonas aerugenosa* has different implications than does a colony of *Staphylococcus albus*. The former should probably be cause for rejection of the lot. The known fungal infection hazard of patients receiving total parenteral nutrition should require that all fungal isolates from such fluids be carefully identified and that fluids containing any *Candida* species be rejected.

Following are suggestions for inclusion in a contamination control program for large-scale manufacturers:

An ongoing determination of the microbial flora of the un-
sterilized product and the environment of the manufacturing plant.

The regular use of biological indicator tests (ie, seeding of selected samples of the actual product with bacteria and/or spores relatively resistant to the sterilizing process used.[8-10] These are then processed with each lot and evaluated. The regulations only recommend, but do not demand their use.

Meticulous physical and chemical monitoring of the sterilization process.

Terminal sampling, but for a new reason. Since the outbreak mentioned above was due to contamination occurring *after* the bottles had been sterilized, terminal sampling should be carried out at a point just prior to the departure of the bottles from the plant to monitor for such posttreatment contamination. Sample size should be somewhat larger, anaerobic bac-
teriology improved, and all recovered organisms carefully identified.

Public disclosure, in a standardized protocol, of the microbial safety program. This protocol should be available to con-
sumers upon request.

In-use testing. All new products and any design changes should be tested not only in the manufacturer's laboratory, but un-
der actual *in-use* situations in hospitals.[11] It is at the bedside that design flaws are stressed and revealed. It is unfortunate that a nationwide epidemic had to occur before we learned the lesson that even minor design changes may carry with them major infection hazards. In-use testing should be introduced rapidly into the appropriate regulations. Because of the septic hazard already demonstrated, this would be par-
ticularly appropriate for new total parenteral nutrition kits.

DELIVERY TO THE PATIENT

We need better records of intravenous therapy in our hospitals. In most institutions, one cannot reconstruct from the patient's chart such details of intravenous therapy as the extremity used for the site of the intravenous infusion, the type of needle or catheter used, how often the site was changed, who inserted the intravenous needle, whether antibiotic ointment was used, and so on.

In order to better monitor TPN therapy at the Vanderbilt University Hospital, Meng employs a part-time TPN nurse. Her duties are roughly analogous to those of our nurse-epidemiologist, and we are now in the process of coordinating her activities. Having a well-defined staff responsible for parenteral nutrition in the institution is the only way a standardized approach regarding both nutrition and safety can be effected.

Accurate infection surveillance is essential in defining the hazard to the patient. Some institutions have included routine periodic blood cultures, but their usefulness is debated. Ward personnel should be trained to recognize early sepsis. At the first signs, a rigorous fever work-up should be done, including a careful history and physical examination, urinalysis, white blood cell and differential counts, appropriate x-rays, and several blood cultures spread over time (the longer the better, consistent with good patient care). While it is recognized that every episode of sepsis in a patient receiving total parenteral nutrition does not originate from the catheter,[5] this clinical distinction is usually difficult to make. When doubt exists, the catheter should be removed. Before removal, a blood culture should be drawn through the catheter. The site of insertion should be cleaned, the catheter withdrawn, and the catheter tip cultured.

Monitoring of infection rates within the hospital will alert the parenteral nutrition staff to changing practices which carry an increased risk of blood-stream infection. It should be advantageous to include a consultant on infectious diseases on the hospital parenteral nutrition staff. Such a person might not be a member of the staff's nucleus, but an informed and interested source, ready to help with patient consultations and program design.

Nationwide surveillance of hospital-acquired infection is now being carried out by the Hospital Infection Unit, Epidemiology Program, at the Center for Disease Control, Atlanta. It provides the surest mechanisms for detecting problems with contaminated fluids in nationwide use.

An imperative part of surveillance is getting information back into the hands of those who need to know. At present there exists no reliable method which assures that workers in the field are apprised of all pertinent new information. The methods used during the outbreak of gram-negative sepsis mentioned earlier[6, 7] were imperfect.[12]

Therefore, I propose that the American Hospital Association provide authorities at the Center for Disease Control with an annually revised list of the names and addresses of the following key people in each hospital: the administrator, the associate administrator directly responsible for infection control, the chairman of the Infection Control Committee, the hospital-epidemiologist, the nurse-epidemiologist, and the hospital pharmacist. These people should be informed (perhaps using color-coded envelopes similar to those now used for notification of drug reactions) of every "voluntary recall" of contaminated "sterile" products. Such notification would enable them to survey hospital storerooms quickly for the contaminated product and to institute appropriate epidemiologic investigation. It seems necessary to notify several people in each institution because, through oversight, vacations, mail-room snafus, and so on, a single letter might go unread.

In conclusion, total parenteral nutrition therapy has passed the "interesting but innovative" stage of development and has entered a period of logarithmic acceptance and exploitation. Nevertheless, we still have not comprehensively documented the infection hazard associated with this therapy.

References

1. Curry CR, Quie PG: Fungal septicemia in patients receiving parenteral hyperalimentation. *N Eng J Med* **285:**1221-1225, 1971.

2. Ashcraft KW, Leape LL: *Candida* sepsis complicating parenteral feeding. *JAMA* **212:**454-456, 1970.

3. Wilmore DW, Groff DB, Bishop HC, Dudrick SJ: Total parenteral nutrition in infants with catastrophic gastrointestinal anomalies. *J Pediatr Surg* **4:**181-189, 1969.

4. Filler RM, Eraklis AJ: Care of the critically ill child: Intravenous alimentation. *Pediatrics* **46:**456-461, 1970.

5. Dillon JD, Schaffner W, Van Way CW, Meng HC: Septicemia and total parenteral nutrition: Distinguishing catheter-related from other septic episodes. *JAMA* **223:**1341-1344, 1973.

6. Center for Disease Control: Nosocomial bacteremias associated with intravenous fluid therapy—USA. *Morbidity and Mortality Weekly Report* (supplement) **20:**81-82, March 12, 1971.

7. Felts SK, Schaffner W, Melly MA, Koenig MG: Sepsis caused by contaminated intravenous fluids: Epidemiologic, clinical, and laboratory investigation of an outbreak in one hospital. *Ann Intern Med* **77:**881-890, 1972.

8. Bruch CW: Sterility or microbial control of commercially supplied items, in *Proceedings of the International Conference on Nosocomial Infections, Center for Disease Control*, 1970.

9. Marinaro A: Development of a biological indicator control program. *Bull Parenteral Drug Association* **25:**75-77, 1971.

10. Miller WS: Types of biological indicators used in monitoring sterilization processes. *Bull Parenteral Drug Association* **25:**80-86, 1971.

11. Center for Disease Control: Follow-up on septicemias associated with contaminated Abbot intravenous fluids, *Morbidity and Mortality Report* **20:**91-92, 1971.

12. Duma RJ: First of all, do no harm, editorial. *N Eng J Med* **285:**1258-1259, 1971.

Chapter 9

The Problem of Sepsis

Donald A. Goldmann, M.D. and Dennis G. Maki, M.D.

Infection is an important complication of TPN therapy, and fungal septicemia has been a particularly serious problem. Fortunately, the risk of TPN-associated sepsis may be reduced substantially if vigorous infection control procedures are followed in the preparation and administration of TPN fluid.

In a controversial report appearing in the *New England Journal of Medicine* in 1971, Curry and Quie dramatically focused attention on the risk of sepsis complicating total parenteral nutrition (TPN) therapy.[1] Reviewing the charts of 33 cases of fungal septicemia occurring at the University of Minnesota Hospital during an 18-month period, they found that 22 patients had developed infection while receiving TPN. Even more alarming was the observation that 18 of these 22 patients with fungal septicemia died, and that this complication was the primary cause of death in 15. These findings prompted a prospective study in which it was found that 13 of 49 patients receiving TPN therapy developed fungal septicemia. Responding editorially in the same issue of the *Journal*,[2] Dr. Richard Duma invoked the dictum attributed to Hippocrates, "As to diseases, make a habit of two things—to help, or at least to do no harm." Duma stated that the risks of TPN therapy "appear unacceptably high," and asked that a "knowledgeable, medically expert group" evaluate TPN devices and equipment prior to licensing them for use. The Hospital Infections Section of the Center for Disease Control, which provides a consultative service for American hospitals, soon began to receive queries from members of the medical community who wanted to know if they could safely continue administering TPN. Clearly, we must address ourselves to the problem of infection. We must decide whether the risks are indeed acceptable.

Although the TPN literature is growing rapidly, most programs are still in their infancy, and few in-depth studies of TPN-associated infection have been performed. Fortunately, an extensive, although not altogether satisfactory, body of information has been accumulated concerning the problem of infection in conventional IV therapy. A selective review of these investigations is helpful in understanding the etiology and control of TPN-associated septicemia. This is not surprising since the apparatus and techniques generally used to deliver TPN and conventional IV solutions are basically similar. In particular, percutaneous plastic catheters have been employed extensively in the administration of both types of therapy. A review of microbiological aspects of infusions through polyethylene catheters follows, therefore, with special reference to points relevant to TPN therapy.

CATHETER-RELATED INFECTION

The indwelling plastic catheter was introduced in 1945[3] and—as with many medical novelties—was immediately abused. The time-consuming task of encouraging reluctant patients to drink was eschewed in favor of the convenience of IV supplementation. Plastic catheters were too often used instead of stainless steel needles because of the erroneous belief that they could be left in place indefinitely with minimal risk. Although several scattered early reports pointed out the danger of septic phlebitis,[4-10] not until the past decade has there been sufficient appreciation of the complications associated with plastic catheters and IV therapy in general. The 1962 edition of the American Hospital Association's *Control of Infections in Hospitals* did not mention infusion therapy as a potential cause of infection,[11] and the first prospective investigation of the problem did not appear until 1963.[12] Numerous studies have been performed subsequently, nearly all focusing on the most distal portion of the administration system, the cannula. Collins et al found that plastic catheters were associated with a 39% incidence of phlebitis.[13] Moreover, the tips of 34% of plastic catheters were colonized at the time of removal, and septicemia attributable to IV therapy developed in 2% of patients with these catheters. Similarly alarming rates of colonization and sepsis were noted in other reports.[12,14-23]

Virtually all investigators agree that the likelihood of colonization and septicemia increases the longer a polyethylene catheter stays in place; very few septicemias are seen if catheters are removed within 48 hours. This important fact has led to the generally accepted recommendation that catheters be routinely changed within 48 hours after placement.[10,12,13,16,19,24,25] Catheters left in for prolonged periods, as for TPN therapy, are clearly associated with an increased risk of infection unless they are inserted and maintained with special care.

Skin flora at the catheter site is often responsible for colonization of the catheter tip. Although many investigators have failed to disinfect the catheter site prior to removing the catheter, thereby risking contamination with skin flora at the time of catheter withdrawal, two well-controlled investigations in which the site was carefully disinfected before catheter removal have demonstrated that the organisms colonizing skin and catheter tip are often identical.[18,26] Theoretically, cutaneous organisms might gain access to the tip of the catheter during insertion or later on by migrating along the moist film between catheter and subcutaneous tissue. It is, therefore, imperative that the IV site be prepared with an effective antiseptic before catheter insertion.

Tincture of iodine (2% iodine in 70% alcohol) is a safe, inexpensive, effective agent,[27-30] but a history of iodine allergy must be sought before use. The iodine solution should be allowed to dry 30 seconds before being removed with 70% alcohol.[31] An iodophor may be substituted in patients with sensitive skin[27,28,32] but should not be washed off since its effectiveness may be due in part to prolonged release of free iodine.[27,28] If necessary, 70% alcohol may be used in iodine sensitive individuals, provided the skin is scrubbed very thoroughly.[33-35] Of course, antiseptics alone will not guarantee freedom from contamination during catheter insertion and maintenance; careful hand-washing and aseptic technique are equally crucial.

Some time-honored surgical preparation traditions are of debatable value. For example, the practice of shaving the catheter site seems to have gained wide acceptance without undergoing the scrutiny of a controlled clinical trial. It is certainly desirable to remove hair from an area where adhesive tape is to be applied. Theoretically, however, the nicks and abrasions caused by even the most deftly guided razor provide foci for the initiation of skin infection. In an intriguing study, Seropian and Reynolds have shown that when hair is removed with a depilatory instead of a razor prior to surgery, the incidence of surgical wound infection is reduced tenfold.[36]

Since cutaneous bacteria are important in the genesis of catheter-related infection, daily application of antimicrobial ointment to the catheter site theoretically should be beneficial. Some studies have suggested that topical preparations containing antibiotics may reduce the rate of catheter colonization, but too few patients were included in these investigations to demonstrate protection against septicemia.[14,17,19,37,38] An observation of particular significance in a discussion of TPN emerged from these studies: Antibiotic ointment may predispose to catheter colonization with fungi.[16,17,19] Therefore, use of a topical antiseptic, such as an iodophor ointment, should be considered, although clinical trials have not yet been performed to demonstrate the safety and efficacy of such agents.

From the preceding discussion it is apparent that meticulous care of polyethylene catheters is essential if infection is to be controlled. This contention is supported by clinical trials employing scrupulous technique in the insertion and maintenance of plastic catheters.[24,39,40] Although these studies were not controlled, rates of catheter colonization were reduced to 5% or less, and the incidence of sepsis to nearly zero. Uniform attention to the details of aseptic technique cannot be accomplished by a hodgepodge of professionals, each with his own idea of what constitutes safe practice. Studies suggest that catheter asepsis is most efficiently and effectively maintained by specially trained IV teams following an established protocol,[39-41] a point which is especially pertinent to the complex care of TPN systems.

Although inadequate asepsis at the catheter site is a frequent cause of catheter colonization, other mechanisms should be considered. A transient septicemia spawned by an anatomically distant site of infection might seed the fibrin clot which quickly forms around the intravascular segment of plastic catheters,[42,43] and pathology examinations have demonstrated organisms trapped within such thrombi.[44] In fact, some investigators have found that when catheters are inserted in infected patients, the organism responsible for the infection is often isolated subsequently from the catheter.[23,41] Of course, organisms from such infections could reach the catheter via the hands of hospital personnel as well as through the bloodstream.

CONTAMINATION OF INFUSION FLUID

Another potential cause of catheter colonization and septicemia is contaminated IV fluid. Until recently, few investigators considered this possi-

322

bility.[45] None of the studies of catheter colonization discussed so far included IV fluid cultures; therefore, the results of these investigations must be interpreted with caution. It is now clear that contaminated IV fluid is often the real culprit in "catheter-induced" septicemia. Four recent epidemics of septicemia attributed to the infusion of intrinsically contaminated solutions have dramatically emphasized the importance of culturing IV fluid when a patient receiving IV therapy develops sepsis of unclear origin.[46-49]

Investigations conducted during a nationwide outbreak of sepsis associated with infusion of contaminated IV products revealed that some common hospital pathogens (specifically, members of the genus *Klebsiella* proliferate rapidly in dextrose-containing IV fluids, increasing by more than 5 logs in 24 hours.[50] Moreover, contamination of IV fluid occurs frequently during administration.[50,51] Should contamination occur, the patient can be protected from the infusion of enormous numbers of pathogens if IV bottles are not left in use more than 24 hours after opening. Since IV administration tubing contains a reservoir of fluid in which organisms can proliferate despite high rates of flow, it should be changed every 24 hours.[46,50]

Center for Disease Control studies of the growth of microorganisms in conventional IV fluids have been extended to TPN solutions.[52,53] It has been found that *Candida albicans, Torulopsis glabrata, Serratia marcescens, Klebsiella pneumoniae,* and some strains of *Staphylococcus aureus* proliferate exuberantly in solution prepared with casein hydrolysate and dextrose (Hyprotigen, McGaw*), whereas other bacteria tested grow poorly. *Candida* and *Torulopsis* also proliferate in synthetic amino acid-dextrose solution (Fre-Amine, McGaw*), although more slowly than in casein hydrolysate-dextrose solution, and the bacteria tested do not grow at all. Because some pathogens multiply in both of these solutions, and contamination of TPN fluid can occur during preparation and administration,[54,55] TPN fluid should be used as soon as possible after preparation. Administration tubing should be changed every 24 hours.

It has been suggested that in-line membrane filters might be useful in preventing contaminated TPN or conventional IV fluid from reaching the patient.[56] Although a 0.22μ filter is theoretically capable of trapping bacteria and fungi, it cannot block the passage of endotoxin. Moreover, insertion and manipulation of filters provide yet one more opportunity for a break in aseptic technique. Controlled clinical trials to evaluate the effectiveness of membrane filters in reducing the risk of sepsis from contaminated fluid have not yet appeared.

PRINCIPLES OF INFECTION CONTROL

Based on the investigations and theoretical considerations outlined above, infection control recommendations have been formulated for TPN therapy.

Since TPN catheters must often be left in place for prolonged periods of time in debilitated patients, TPN therapy must be

---

*Use of trade names is for identification only and does not imply endorsement by the Center for Disease Control.

administered using strict infection control precautions that would be impractical and probably inappropriate for conventional IV therapy.

TPN should be administered by a specially trained team following a written protocol.

TPN fluid should be mixed under a laminar flow hood and used immediately; if storage is absolutely necessary, refrigeration at 4°C is useful in suppressing the growth of contaminants.[53]

Surgical aseptic technique is required for the insertion and care of TPN catheters. The catheter site should be prepared with an effective antiseptic, the catheter secured, and a sterile dressing applied. The use of an antiseptic ointment may be considered.

Periodic inspections of the catheter site are necessary to detect inflammation or purulence; the site may be carefully cleaned on these occasions.

Administration tubing should be changed every 24 hours.

The TPN system should not be used for sampling blood, measuring central venous pressure, or administering "piggyback" medications.

Should septicemia of obscure origin develop in a patient receiving TPN, the TPN fluid and patient's blood should be cultured immediately and strong consideration given to prompt removal of the catheter.

These recommendations have been published in detail.[52]

TPN programs employing sound infection control techniques similar to these have generally experienced a much lower incidence of TPN-associated infection than that reported by Curry and Quie (Table 1). A Center for Disease Control survey of 31 such programs with a combined experience of 2,078 patients revealed a 7% incidence of TPN-associated septicemia.[52] In another study, when catheters were inserted and maintained following a strict infection control protocol sepsis was associated with only 3%, whereas a 20% septicemia rate was noted when catheter care was not adequately regulated.[57]

Table 1.— Incidence of Septicemia Associated With Total Parenteral Nutrition (selected reports)

First Author	Reference	Number of Patients	Rate of Septicemia— All Pathogens (percent)	Rate of Candidemia (percent)
Dudrick	58, 59	47	6	4
Ryan	57	355*	7	3
Freeman	60	111	7	7
Owings	61	66	0	0
Parsa	62	307	9	2
Sanderson	63	100	1	0
Dillon	64	122	4	2
CDC	52	2,078	7	4

FUNGAL SEPTICEMIA

Careful technique can reduce the incidence of TPN-associated infection, but fungal septicemia, especially candidemia, has been a persistent problem even in some of the most successful programs.[52,57-60,62,64-68] This is in contrast to the relative rarity of fungal septicemia in patients receiving conventional IV infusions, although Vic-Dupont et al reported a significant incidence of this complication.[69] It is not known why *Candida* infection occurs so frequently in TPN patients, but several factors seem important:

> Patients requiring TPN are usually debilitated and often have a compromised immunologic response; they would be prime candidates for fungal infection even if they did not receive TPN. Moreover, such patients are frequently treated with broad spectrum antibiotics, radiation, steroids, and immunosuppressives, all of which predispose them to fungal septicemia.[70-73] In Curry and Quie's retrospective series, 18 of 22 patients with fungal septicemia were receiving broad spectrum antibiotics, and two were on steroids. Six had conditions sometimes associated with a depressed immunologic system, and all were extremely ill.

> *Candida* and *Torulopsis* proliferate more rapidly than most of the bacterial strains tested in casein hydrolysate-dextrose solution and are the only pathogens tested capable of growth in synthetic amino acid-dextrose solution.[52,53] In contrast, *Candida* grows much more slowly than some bacteria in conventional dextrose-containing IV solutions.[50]

> Antibiotic ointments, which may predispose to catheter site colonization with fungi,[16,17,19] have been used liberally in the maintenance of TPN catheters. Moreover, the occlusive dressings used in the care of TPN catheters alter the microbiologic flora of the skin and may favor the proliferation of fungi.[74]

CONCLUSION

Enthusiasm for the therapeutic potential of TPN must be tempered by awareness of the risk of TPN-associated sepsis. Indiscriminate use of TPN therapy is reprehensible. The basic principles of infection control must be disseminated as widely as possible, and further clinical trials should explore ways to reduce the hazard of infection.

References

1. Curry CR, Quie PG: Fungal septicemia in patients receiving total parenteral hyperalimentation. *N Eng J Med* **285:**1221-1224, 1971.

2. Duma RJ: First of all do no harm, editorial. *N Eng J Med* **285:**1258-1259, 1971.

3. Meyers L: Intravenous catheterization. *Am J Nurs* **45:**930-931, 1945.

4. Neuhof H, Seley GP: Acute suppurative phlebitis complicated by septicemia. *Surgery* **21:**831-842, 1947.

5. Moncrief JA: Femoral catheters. *Ann Surg* **147:**166-172, 1958.

6. Bansmer G, Keith D, Tesluk H: Complications following use of indwelling catheters of inferior vena cava. *JAMA* **167:**1606-1611, 1958.

7. Phillips RW, Eyre JD Jr: Septic thrombophlebitis with septicemia. Report of three cases due to *Staphylococcus aureus* infection after intravenous use of polyethylene catheters for parenteral therapy. *N Eng J Med* **259:**729-731, 1958.

8. Indar R: The dangers of indwelling plastic cannulae in deep veins. *Lancet* **1:**284-286, 1959.

9. McNair TJ, Dudley HA: The local complications of intravenous therapy. *Lancet* **2:**365-368, 1959.

10. Crane C: Venous interruption for septic thrombophlebitis. *N Eng J Med* **262:**947-951, 1960.

11. Colbeck JC (ed): *Control of Infections in Hospitals.* Chicago, American Hospital Association, 1962.

12. Druskin MS, Siegel PD: Bacterial contamination of indwelling intravenous polyethylene catheters. *JAMA* **185:**966-968, 1963.

13. Collins RN, Braun PA, Zinner SH, et al: Risk of local and systemic infection with polyethylene intravenous catheters. *N Eng J Med* **279:**340-343, 1968.

14. Moran JM, Atwood RP, Rowe MI: A clinical and bacteriologic study of infections associated with venous cutdowns. *N Eng J Med* **272:**554-559, 1965.

15. Brereton RB: Incidence of complications from indwelling venous catheters. *Del Med J* **41:**1-8, 1969.

16. Zinner SH, Denny-Brown BC, Braun P, et al: Risk of infection with intravenous indwelling catheters: Effect of application of antibiotic ointment. *J Infect Dis* **120:**616-619, 1969.

17. Norden CW: Application of antibiotic ointment to the site of venous catheterization: A controlled trial. *J Infect Dis* **120:**611-615, 1969.

18. Banks DC, Yates DB, Cawdrey HM, et al: Infection from intravenous catheters. *Lancet* **1:**443-445, 1970.

19. Levy RS, Goldstein J, Pressman RS: Value of a topical antibiotic ointment in reducing bacterial colonization of percutaneous venous catheters. *J Albert Einstein Med Ctr* **18:**67-70, 1970.

20. Glover JL, O'Byrne SA, Jolly L: Infusion catheter sepsis: An increasing threat. *Ann Surg* **173:**148-151, 1971.

326

21. Bernard RW, Stahl WM, Chase RM: Subclavian vein catheterization: A prospective study. II. Infectious complications. *Ann Surg* **173:**191-200, 1971.

22. Freeman R, King B: Infective complications of indwelling intravenous catheters and the monitoring of infections by the nitrobluetetrazolium test. *Lancet* **1:**992-993, 1972.

23. Mogensen JV, Frederiksen W, Jensen JK: Subclavian vein catheterization and infection. A bacteriologic study of 130 catheter insertions. *Scand J Infect Dis* **4:**31-36, 1972.

24. Bolasny BL, Martin CE, Conkle DM: Careful technique with plastic intravenous catheters. *Surg Gynecol Obstet* **131:**1030-1032, 1971.

25. Bentley DW, Lepper MH: Septicemia related to indwelling venous catheter. *JAMA* **206:**1749-1752, 1968.

26. Balagtas RC, Bell CE, Edwards LD, et al: Risk of local and systemic infections associated with umbilical vein catheterization: a prospective study in 86 newborn patients. *Pediatrics* **48:**359-367, 1971.

27. White JJ, Wallace CK, Burnett LS: Skin disinfection. *Johns Hopkins Med J* **126:**169-176, 1970.

28. Gershenfeld L: Iodine, in Lawrence CA, Black SS (eds): *Disinfection, Sterilization, and Preservation.* Philadelphia, Lea & Febiger, 1968, pp 329-347.

29. Lowbury EJ, Lilly HA, Bull JP: Disinfection of the skin of operation sites. *Br Med J* **2:**1039-1044, 1960.

30. Price PB: Surgical antiseptics, in Lawrence CA, Black SS (eds): *Disinfection, Sterilization, and Preservation.* Philadelphia, Lea & Febiger, 1968, pp 532-542.

31. Selwyn S, Ellis H: Skin bacteria and skin disinfection reconsidered. *Br Med J* **1:**136-140, 1972.

32. Joress SM: A study of disinfection of the skin: A comparison of providone-iodine with other agents used for surgical scrubs. *Ann Surg* **155:**296-304, 1962.

33. Spaulding EH: Alcohol as a surgical disinfectant. *Assoc Oper Rm Nurses J* **2:**67-71, 1964.

34. Morton HD: Alcohols, in Lawrence CA, Black SS (eds): *Disinfection, Sterilization, and Preservation.* Philadelphia, Lea & Febiger, 1968, pp 237-251.

35. Lee S, Schoen I, Malkin A: Comparison of use of alcohol with that of iodine for skin antisepsis in obtaining blood cultures. *Am J Clin Pathol* **47:**646-648, 1967.

36. Seropian R, Reynolds BM: Wound infections after preoperative depilatory versus razor preparation. *Am J Surg* **121:**251-254, 1971.

37. Crenshaw CA, Kelly L, Turner RJ, et al: Bacteriologic nature and prevention of contamination to intravenous catheters. *Am J Surg* **123:**264-266, 1972.

38. Crenshaw CA, Kelly L, Turner RJ, et al: Prevention of infection at scalp vein sites of needle insertion during intravenous therapy. *Am J Surg* **124:**43-45, 1972.

39. Corso JA, Agostinelli R, Brandriss MW: Maintenance of venous polyethylene catheters to reduce risk of infection. *JAMA* **210:**2075-2077, 1969.

40. Fuchs PC: Indwelling intravenous polyethylene catheters: Factors influencing the risk of microbial colonization and sepsis. *JAMA* **216:**1447-1450, 1971.

41. Henzel JH, DeWeese MS: Morbid and mortal complications associated with prolonged central venous cannulation. *Am J Surg* **121:**600-605, 1971.

42. Nejad MS, Klaper MA, Steggerda FR, et al: Clotting on the outer surfaces of vascular catheters. *Radiology* **91:**248-250, 1968.

43. Hoshal VL Jr, Ause RC, Hoskins PA: Fibrin sleeve formation on indwelling subclavian central venous catheters. *Arch Surg* **102:** 353-358, 1971.

44. Anderson AO, Yardley JH: Demonstration of *Candida* in blood smears. Letter to the Editor. *N Eng J Med* **286:**108, 1972.

45. Michaels L, Ruebner B: Growth of bacteria in intravenous infusion fluids. *Lancet* **1:**772-774, 1953.

46. Center for Disease Control. Nosocomial bacteremias associated with intravenous fluid therapy. *Morbidity Mortality Weekly Rep* **20** (special supplement to No. 9), March 1971.

47. Phillips I, Eykyn S, Laker M: Outbreak of hospital infection caused by contaminated autoclaved fluids. *Lancet* **1:**1258-1260, 1972.

48. Report of the committee appointed to inquire into the circumstances, including the production, which led to the use of contaminated infusion fluids in the Devenport Section of Plymouth General Hospital: London, Her Majesty's Stationery Office, 1972.

49. Center for Disease Control. Septicemias associated with contaminated intravenous fluids. *Morbidity Mortality Weekly Rep* **22(11):**99, 1973.

50. Maki DG, Rhame FS, Mackel DC, et al: Nosocomial septicemias subsequent to contaminated intravenous fluid. Read before the American Society for Microbiology, Minneapolis, 1971.

51. Duma RJ, Warner JF, Dalton HP: Septicemia from intravenous infusions. *N Eng J Med* **284:**257-260, 1971.

52. Goldmann DA, Maki DG: Infection control in total parenteral nutrition. *JAMA* **223:**1360-1364, 1973.

53. Goldmann DA: Prevention of infection in hyperalimentation therapy. Read before the Ninth International Congress of Nutrition, Mexico City, 1972.

54. Hak LJ, Long JL, Ruberg RL, et al: Contamination incidence in IV solutions with additives. Read before The American Society of Hospital Pharmacists, San Francisco, 1971.

55. Deeb EN, Natsios GA: Contamination of intravenous fluids by bacteria and fungi during preparation and administration. *Am J Hosp Pharm* **28:**764-767, 1971.

56. Wilmore DW, Dudrick SJ: An in-line filter for intravenous solutions. *Arch Surg* **99:**462-463, 1969.

57. Ryan JA, Abel RM, Abbott WM, et al: A prospective study of sepsis in prolonged venous hyperalimentation. Read before the Ninth International Congress of Nutrition, Mexico City, 1972.

328

58. Dudrick SJ, Groff DB, Wilmore DW: Long-term venous catheterization in infants. *Surg Gynecol Obstet* **129:**805-808, 1969.

59. Wilmore DW, Dudrick SJ: Safe long-term hyperalimentation. *Arch Surg* **98:**256-258, 1969.

60. Freeman JB, Lemire A, MacLean LD: Intravenous alimentation and septicemia. *Surg Gynecol Obstet* **135:**708-712, 1972.

61. Owings JM, Bomar WE, Ramage RC: Parenteral hyperalimentation and its practical implications. *Ann Surg* **175:**712-719, 1972.

62. Parsa MH, Habif DV, Ferrer JM, et al: Intravenous hyperalimentation: Indications, technique, and complications. *Bull NY Acad Med* **48:**920-942, 1972.

63. Sanderson I, Deitel M: Intravenous hyperalimentation without sepsis. *Surg Gynecol Obstet* **136:**577-585, 1973.

64. Dillon JD, Schaffner W, VanWay CW III, Meng HC: Septicemia and total parenteral nutrition; distinguishing catheter-related from other septic episodes. *JAMA* **223:**1341-1344, 1973.

65. Boeckman CR, Krill CE: Bacterial and fungal infections complicating parenteral alimentation in infants and children. *J Pediatr Surg* **5:**117-126, 1970.

66. Filler RM, Eraklis AJ: Care of the critically ill child: intravenous alimentation. *Pediatrics* **46:**456-461, 1970.

67. McGovern B: Intravenous hyperalimentation. *Milit Med* **135:**1137-1145, 1970.

68. Ashcraft KW, Leape LL: *Candida* sepsis complicating parenteral feeding. *JAMA* **212:**454-456, 1970.

69. Vic-Dupont V, Cartier F, Margairaz A, et al: Les septicémies: Complications des cathétérismes veineux de perfusion. *Bull Société Médicale des Hôpitaux de Paris* **117:**89-102, 1966.

70. Seelig MS: The role of antibiotics in the pathogenesis of *Candida* infections. *Am J Med* **40:**887-917, 1966.

71. Klainer AS, Beisel WR: Opportunistic infections: A review. *Am J Med Sci* **258:**431-456, 1969.

72. Frenkel JK: Role of corticosteroids as predisposing factors in fungal diseases. *Lab Invest* **11:**1192-1208, 1962.

73. Rifkind D, Marchioro TL, Schneck SA, et al: Systemic fungal infections complicating renal transplantation and immunosuppression therapy; clinical microbiological, neurologic and pathologic features. *Am J Med* **43:**28-38, 1967.

74. Pillsbury DM: *A Manual of Dermatology.* Philadelphia, WB Saunders Co, 1971, p 149.

Chapter 10

Preparation and Guidelines to Utilization of Solutions

W. Arthur Burke, Pharm.D.

This paper includes a prototype format for developing a TPN protocol and describes how the pharmacist contributes to safety in his management of TPN through utilization of effective communications and his total involvement. He observes aseptic techniques in preparation of formulations, which are accurately labeled and available through a comprehensive Nutritional IV Request form. His knowledge of compatibility of additives aids in consideration of the patient's total medication regime, from which he develops a Patient Profile Record system. He recognizes the need for in-house education, also for development and maintenance of a TPN staff or team.

Key words comprising the element of safety are involvement, communication, and awareness. Safety in the major aspects of hyperalimentation —in the administration of nutrient solutions, monitoring of the patient, preparation of nutritional formulas—depends upon total involvement and good communication among the nurse, pharmacist, and physician. Safety requires awareness by all three of the potential problems, principles, and purpose of this procedure. Each must be acutely sensitive to the significance of the contributions of the other group members.

Some of these roles and some unusual pharmacist involvement will be elucidated in the following discussion of our work at the Wilmington Medical Center.

PREPARATION OF IV SOLUTIONS

The Pharmacy IV Additive service in this institution prepares all intravenous (IV) nutritional solutions and thus is involved indirectly in the therapy of every patient treated by hyperosmolar alimentation (HA). This presents a logical avenue for clinical involvement, for direct patient monitoring, and for our services as a focal point for information about this nutritional technique. From this direct involvement with hundreds of patients, we correlate observations and clinical findings, compile meaningful data, and develop flexibility and expertise. Hence we are equipped to improvise and tailor solutions to fit specific patient needs, functioning ultimately as a consultant specialist.

A starting point for safe total parenteral nutrition is the careful preparation of nutritional solutions. The busy patient care area, with its many distractions, excess traffic, and, frequently, inadequate lighting, is not the optimum site for careful calculation, compounding, and inspection of a medication as critical as intravenous solutions. The environmental conditions of patient care areas have been compared with centralized admixture labs to determine the effect of air inoculum on sterile solutions. These studies demonstrate that the ambient air in patient care areas does not provide a satisfactory environment for the compounding of sterile admixtures. Contamination rates of 10% to 18% have been reported.

The first criterion for safety, therefore, is that IV nutritional solutions should be prepared and all additions and manipulations performed by knowledgeable personnel, utilizing aseptic technique, in the clean air environment created by a laminar air flow unit. To enhance stability and retard the possibility of bacterial and fungal contamination and growth, the completed basic solution is stored under refrigeration at 5°C.

The original IV solutions from the Pharmacy Department at the hospital of the University of Pennsylvania were prepared by dissolving anhydrous dextrose in a protein hydrolysate solution, bacterial filtering of this solution, and repackaging in screw-cap bottles. This procedure required scrupulous technique and considerable equipment and probably could not be carried out by more than a half-dozen institutions in the country. With the demise of the screw-cap intravenous containers, the only system presently available in rigid, glass containers by all manufacturers is the vacuum or closed system.

THE TPN KIT

For the small institution with limited facilities and an occasional nutrition patient or for patients maintained at home, the TPN Kit (also called HA, or hyperosmolar alimentation kit) is available. The kit consists of:

A bottle containing a concentrated protein source, either as protein hydrolysate or as crystalline amino acids;
A separate bottle containing a concentrated carbohydrate, generally 40% to 50% dextrose in water; and
The necessary fluid transfer and administration sets.

To insure stability, the basic nutritional solution is prepared, shortly before use, by aseptically transferring the contents of one bottle to the other. This is performed by means of a sterile transfer set, utilizing the vacuum of one of the underfilled bottles to effect transfer. All manipulations ideally should be accomplished within a laminar air flow hood. These kits are convenient to use and the resultant formulas are effective for most patients.

In our 1,200-bed complex, we help monitor, at any given time, from 5 to 18 patients receiving TPN. We utilize from 15 to 65 units of nutritional fluid every day. The average is approximately 45 units. We can prepare the nutritional solutions at about one-third the cost of kits purchased from an outside agency; also, we lose some flexibility in modifying solutions from these kits to specific situations. Our method assures the patient receiving three or four units per day of nutritional solutions that these will be tailored to his needs at a significant saving.

The following procedure, which can be employed by any institution, illustrates a safe technique for preparing the basic nutritional formula.

CLOSED, NO-WASTE TECHNIQUE

Supplies for Basic Formulation

3x1 liters Amigen 5%/D-5%
3x500 ml dextrose 50% (D-50)
(Same lot number for both)
1 liter plasma collecting
    vacuum bottle

1 double needle "blood
collection" set (sterile tubing with 18- and 15-gauge
needles) for fluid transfer

Any commercially manufactured solution can be used (see Fig 1).

YIELD: 4 units of the classic HA adult formula

NUTRITIVE VALUE: 725 nonprotein kilocalories (calculated as 3.4 kcal/gm glucose monohydrate); 4.5 gm protein nitrogen per 1,100 ml.

STEP 1: Calibrate the plasma vacuum bottle into 250-ml increments (Fig 2). For the fluid transfer set, use a short, sterile tubing with an 18-gauge and 15-gauge needle fastened at either end. Insert the larger 15-gauge needle into the plasma vacuum bottle and the 18-gauge needle into the Amigen bottles, since it causes less "coring." Coring is a phenomenon that can occur when a needle is inserted through a solid rubber stopper. The "heel" of the needle, passing through, can cut out a piece of rubber, which generally is deposited where it is not wanted, right in the solution! We routinely use an administration set with a nylon mesh filter to control this problem. Tests indicate that the core particles are sterile.

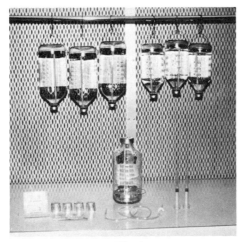

Fig 1

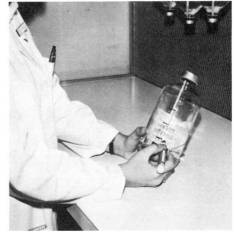

Fig 2

STEP 2: Remove 250 ml from each of the 3 Amigen bottles. The rubber closure seals itself when the needle is removed; therefore, there is little opportunity for airborne contamination. This step yields 4 bottles (Fig 3), each containing 750 ml of Amigen 5%/D-5%.

STEP 3: At this point, insert the 15-gauge needle from the vacuum bottle into the D-50% bottle. This allows use of the smaller 18-gauge needle for the Amigen bottles to minimize coring. Insert a syringe into the airway of the D-50% bottle to facilitate fluid transfer by breaking the resisting vacuum in that unit. Using the graduations of the inverted D-50% as a guide, transfer 350 ml of D-50% to the 750 ml of Amigen 5%/D-5% (Fig 4).

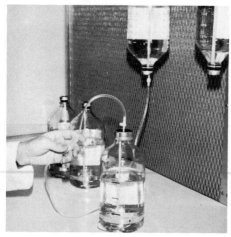

Fig 3

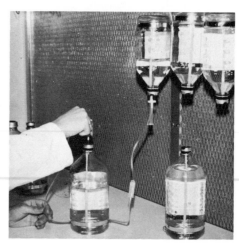

Fig 4

STEP 4: Transfer the 150 ml of D-50% remaining in the first bottle to the next Amigen bottle. Then start a new D-50% for the additional 200 ml.

STEP 5: Repeat the process until all of the Amigen 5%/D-5% units have had 350 ml of D-50% added (Fig 5). (Note: When preparing 60 units at one time, as we do, 45 liters of Amigen 5%/D-5% and only 42x500 ml D-50% are required. There is no waste.)

STEP 6: Examine the finished TPN units. Take samples for bacteriologic survey and cap them, using an alcohol sponge and an aluminum overseal. The units are then labeled (Fig 6) with a storage label and refrigerated. An experienced pharmacist or trained technician can prepare about 24 basic HA units in 30 minutes.

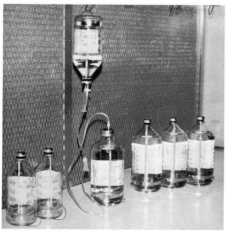

Fig 5

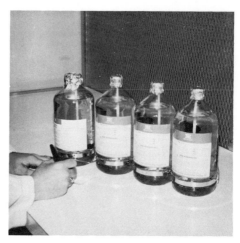

Fig 6

DIFFERENCES IN SOLUTIONS

A prime responsibility of the pharmacist on a nutritional unit is to be totally knowledgeable of differences in the various solutions and the clinical significance, if any, of these differences. Formulas prepared from fibrin hydrolysates and some of the crystalline amino acid solutions are deficient in magnesium, calcium, and phosphorus and will require addition of these ions, whereas formulas prepared from casein hydrolysate (as the protein source) provide, per unit, about 1.5 mEq Mg, 4 mEq Ca, and about 22 mEq PO_4. Some addition may be required, but generally not as much as with the crystalline amino acid solutions.

Gross differences in the inherent electrolyte content of solutions from various manufacturers can produce unexpected deviations in the patient's chemistry unless good communication exists between the physician and the pharmacist. Definite ordering policies must be established, as we shall see later. Differences in various amino acid concentrations can produce undesirable effects (eg, variations in aspartic and glutamic acid content can produce nausea and vomiting). Perhaps these two amino acids should be deleted in an ideal formulation.

One synthetic amino acid formula tended to produce acidosis, a consequence, we soon realized, of the L-form amino acids, a few of which were present as the hydrochloride salt. Addition of sodium ions as the bicarbonate remedied the problem but created new ones with the other additives.

ADDITIVE COMPATIBILITY

What about additives in the nutritional formula? If you rely solely on the published data available, you will find that few additives are compatible with protein hydrolysates. A list of commonly used additives follows, with clinically significant data based solely on my own experience. I strongly urge each clinician to conduct his own tests before concluding that any drug is safe to add.

Albumin, though unanimously listed as incompatible, appears to be stable and clinically effective for at least 24 hours.

Calcium is not compatible with sodium bicarbonate. The chloride salt of calcium precipitates quickly in the presence of magnesium sulfate. The glucoheptonate salt, despite reports in the literature, appears to react more slowly and, in usual concentrations, does not show evidence of precipitation for several days. The gluconate salt may cause an apparent false depression in serum and urine magnesium levels when the Titan yellow method for determining magnesium is used. It does not interfere with the phosphate precipitation or flame photometric method of measuring serum or urine magnesium. Knowing how laboratory tests are performed is important because of possible drug interference.

Dextrose in high concentration is incompatible with whole blood; it causes clumping of RBC.

Digitalis is not usually added to HA solutions. It is incompatible! If it should be used concomitantly with HA solutions containing excess calcium, caution is required, especially in pediatric cases. If necessary to digitalize, discontinue the nutritional feeding or use a calcium-free solution. Wait 8 to 10 hours before digitalizing, since calcium half-life is three hours. Serious consequences have occurred when this precaution was not observed.

Insulin is not stable in presence of sodium bicarbonate. Five to eight units of regular insulin per bottle of HA solution produce a clinical response, despite reported glass and plastic adsorption of insulin—23% to 27%—in regular IV solutions. Possibly some degree of protein binding with nutrient solution carries the insulin into the patient. At any rate, adding insulin *to the bottle* appears to be the safest way to cover urine sugar spillage. If the nutritional solution is interrupted or discontinued, so is the extra insulin.

Magnesium sulfate can be added with calcium glucoheptonate. The most common problem regarding magnesium sulfate seems to occur with the calculations. The USP salt is $MgSO_4 \bullet 7H_2O$; 2 ml of 50% magnesium sulfate (USP) contain approximately 8 mEq Mg (not 16 mEq as frequently reported). The importance of magnesium is too frequently overlooked. We have been using 8 to 10 mEq per HA unit.

Sodium bicarbonate decreases activity of insulin and B-complex with vitamin C; it also precipitates calcium salts.

Vitamin K_1 produces some inactivation by ascorbic acid and vitamin B_{12}.

Vitamin B_{12} produces some inactivation by ascorbic acid, vitamin K, and high concentrations of dextrose.

Folic Acid precipitates with calcium salts.

Patient medication profile system Since side effects of many drugs may be significant in the patient receiving TPN, it is necessary to be aware of the patient's total medication regimen. A *patient medication profile system* is valuable. Basic to its development is consideration of the side effects of drugs. For example:

Alcohol may increase magnesium excretion and depress serum magnesium levels.

High doses of insulin may cause a drop in serum magnesium levels.

With Amphotericin B, low magnesium and very low serum potassium levels can be anticipated (potassium may be as low as 2 mEq). Expecting this and compensating for it can minimize potential problems. The drug also produces an increased BUN and creatinine.

STABILITY OF SOLUTIONS

How stable are these solutions? My experience and chemical and chromatographic analyses suggest that the basic formulation before inclusion of additives (as prepared above) appears to be stable for at least six months when properly refrigerated.

At room temperature, stability is shortened to about 8 to 10 weeks before some degree of darkening starts to occur. The solution, with electrolytes and vitamins added, appears to be relatively unchanged and stable for about 21 days of refrigeration, except for vitamin C loss. I am not suggesting that these solutions should be routinely used when this old; I am saying only that they appear to be stable for these periods. When our unit's patient census was low, we have used solutions which were 7 to 10 days old. No detectable difference in patient response was observed. For obvious legal reasons, commercial kits indicate that solutions should not be used after 8 to 12 hours. For legal reasons one should comply.

LABELING

Uniform labeling of these nutritional solutions is essential and can be helpful to the person who must administer them. We employ a basic format that indicates:

Patient information (location, time solution needed, date, etc.);

Desired volume per hour;

Approximate drop rate per minute (Note: This can vary with the type of administration set used and is dependent upon the fluid viscosity; therefore, periodic determinations are advisable.);

Total mEq content of the major electrolytes; and

Approximate total volume per unit.

We use an unsophisticated method to maintain a uniform format: a rubber stamp. When the stamp is made, be sure it is spaced to coincide with your typewriter. This may seem trivial, but it can save much time and aggravation when typing labels.

COMMUNICATIONS FORM

Following is a prototype of what I consider a meaningful communications form (Fig 7):

NUTRITIONAL IV REQUEST

PATIENT_____ ROOM NO _____

DATE _____ DR _____

A. **FIXED FORMULATIONS** (Description and Administration Route)
Indicate 24 hour quantity

H A (Basic formula) $\left\{ \begin{array}{l} \text{Prot hyd 3.4\%} \\ \text{Dextrose 20\%} \end{array} \right\}$ CVP

Provides: Pro 28 gm (4.5 gm N)
725* (850) Nonprotein kcal/1,100 ml   _____ ml

Syn Am Ac $\left\{ \begin{array}{l} \text{Cryst am ac 4.25\%} \\ \text{Dextrose 25\%} \end{array} \right\}$ CVP

Provides: Pro 39 gm (6.25 gm N)
850* (1,000) Nonprotein kcal/1,000 ml   _____ ml

AFA-800 $\left\{ \begin{array}{l} \text{Prot hyd 5\%} \\ \text{Fructose 12.5\%} \\ \text{Alcohol 2.4\%} \end{array} \right\}$ Peripheral

Provides: Pro 37.5 gm (6 gm N)
670* (700) Nonprotein kcal/1,000 ml   _____ ml

B. **SPECIAL or PEDIATRIC FORMULATION**
Indicate amount per 24 hours

Indicate source:

Protein _____gm   Protein hydrolysate _____

or: _____gm N   Synthetic am ac _____

     Essential am ac only_____

Nonprotein   Indicate source:

Kcalories_____   Dextrose_____

     Fructose _____

     Alcohol _____

Total Volume: _____ ml per 24 hours

C. **ELECTROLYTES AND ADDITIVES**
Indicate total per bottle or per 24 hours

KCl _____mEq   Reg. insulin_____units

NaCl_____mEq   Alcohol 7 kcal/gm _____gm

$MgSo_4$ (2cc 50%—8.1 mEq Mg) _____mEq   MVI_____ ml

CaGluc (10cc 10%—4.5 mEq Ca) _____mEq   SBF _____ ml

$NaHCO_3$ _____mEq   Heparin_____units

K Phos _____mEq   Specific L-amino acids

    _____ mg/liter

*Calculated as 3.4 kcal/gm glucose monohydrate. Figures in parentheses are rounded
values using 4 kcal/gm glucose.

Fig 7

Let us take a closer look at each section.

A. FIXED FORMULATIONS (Description and Administration Route)
   Indicate 24 hour quantity

HA (Basic formula) { Protein hydrolysate 3.4% / Dextrose 20% } CVP
   Provides: Protein 28 gm (4.5 gm N)
            725* (850) Nonprotein kcal/1,100 ml   _____ ml

Syn Am Ac { Crystalline amino acids 4.25% / Dextrose 25% } CVP
   Provides: Protein 39 gm (6.25 gm N)
            850* (1,000) Nonprotein kcal/1,000 ml   _____ ml

AFA-800 { Protein hydrolysate 5% / Fructose 12.5% / Alcohol 2.4% } Peripheral
   Provides: Protein 37.5 gm (6 gm N)
            670* (700) Nonprotein kcal/1,000 ml   _____ ml

*Calculated as 3.4 kcal/gm glucose monohydrate. Figures in parentheses are rounded values using 4 kcal/gm glucose.

This allows the physician a choice of available fixed formulations for general use and a choice of administration routes, depending on the patient's condition. He need only indicate a 24-hour quantity plus additional electrolytes.

B. SPECIAL or PEDIATRIC FORMULATION
   Indicate amount per 24 hours

Protein _____ gm   Indicate source:
                                   Protein hydrolysate _____
or: _____ gm N   Synthetic amino acids _____
                                   Essential amino acids only _____

Nonprotein   Indicate source:
Kilocalories _____   Dextrose _____
                                   Fructose _____
                                   Alcohol _____
Total Volume: _____ ml per 24 hours

The physician can tailor or modify the entire diet to meet individual needs. He can indicate the source of the protein for specific formulations. By using specific crystalline amino acids he may enhance the tyrosine content in pediatric deficiencies or control the content of various amino acids (eg, branched-chain amino acids for a baby with maple syrup urine disease). He can also select the nonprotein caloric source. The possibilities are limitless.

338

C. ELECTROLYTES AND ADDITIVES
Indicate total per bottle or per 24 hours

KCl _____mEq

NaCl _____mEq

MgSo₄ (2cc 50%—8.1 mEq Mg) _____mEq

CaGluc (10cc 10%—4.5 mEq Ca) _____mEq

NaHCO₃ _____mEq

K Phos _____mEq

Reg insulin _____ units

Alcohol 7 kcal/gm _____gm

MVI_____ ml

SBF _____ ml

Heparin _____units

Specific L-amino acids

_____ mg/liter

Ordering electrolytes as the total mEq desired per bottle, or per 24 hours, eliminates ambiguity and allows greater flexibility in use of different base solutions, whether through design or through necessity. Remember that variations in the electrolyte content exist in different solutions.

Good labeling, meaningful order form or method, and clearly defined ordering policies can do much to enhance in-house safety.

NUTRITIONAL TEAM

At the medical center, there is no official nutritional team, though I believe this is the best method for maximum control; to promote in-house safety, however, I do have probably the world's largest unofficial team.

When a new patient is to receive total parenteral nutrition, we notify the nurse epidemiologists. They monitor the patient for early signs of sepsis and forward a report of their findings on each patient. The environmental control technician recovers equipment, final filters, and nutritional solutions for bacteriological survey. The IV nurses, during their rounds, ascertain that a specific administration set with a nylon mesh filter is being used. They check use of final filters where indicated.

Continuing in-service education lectures and demonstrations on the principles of hyperosmolar alimentation and aseptic techniques inform the nurse who is inexperienced in this field, increase her awareness that success depends largely on her efforts, and serve to update our procedures for all nurses.

We insert a "Reference and Guide for Nursing" in the chart of each patient receiving intravenous alimentation. Every institution in which TPN is utilized should have, if not a special nursing team, at least, as an alternative, a fully trained supervisor to perform these in-service education functions and vital follow-up.

You might be wondering, at this point, "Are all of these precautions necessary?"

With our unofficial and unorthodox approaches and efforts, our fungemia attack rate, for more than 650 patients since July 1969, is less than 2%. Hence, safe parenteral nutrition is possible with proper precautions.

Where do we go from here? What does the future hold for total parenteral nutrition, and, in particular, how can the nutritional solutions themselves be made safer?

I was intrigued with the drawing of a proposed plastic container for mixing of components of parenteral diets in an excellent article by Dudrick and Rhoads, "New Horizons for Intravenous Feeding," (*JAMA* **215:**939 (947), 1971). This suggests a totally closed unit with compartmentalized areas for the additives. These are squeezed to introduce the electrolytes and vitamins to the nutritional fluid in a totally nonair-dependent system.

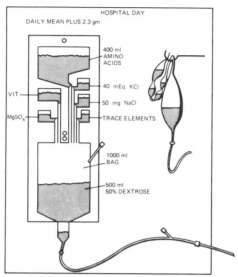

Fig 8

My first impression was, "Wow, that's pretty far out!" And like any other innovative idea, it took a while to develop. But that "far out" idea, at least the plastic bag part, is what we are now using in the medical center for our nutritional formulas (see Fig 9).

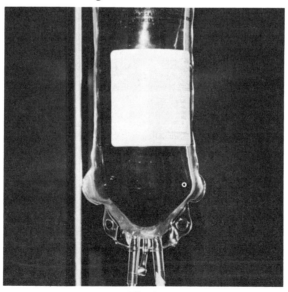

Fig 9

340

This HA unit is a nonair-dependent, soft plastic container that collapses as the fluid is administered to the patient, thereby eliminating the possibility of airborne contaminants entering the unit. It eliminates the problems of coring and the mess and potential hazard of fluid leaking from an airway. Because the bag can expand, it can accommodate an unlimited volume of additives. The PL-146 polyvinyl formulation used in the Travenol Viaflex bags represents the safest plastic formulation presently available.

We developed an improved technique for preparing HA solutions in Viaflex, one that offers the ultimate in safety and flexibility. We think of it as the prototype of Dudrick's and Rhoads' "package of the future." Commercially manufactured solutions can be used in this preparation.

PREPARATION OF HA SOLUTIONS IN VIAFLEX

Supplies (Fig 10)

3x1 liters Amigen 5/D-5
 (Am-5/D-5)
3x500 ml dextrose-50% (D-50%)
 (same lot numbers for both)
4 empty, sterile 1 liter plastic bags
 (Viaflex, Baxter Labs PL-146)

Vacuum unit (Viavac) and pump. Y-type administration set and 19-gauge needle (allows latex disc of bag to positively reseal)

YIELD: 4 units of basic HA adult formula.

STEP 1: Number the AM-5/D-5 bottles sequentially, calibrate them (Fig 11) in the inverted position, in 750 ml increments (ie, 750 ml from bottle #1, then the 250 ml balance of bottle #1 is added to 500 ml from #2, etc.).

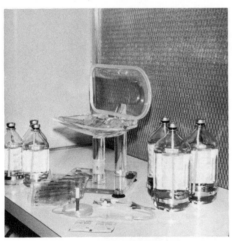 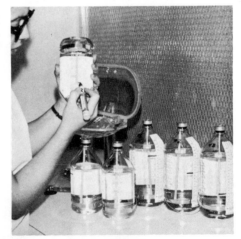

Fig 10   **Fig 11**

STEP 2: Number the D-50% bottles sequentially in the inverted position and calibrate in increments of 350 ml (in the same manner as above).

To prevent fluid from dripping from the airway of the bottle when inverted, the Y set is clamped shut and pushed through the previously prepared latex disc. (Do not remove the latex disc.)

STEP 3: Prepare the "injection port" of the plastic bag and insert the 19-gauge needle. Place the empty bag in the vacuum unit (Fig 12) and rotate to the vertical "vacuum" position. Open the roller clamp to permit transfer of fluid into the bag, *then* insert needle into air vent of Amigen bottle to facilitate transfer. When 750 ml have run into the bag, clamp the roller on the Amigen to shut it.

STEP 4: Run 350 ml of D-50% into the bag; again, insert needle to facilitate transfer. When the HA unit is completed, shut off main roller clamp closest to bag.

STEP 5: Prepare the next bag and remove the needle from the completed unit and insert immediately into the next empty bag. This prevents the needle from being contaminated. Remove the completed TPN unit and place the next empty bag into the vacuum unit.

STEP 6: Run the remaining solutions from the first bottles into the bag (Fig 13). While they are running, prepare the next set of bottles. Insert the administration set *through* the latex and continue the pattern as before (ie, the fluid is removed from each bottle down to the next calibration). Numbering and marking in this fashion reduces possible errors during transfers, and the procedure can be performed by a specially trained technician.

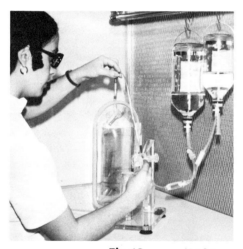

Fig 12

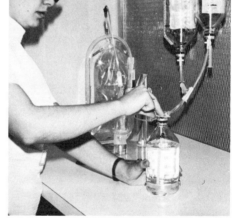

Fig 13

This sequence is followed until all of the bags have been completed (Fig 14).

STEP 7: Identify the completed units with a storage label and refrigerate the units (Fig 15).

To speed up preparation time, two vacuum units may be monitored by one operator. With a good vacuum pump, these plastic bags are completed in about 3.5 minutes each. A new type will be released that requires no needles and can be filled in about 30 seconds.

Though not shown here, an in-line membrane filter can be used to provide additional protection from particulate contamination, especially with formulations for pediatric use.

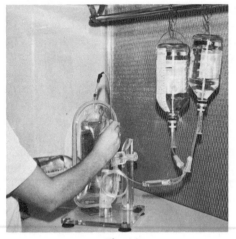

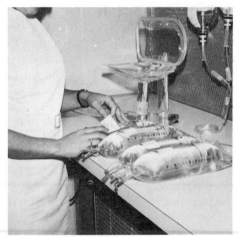

Fig 14   Fig 15

We conducted a study to determine the efficacy of final filters. In a pediatric intensive care unit, we detected a 22% contamination rate of the proximal surface of in-line final filters (0.45μ) on regular IV solutions. The distal surfaces were negative, indicating that the final filter was effective. An interesting aspect of the study is that the predominant organism was diptheriod, a common skin organism, suggesting touch-contamination upstream of the filter, possibly during IV tubing changing and manipulation.

Poor technique can be a significant factor in bacterial and fungal septicemia. Strict procedural and technique policies for handling sterile solutions and related accessories must be established and enforced in every institution. The intravenous route for supplying medications or nutrients is potentially hazardous; yet because it is used so frequently, it is one of the most taken-for-granted routes of administration. Also, the patient's medications can produce significant changes in body chemistry and electrolyte patterns.

DEVELOPING A TPN PROTOCOL

The institution, person, or persons responsible for a nutritional team must develop or adopt a protocol or physician's guide to encourage the rational and safe use of parenteral alimentation. Too frequently problems develop because TPN is handled as an adjunct to conventional IV therapy. The "life-line" catheter is used as a convenient, multipurpose access to the patient. Vital laboratory tests are not performed routinely. Subtle changes go undetected until heroic efforts are required to correct them.

With these problems in mind, I have prepared a protocol or format which may be adapted to individual situations.

Following is a proposed list of guidelines to encourage rational and safe use of total parenteral alimentation. The ramifications of this intravenous nutritional procedure are too involved to present here in an outline form. This proposed protocol is based upon guidelines observed by medical centers in Philadelphia employing this feeding technique; modifications of procedures and tests suggested by Dudrick et al; and compilations of data obtained in the Wilmington Medical Center and other institutions.

TPN Protocol

1. Carefully evaluate patient as a candidate for TPN and set specific objectives for therapy.
2. The following tests should be performed. As a starting reference, perform the following tests: SMA-12; Electrolytes including magnesium; CBC; Hct.
3. At initiation of TPN, correct anemia and/or plasma protein deficit.
4. Insert catheter to superior vena cava and confirm placement radiographically.
5. Write complete order specifying
   (a) volume of TPN solution per 24 hours;
   (b) total mEq of essential electrolytes, as indicated by laboratory work, per TPN unit bottle *or* per 24 hours;
   (c) other additives and quantities.
   NOTE: TPN solutions decrease serum potassium levels.
6. Laboratory work
   (a) perform daily studies until patient is stabilized (5 to 7 days):
      (1) fractional urines q6h, sliding scale insulin for more than 2+ glucose or more than trace acetone;
      (2) blood sugar;
      (3) electrolytes and CO_2, pH, and pCO_2;
      (4) accurate input/output (I/O);
      (5) body weight.
   NOTE: After one week: CBC, prothrombin, creatinine, Hct, pH, SMA-12, magnesium, phosphorus.
   (b) proceed with routine laboratory work after patient is stabilized and tolerating HA formula (receiving 2,500 to 5,000 ml/24 hours):
      (1) daily: fractional urines (see above), I/O, body weight, clinical evaluation by MD (physical examination);
      (2) two to three times weekly: electrolytes, change catheter dressing (Monday, Wednesday, Friday);
      (3) once weekly: CBC, prothrombin, creatinine, Hct, pH, SMA-12, magnesium, phosphorus;
      (4) on each Monday and Friday add 2.5 mg folate and 100μg B_{12}.

When ancillary fluids are needed, solutions providing additional dextrose can result in sugar spillage into the urine and produce some diuresis; 0.45% saline can be used for supplementing fluid intake without contributing to the problem of extra dextrose.

In an emergency (eg, bottle breaks, catheter clots at night) use $D_{10}W$ or D_5W until more HA solution is obtained.

Avoid sudden discontinuing of the solution. Taper off (eg, from 4 U/day, decrease to 2 U/one day, then decrease to regular IV fluids if indicated, or discontinue).

To reduce contamination potential, no TPN unit should hang longer than 12 hours. Discard old fluid and hang new unit. Record amount received by patient on input/output sheet.

TPN PROTOCOL DISCUSSION

First, carefully evaluate patient as a candidate for TPN. (See also p 342.) TPN should not be considered a short-term therapy. One to two weeks of continuous infusion at an input sufficient to achieve positive nitrogen balance is generally necessary for any significant patient improvement or true weight gain or tissue repair. To treat a patient with HA for only a few days is probably not a rational use of this procedure. Many patients with sufficient upper GI and small bowel function (as little as 1 to 30 cm small bowel reported) may be adequately nourished by one of the oral, low-residue, elemental amino acid/carbohydrate diets (eg, Vivonex-100 H-N). Set specific goal for therapy (eg, heal fistula, until x-rays improve; personal goal of patient; one-month period) so that some appropriate end point can be anticipated.

Second, have sufficient body chemistry data as a starting reference before initiating TPN. The results to the following tests should be available before initiating TPN: SMA-12; electrolytes including magnesium; CBC, Hct.

Correct anemia and/or hypoalbuminemia at onset of TPN therapy so that HA fluids will be utilized for tissue production rather than for serum protein replacement.

Markedly impaired renal function and severe azotemia and/or severe liver disease may preclude use of conventional hyperalimentation solutions. Special formulas may be required.

Third, insert indwelling catheter and initiate catheter care. The HA solution is extremely hypertonic (exerting between 1,800 to 2,000 mOsm); consequently, it *cannot* be given peripherally for any extended period.

The preferred route for children of 5 kg or more and adults is via indwelling catheter inserted into the subclavian vein and directed into the *superior* vena cava. Use of the percutaneous puncture technique outlined by Dudrick et al is convenient, rapid, and appears to reduce the incidence of contamination. Familiarity with this technique is vital in avoidance of the potential hazards (eg, pneumothorax, misdirection of catheter, etc.).

In infants weighing less than 5 kg and in children, the right external jugular is preferred because of the direct approach into the superior vena cava. (The left approach gives possibility of occluding the thoracic duct although it has been done successfully with caution.)

Long catheters from peripheral veins increase the risk of mechanical and chemical irritation of the intima of the peripheral veins and present a slight increase in the incidence of sepsis; but they have been used successfully in some cases where difficulty was experienced with the primary routes.

The superior vena cava appears to be a safer route. Infusion of *slightly* hypertonic solutions via catheter into the *inferior* vena cava has been accompanied frequently by thrombosis and pulmonary embolism.

Whichever route or technique is employed, it is advisable, especially if any difficulty during catheter insertion is encountered, that the catheter tip be located and identified by chest x-ray. Use of a radio opaque catheter simplifies visual identification.

Experience indicates that meticulous care of the catheter site (see p 320) and regular change of IV tubing, down to the catheter, have significantly reduced incidence of bacterial and fungal sepsis. All tubing and catheter connections should be scrupulously prepared with Betadine solution *before* and *after* changing IV tubing, and the connection sites protected from direct contact with the patient's skin by sterile gauze. A suggested schedule of Monday, Wednesday, and Friday may simplify and encourage follow-through of this *important* routine step.

Do not draw blood or give blood via the HA catheter. If, for any reason, the catheter plugs up, it should be *removed* and a new catheter inserted. *Caution:* The obstructed catheter should *not* be cleared by irrigation. Catheters should be changed at least every two weeks. Since this catheter is essentially the patient's life-line, it is wisest to restrict use to delivery of nutritional solutions *only*. It should not be used to monitor central venous pressure or administer other drugs, unless absolutely necessary.

USE OF FILTER SETS

Administration sets containing a nylon-mesh "blood filter" chamber are to be used routinely when HA solutions are being administered by gravity (ie, without aid of an infusion pump) to adult patients. When more efficient filtration is indicated (ie, for all pediatric patients; with IV infusion pump), an 0.45-μ "final filter" will be provided. This is secured to the distal end of the IV set between the tubing and catheter. All IV sets and accessories are replaced *daily*.

THE TPN ORDER

A complete order should be written specifying: volume of solution per 24 hours, *total mEq* of essential electrolytes desired *per TPN bottle*, other additives and quantities.

Parenteral hyperalimentation is efficient and effective when the HA solutions are given continuously. Brief interruptions, if necessary for administration of other medications (see catheter care), do not disrupt the nutritional regimen significantly. Too frequently parenteral alimentation has appeared ineffective because inadequate daily volume has been given.

A choice of formulations to satisfy the individual patient's nutritional requirements is desirable. The Protocol should describe those formulas available for in-house use. Following is an example:

Two basic formulations are available:

The basic formulation most commonly used is designated HA. It consists of 1,100 ml and provides:
Dextrose 212 gm (about 20%)
Protein 28 gm (8 essential amino acids plus histidine (approximately 4.5 gm N)

Potassium	. . 13 mEq	Calcium	. . .	5 mEq
Sodium	. . . 25 mEq	Chloride	. . .	16 mEq
Magnesium	. . 1.5 mEq	Phosphate	. .	22 mEq

Yields approximately 725* (850) nonprotein kilocalories.

A newer, more concentrated formula designated as *Neo HA* consists of 1,000 ml and provides:
Dextrose 250 gm (about 25%)
Protein 37.5 gm (approximately 6 gm N)

Potassium	. . 15 mEq	Calcium	. . .	5 mEq
Sodium	. . . 30 mEq	Chloride	. . .	22 mEq
Magnesium	. . 2 mEq	Phosphate	. .	30 mEq

Yields 850* (1,000) nonprotein kilocalories.
*See p 336.

Added to these basic formulations are essential multiple vitamins and additional electrolytes as indicated by the patient's lab values.

LABORATORY WORK

Perform routine laboratory work as outlined. Serious and fatal consequences have resulted when recommended tests were not performed for extended periods.

Prolonged intravenous alimentation can produce some degree of erythroid hypoplasia and gradual downward deviation of the hematocrit.

Early detection of electrolyte and blood chemistry changes allows safe minor adjustments in the nutritional formula and avoids resorting to heroic measures to correct a gross deficiency.

NURSING IMPLICATIONS AND GUIDE

Maintain a constant and correct flow rate of infusion calculated for the amount of fluid ordered per 24 hours. Too rapid administration can cause nausea, vomiting, twitching, and convulsions; it can also result in hyperosmolar diuresis and dehydration. Hypertonic solutions, given too rapidly, can produce an acidotic state.

Check the flow rate frequently and make minor adjustments if necessary. Don't try to "catch up" if the flow schedule falls behind. The IV label has the calculated milliliter-per-hour rate and approximate drops-per-minute rate.

Don't forget that the positioning of the patient (sitting, walking, etc.) can influence the drip rate.

Check the IV tubing for kinks.

Keep strict input and output record.

Do fractional urines every six hours; report 4+ sugar and any acetones to the physician.

Use aseptic technique when changing HA bottles and when necessary to make addition (eg, insulin) to bottle, do so just before hanging unit.

Because of potential incompatibilities (see p 333), other medication should not be added to HA formula. If additions are necessary (eg, electrolytes), call pharmacy to check compatibility and make additions just prior to hanging TPN unit.

Once a patient is placed on a TPN regimen, his formula will be sent daily, automatically.

Keep this TPN solution refrigerated until needed. If not used within 48 hours, return to pharmacy.

Be sure the subclavian dressing is kept dry and check the area of the catheter to note swelling of neck or face, distension of neck veins, pain in arm or shoulder, leakage, prominence of arm and hand vein. Report any positive findings to physician.

Notify the physician if patients do not tolerate (nausea and vomiting) the HA solution or spike a temperature.

Call physician if patient has sudden temperature elevation.

Administer the TPN solution using a Blood Filter IV set.

Don't use careless sterile technique. HA solution is an excellent medium for microorganisms.

Don't draw or administer blood through the TPN infusion catheter. An alternate route should be used.

Notify pharmacy immediately if there is any change in TPN order. Pharmacy will call every day to check the order status and any problems and will generally send a 24-hour supply of TPN solution daily.

Chapter 11

Hospital Practice of Total Parenteral Nutrition

Robert L. Ruberg, M.D.

Major areas of problems encountered in the administration of parenteral nutrition solutions include patient-solution incompatibilities, metabolic aberrations, mechanical malfunctions, and infections. Discussion of these four areas is used as a basis for constructing a system of administrative principles and guidelines for total intravenous nutrition.

The final step in delivery of parenteral nutrition solutions is the administration of such preparations to individual patients. Despite the fact that this is the last stage, it is, by no means, the least important. The theoretically perfect solution—one which is nutritionally balanced, accurately formulated, bacteriologically sterile, and chemically pure—can still produce serious complications if not administered to the patient in the proper manner. Hence, a critical appraisal of the various complications which may occur in patients receiving high-calorie parenteral nutrition solutions is essential to facilitate construction of a rational series of criteria for safety and to formulate principles of administration for the delivery of total parenteral nutrition solutions to patients. At this point, one assumption will be made: that the patient who is to receive the nutritional solution already has in place a functioning, properly positioned central venous catheter.

COMPLICATIONS IN THE PRACTICE OF TPN

Four major areas in which problems may arise during the course of total parenteral feeding are:

Patient-versus-solution incompatibility,
Metabolic alterations,
Mechanical malfunction, and
Infection.

Patient-Versus-Solution Incompatibilities

Problems of patient-versus-solution incompatibility are rare phenomena. In our experience at the University of Pennsylvania, these reactions have taken two different forms. One manifestation is fever; the other presents a more typically allergic picture. The febrile pattern usually appears shortly after the initiation of infusion, within 15 to 30 minutes. The patient's oral temperature may rise to 103°F or more, accompanied by a shaking chill. If the infusion is stopped, the patient quickly defervesces, and repeated attempts at infusion with the same solution will have identical results.

In several patients, we have observed a more delayed reaction, the appearance of hives, wheals, and other typical signs of allergy; these also disappear when the solution is stopped and return with subsequent challenge.

To date, we have seen the febrile and allergic patterns only with hydrolysate solutions. In five of our cases, the patients were successfully switched to crystalline amino acid solutions without further complication.

Metabolic Alterations

The most common metabolic alteration results from the high level of glucose used in most parenteral nutrition solutions. Two opposite extremes of this problem may occur: Hyperosmolar nonketotic hyperglycemia, resulting from reduced glucose tolerance, an improper nutrition regimen with excessive glucose, or accidental rapid infusion of standard solution; and severe hypoglycemia, usually resulting from inappropriate insulin administration or sudden cessation of the concentrated glucose infusion. Lesser degrees of hypo- or hyperglycemia also have deleterious effects and may be avoided through the proper practice of parenteral feeding. The use of partial substitutes for glucose calories (eg, sugar alcohols or fat) might ultimately reduce the incidence of these aberrations.

Another area of metabolic alteration is acid-base imbalance. With hydrolysate solutions, acid-base balance problems are infrequently seen and easily corrected. With the newer crystalline amino acid solutions, however, hyperchloremic metabolic acidosis can occur unless care is taken to avoid the addition of chloride-containing compounds to the base solution. If the routine solution additives (eg, sodium chloride and potassium chloride) are made in the usual fashion, a hyperchloremic acidosis will result. To circumvent this problem, we have been adding sodium as bicarbonate and potassium as acetate. Nevertheless, these newer solutions provide more of a challenge in maintaining acid-base equilibrium.

As in routine intravenous therapy, electrolyte imbalance can appear in patients receiving total parenteral alimentation. Administration of potassium ion poses a special problem with high calorie solutions. Because of the high level of glucose delivered intravenously, there is a shift of circulating potassium into cells. Also, if—as we postulate—there is active synthesis of cellular mass, potassium as the major intracellular ion is needed in greater than usual amounts. As a result, adult patients on intravenous hyperosmolar alimentation usually require at least 100 mEq of potassium per day, and sometimes more than 200 mEq/day. Frequent determination of the serum potassium ion concentration is vital, therefore.

We have demonstrated incidence of hypophosphatemia in patients receiving hyperalimentation with a variety of solutions. Serious consequences of hypophosphatemia have been documented, including decreased levels of adenosine triphosphate and 2,3-diphosphoglycerate, a leftward shift of the oxygen-hemoglobin equilibrium curve, and a specific metabolic block in the glycolytic pathway. These effects can and should be prevented through the routine inclusion of calcium and phosphorus in total parenteral nutrition mixtures. The serum phosphorus level must be monitored in order to judge adequacy of replacement.

The evidence for assuring levels of other minerals and trace elements is not as clear as in the case for calcium and phosphorus. Magnesium is generally included in parenteral feeding mixtures, and occasional checks of serum magnesium levels may aid in recognizing serious deficiency. Ultimately it may be necessary to monitor serum levels of certain vitamins as well as trace elements (eg, zinc and copper).

Finally, because of the generally high volumes of nutritional infusion given, fluid overload may occasionally occur, particularly in debilitated patients. Appropriate use of diuretics plus alterations in infusion rate can minimize this problem when recognized early.

Mechanical Malfunction

One frequent source of mechanical malfunction is the central venous catheter. Air embolization is a significant risk in the patient with an indwelling central infusion line. At any time that the catheter is dressed, tubing replaced, or bottles changed, the patient is exposed to potential air embolization. For this reason, it is safest to place the patient in the reclining position whenever tubing manipulations are carried out.

Generally, the serious incidents of air embolization occur when the integrity of the infusion system is *accidentally* disrupted. A patient may try to get out of bed when his tubing is caught in the bedrails, inadvertently disconnect his tubing from the central venous catheter, and suffer a significant or even fatal air embolus. Several precautions must be taken to prevent such a catastrophe. All tubing connections can be tightened maximally and reinforced with adhesive tape. A minimal number of tubing segments should be used; stopcocks and other extraneous connectors in the tubing system should be avoided. The patient should be cautioned *not* to manipulate his infusion apparatus in any way. Through meticulous attention to detail, air embolization can be prevented.

Another more common mechanical malfunction—and potentially as dangerous—is the inadvertent rapid infusion of the hyperosmolar nutritional solution. The rapid infusion of a large portion of the nutritional fluid can result in significant metabolic alteration leading to coma. A hyperosmolar state is rapidly achieved, and an osmotic diuresis may ensue with the resultant loss of fluids and electrolytes. Headache, nausea, vomiting, and seizures have been observed after such rapid inadvertent infusion. Where gravity flow is utilized for infusion, a flow rate which is relatively constant over 24 hours must be maintained. Frequent confirmation of the accuracy of flow rate is necessary. Where infusion pumps are available, this problem is eliminated, though admittedly replaced by other problems related to the mechanics of the pumps. A perfectly adequate infusion program can be maintained with gravity drip infusion.

Again, the opposite extreme of flow-rate abnormality can result in serious deleterious effects. A sudden cessation of flow will occasionally produce a significant rebound hypoglycemia. To avoid hypoglycemia if infusion is interrupted, it is generally safer to provide exogenous insulin, when required, via the intravenous route rather than subcutaneously. In patients receiving no exogenous insulin, circulating endogenous insulin levels rarely cause significant hypoglycemia where infusion is abruptly stopped.

The usual cause of this phenomenon is clotting of the infusion catheter, though occasionally other mechanical malfunctions—catheter displacement or tubing leakage—can have the same effect. The maintenance of a constant flow rate with careful catheter and tubing care can minimize the incidence of either of these effects. Clearly, when infusion is interrupted, glucose must be provided quickly, either through reinstitution of the intravenous infusion or oral feeding where possible.

Infection

Perhaps the most controversial of these four problem areas is infection. In the majority of cases, fever in patients receiving intravenous hyperosmolar alimentation results from infection elsewhere in the body. Occasionally this is difficult to identify. As a result, it becomes necessary to remove a parenteral-feeding catheter as a precautionary measure. Infection may result from contaminated bottles or tubing, as well. Infections from these sources generally respond to bottle and tubing change. If fever persists, catheter infection must be suspected.

The incidence of catheter infection varies widely according to different investigators. In a prospective study of contamination, the data, as yet in the preliminary stage, point to a *primary catheter infection* rate of approximately 4% in over 150 consecutive cultured catheters. Primary catheter infection signifies a positive catheter culture obtained in a patient with no known pre-existing source of infection. The overall positive catheter culture rate was approximately 12%. In one third of these, the organism found on the catheter had been isolated previously from another source (eg, urinary tract or wound infection) in the same patient. In another one third—also patients with positive cultures—multiple flora infections at other sites were present, although the specific organism found on the catheter was not identified elsewhere. Thus, at least one third of all catheters—possibly as many as two thirds of all catheters—appear to be secondarily infected. In this way we arrive at an incidence of primary catheter infection (ie, where no previous source of contamination has been identified) of 4% of the total number of catheters placed. We feel that this favorable infection rate represents the result of proper care and maintenance of catheters by the physician and nursing personnel.

When present, catheter infection almost invariably becomes evident promptly. The patient's temperature will generally rise to above 102°F. Occasionally, the temperature elevation will not be as high, but a fever of only 100°F accompanied by shaking chill may herald catheter infection. Removal of the infected central venous catheter almost invariably results in prompt defervescence without further sequelae. The incidence of positive catheter cultures *without* fever is low. Only 3% of the catheters removed from afebrile patients in the aforementioned study grew organisms.

In summary, recommendations evolving from this study of central venous catheters are prompt removal of catheters when infection is considered and maintenance of a high level of suspicion in patients with known infection elsewhere. With proper catheter care, the incidence of catheter infection can be kept acceptably low.

CRITERIA FOR SAFETY

The preceding review of the various complications in patients receiving total parenteral nutrition serves as a basis for determining criteria for safety and the principles of administration during hyperosmolar alimentation expressed in the guidelines which follow. These are constructed within the framework of the four problem areas discussed above as they apply to medical and nursing personnel.

From the nursing point of view, a number of guidelines can be stated (see Table 1). To monitor the incidence of incompatibilities, vital signs should be taken at least every four hours in patients receiving high-calorie solutions. In addition, if a sudden change in the patient's condition is noted, temperature and vital signs (given in Table 1) should be repeated immediately.

Table 1.—Nursing Principles

Vital signs q4 h and prn
Accurate daily weights
Strict intake and output
Fractional urines q6 h; notify MD of 4 + glucose.
Maintain constant flow rate (<10% change).
Notify MD of flow rate change.
Notify MD of temperature elevation.
Handle catheter aseptically.

To monitor metabolic status, several nursing procedures should be carried out. The patient must be accurately weighed each day. Where available, bed scales provide easy access to accurate data. Carefully measured intake and output assist in the determination of the state of fluid balance. The urinary glucose spill should also be determined at least every six hours, and the physician in charge notified of 4 + nitroprusside reaction. In addition, the skilled nurse can observe signs and symptoms of electrolyte imbalance and hypo- or hyperglycemia.

The nurse plays a vital role in preventing problems in the third major area, that of mechanical malfunction. The nurse must maintain a constant infusion rate when gravity flow is used. Variations of greater than 10% from the prescribed rate of flow should not be permitted. If accidental slowing occurs, discard extra solution rather than try to "catch up" to a fixed bottle change schedule through rapid infusion. If rapid infusion occurs, or the infusion is suddenly stopped, the physician should be notified promptly so that appropriate therapy can be instituted immediately. When bottle changes and tubing manipulations are carried out, all precautions against air embolus must be observed.

The fourth group of nursing principles concerns approach to, and prevention of, infection. Whenever a temperature elevation occurs, the nurse

354

should notify the physician promptly. When handling the central venous catheter, especially during dressing changes, strict aseptic techniques must be observed at all times to minimize the incidence of infections.

The physician guidelines (see Table 2) also stem from the four major problem areas. The physician must be wary of early patient-versus-solution incompatibilities and carefully review the daily record of vital signs. More importantly, the physician plays an essential role in detecting and correcting metabolic aberrations. The physicians must review the recorded weight and intake and output daily. A daily physical examination gives further information concerning the patient's state of hydration. A daily weight increase—up to a three-quarter-pound average—can be seen with tissue synthesis during hyperosmolar alimentation; but more than this amount clearly suggests fluid overload. Routine laboratory data should be reviewed promptly, and appropriate corrections should be made in the infusion program. Particular attention should be paid to the serum potassium level.

Table 2.—Physician Guidelines

Review vital signs.
Check I and O, daily weight.
  (<3/4 lb weight increase)
Daily physical exam (state of hydration, etc.)
Review electrolytes. Correct when needed.
Check urinary glucose (add insulin for persistent 3+ and 4+
  combined with elevated blood sugar).
Treat over- and underinfusion promptly.
Evaluate fever promptly; (change bottle first, pull catheter
  when indicated).

The physician must follow the urine and blood sugar determinations closely. Occasional 4+ urinary spill can be covered with subcutaneous insulin, but persistent 3+ or 4+ spill should be promptly treated by the addition of insulin to the infusion mixture and/or slowing the rate of solution delivery.

The serious consequences of hypophosphatemia are avoided by following closely the serum phosphorus level and making appropriate adjustments in the infusion mixture.

In the area of mechanical malfunction, the physician generally plays a less important role than the nurse. He must be prepared to treat promptly sudden accidental rapid infusions or inadvertent cessation of flow. He should avoid the use of the central venous catheter for the infusion of blood or blood products, in order to maximize catheter life.

Finally, the physician's most challenging problems often are infections. Because of the multiple medical problems encountered in patients receiving total parenteral nutrition, fevers are not rare. Each temperature elevation must nevertheless be carefully analyzed by the physician. Our basic recommendations are as follows:

Suspect the bottle or tubing, particularly if a new bottle has recently been started.
Change and culture the tubing and bottle, and follow the fever pattern.

If the temperature persists over a few hours, reevaluate and reexamine the patient thoroughly to determine a source of fever *other than* the central venous catheter.

If a source of sepsis other than the catheter is clearly evident, then treat appropriately. If not, remove and culture the central venous catheter. The high calorie infusion may be transferred to another site and preferably at a later date.

The following summarizes a hyperosmolar alimentation laboratory test schedule (see Table 3) suggested for adults: Blood sugar, sodium, potassium, chloride, and CO_2-combining power are measured routinely three times a week. During the early stages of feeding and when significant changes in the regimen are made, these determinations may be carried out daily. In patients receiving solutions which have no phosphorus content, calcium and phosphorus are added to the solution (as noted earlier), and serum levels of calcium and phosphorus are measured up to three times a week. Other determinations, including magnesium, blood urea nitrogen, serum protein, and a complete blood count, are done once a week. Liver and renal function tests often are useful on a weekly basis as well. Blood gases may be needed occasionally if problems with acid-base balance appear. Determinations of trace element and certain vitamin levels may also become routine.

Table 3.—Laboratory Studies

Blood sugar	3 x weekly
Electrolytes	3 x weekly
Ca, P	2-3 x weekly
Mg, Proteins, CBC, BUN	Once weekly
Trace elements	
Vitamins	??
Blood gases	

This system of guidelines and principles should be applicable in all institutions to all patients receiving this potentially lifesaving form of therapy.

PART THREE

Section One

B. Chemical and Physical Safety

12 Migration of Phthalate Ester Plasticizers
Robert J. Rubin, Ph.D., and Rudolph J. Jaeger, Ph.D.
13 Chemicals and Particulate Matter
Kenneth E. Avis, D.Sc.

Colloquium: Safety
Digest of Colloquium
P. William Curreri, M.D., and Robert H. Henry, M.S.

SAFETY AND DELIVERY OF SOLUTIONS

Chapter 12

Migration of Phthalate Ester Plasticizers

Robert J. Rubin, Ph.D., and Rudolph J. Jaeger, Ph.D.

The role of phthalate esters in plasticizing a variety of polymeric materials, giving them the pliability that makes the plastics acceptable for use in parenteral equipment, is discussed, di(2-ethylhexyl)phthalate (DEHP) in particular. Its migration into the circulating blood is considered, also the migration of plasticizers from blood storage packs into stored human and dog blood. Implications of this migration into complex biological solutions suggest reevaluation of the toxicological impact of the esters and the necessity for remedial techniques.

During experiments with the isolated, perfused rat liver, an unidentified compound accumulated in both the liver and circulating blood. Analytical studies utilizing the techniques of nuclear magnetic resonance, infrared and mass spectrometry, established the identity of the compound as glycolyl phthalate. Subsequent studies indicated that it arose in the perfusion system as an hepatic metabolite of a plasticizer that had migrated into the circulating blood from the plastic tubing used in the apparatus. The plasticizer was identified as the butylglycolyl butyl ester of phthalic acid.[1]

The structure of phthalic acid and the nature of the esterification of this acid with various alcohols to form a family of compounds, referred to as phthalate esters, is shown in Figure 1. Examples of this class of compound are dibutyl phthalate (DBP), butylglycolyl butyl phthalate (BGBP), and di(2-ethylhexyl)phthalate (DEHP). The latter compound is also frequently referred to as dioctyl phthalate (DOP). The phthalate esters, as a class, are used widely to plasticize (make supple or pliable) a variety of polymeric plastics. They accomplish this by lessening the intermolecular attractions between adjacent polymeric chains, allowing them to slide over one another, giving to them the characteristic referred to as pliability. The plasticizers are not covalently linked to the polymeric chains but may be looked upon as being dissolved in the polymer. This gives rise to the possibility of migration of the plasticizers from the plastic surface. Further, the plasticizers are not present in trivial or trace amounts. They account for 30% to 40% of the weight of the final plastic. This is particularly so with the polyvinylchloride (PVC) plastics as they are formulated for various medical applications such as bags for blood and parenteral solutions, tubing and intravenous infusion sets. The most widely used plasticizer in these applications is DEHP.

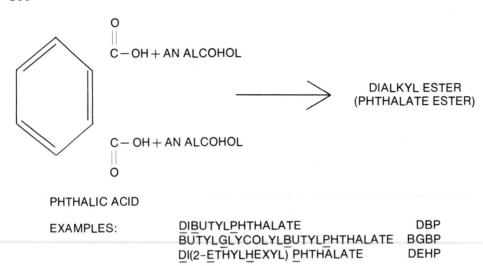

PHTHALIC ACID

EXAMPLES:
DIBUTYLPHTHALATE	DBP
BUTYLGLYCOLYLBUTYLPHTHALATE	BGBP
DI(2-ETHYLHEXYL) PHTHALATE	DEHP

Fig 1. Phthalic acid.

EXPERIMENTAL EVIDENCE OF MIGRATION

Experiments with DEHP-plasticized PVC tubing (medical-surgical grade Tygon S-50HL) in the isolated, perfused liver preparation indicated that this phthalate ester readily migrated into the circulating blood.[2,3] Fifty ml of diluted rat whole blood extracted a total of 2 mg of DEHP after 5 hours of circulation at 37 C. Under identical conditions, a solution of 4% bovine serum albumin extracted approximately 40% of the amount of DEHP extractable by whole blood, a finding with implications for storage of parenteral solutions in plasticized PVC bags. Thus, the migration problem is not related solely to the presence of lipoid substances such as are present in blood. Protein alone is able to extract significant amounts of the plasticizer; but saline was unable to extract any amount of DEHP greater than was seen in the solvent blank.

To further explore the migration of plasticizer from tubing, commercially available hemodialysis units (Travenol) and cardiopulmonary bypass units (Travenol) were set up in the laboratory, and human blood was continuously circulated through them for five to eight hours in a manner simulating clinical use. Levels of DEHP ranging from 5.7 to 9.2 mg/100 ml were noted. Another plasticizer, di(2-ethylhexyl)adipate, was observed to migrate from both types of units. From the hemodialysis unit, it reached blood levels of 2 mg/100 ml in eight hours and 5 mg/100 ml from the bypass unit in five hours.[2]

Attention was turned to a study of the migration of plasticizers from the blood storage packs (Fenwal JA-2C Blood Pack) into stored human and dog blood.[3,4] For both dog and human blood the rate of migration was found to be linear, and amounted to 0.25 mg/100 ml/day at 4°C. At 21 days, the DEHP concentration in human blood ranged from 5 to 7 mg/100 ml. From such data it can be calculated that a whole body exchange transfusion of 21-day-old blood in a 70-kg man (approximately 10 to 12 units of blood) would result in the intravenous administration of 250 to 420 mg of DEHP or a dose of 4 to 6 mg/kg.

We next looked at the distribution of DEHP in various fractions obtained from whole blood stored in plastic packs for 14 days.[2] Approximately 60% of the total extracted plasticizer is found in the density <1.21 fraction of plasma, which indicates that the bulk of the plasticizer is found associated with the lipoprotein fraction of blood. The density >1.21 fraction represents the lipid-free protein fraction of the plasma; the accumulation of approximately 25% of the total plasticizer in this fraction once again emphasizes the affinity of the plasticizer for protein. The red blood cells contained only a small portion of the total plasticizer.

Having followed the migration of DEHP from the plastic pack to the blood, we looked for the plasticizer in the tissues of individuals who received transfusions of various volumes of whole blood of different storage ages.[4] All samples were obtained at autopsy. The time elapsed between transfusion and death was variable and is not precisely known in all cases.

Our studies revealed the presence of DEHP in a number of human tissues, the most frequent being the lung, with concentrations ranging from 13 to 91μg/gm of dry tissue weight. These levels were found in 7 out of 12 lung tissues assayed. Surprisingly enough, DEHP was found in only one of five samples of abdominal fat, although three of the four negatives displayed DEHP in the lung tissue. In addition, no DEHP was detected in the abdominal fat of seven individuals who had received no known blood transfusions. A more complete evaluation of the DEHP tissue levels of individuals with and without a history of blood transfusion is currently underway.[5]

Experiments in which DEHP was administered intravenously to rats confirmed the high affinity of lung tissue for this plasticizer: 27% of the injected dose was found in the lung after 24 hours; another 27% was found in the liver.[2] An experiment with the isolated perfused rat liver suggests further cause for concern about the toxicological implications of the migration of significant quantities of plasticizer into blood. In a perfusion system in which all of the PVC tubing was replaced with nonplasticized silicone rubber tubing, an aliquot of DEHP was added exogenously to the perfusing blood. It was observed that within one-half hour of perfusion the blood level had fallen to 10% of the initial level and that by 4.5 hours the blood was essentially cleared of all DEHP.[2,3] Extraction of the total liver after 4.5 hours of perfusion indicated that approximately 90% of the initial DEHP was accumulated unchanged in the liver. It is this accumulation of unmetabolized DEHP in tissue that may be of toxicological significance.

Whereas blood is stored at 4°C, platelet preparations (platelet-rich plasma:PRP) are currently stored for short periods of time at room temperature. We therefore investigated the migration of DEHP into PRP stored in PVC transfer packs (Fenwal TA-2) for two days at room temperature.[6] We found that the plasma attained levels of 15 mg/100 ml within the two-day storage period, as compared to less than 1 mg/100 ml at this time period, or 5 to 7 mg/100 ml in 21 days for whole blood at 4°C. Thus, the process of migration appears to be highly dependent upon temperature. In addition, it was observed that the platelets reached a level of some 2.5 times the concentration of DEHP in the plasma in which they were bathed, suggesting a preferential uptake of DEHP.

TOXICOLOGICAL SIGNIFICANCE

In general, DEHP and a variety of other phthalate esters have been reported to have a low order of toxicity. Of eight phthalate esters examined in one study, the intraperitoneal LD_{50} dose in mice ranged from 1.5 to 14.2 gm/kg. In rats, the intraperitoneal LD_{50} of DEHP has been reported by several investigators to range from 2 to 31 gm/kg. One report by Hodge in 1943 indicated that a single intraperitoneal dose of 128 gm/kg of DEHP produced death in only 5% of a group of treated mice.[7] Other studies on oral administration of DEHP indicated an LD_{50} of approximately 30 gm/kg in rats and rabbits given a single oral intubation. Ninety-day and two-year feeding studies in rats and one-year feeding studies in guinea pigs and dogs also indicated a low order of toxicity for DEHP. These data have resulted in the Food and Drug Administration's approval of DEHP for use in plastic wrapping for food intended for human consumption.[8]

These toxicological data have at least two shortcomings. First, they pertain mainly to oral and intraperitoneal administration. Few, if any, data are available on the toxicologic potential of intravenous administration of phthalates, such as would be relevant to the situation with intravenous transfusions. Until recently there was little evidence indicating the degree of absorption of the phthalates from the gastrointestinal tract or peritoneal cavity. In the latter case, some data suggest that absorption was rather poor. More complete studies are in progress.[9] The second shortcoming is that the toxicologic evidence deals primarily with gross, overt effect (ie, death, body and organ weights, and histologic changes). It does not take into account more subtle toxicologic effects.

Observation of such subtle effects in our laboratory prompted the question: what is the effect of the plasticizer on the quality of stored blood?

Based on our observations of the enhanced uptake of DEHP by platelets in platelet-rich plasma stored in PVC packs, we looked at platelet adhesiveness and the tendency of platelets to form microaggregates in stored blood. We found a high order of correlation ($r = 0.84$) between the DEHP content of stored blood and the presence of microaggregates.[2] Further work is underway to determine if the DEHP is causally related to the increased platelet aggregation seen in stored blood.[10]

BEHAVIORAL EFFECTS IN ANIMALS

The effect of DEHP on several behavioral parameters in experimental animals was studied. Hypothalamic electrodes were implanted in rat brains.[2,11] These electrodes were localized in the so-called pleasure centers and were set up so that if the rat pressed a bar an electrical stimulus was delivered to the electrode and a "pleasureful" reward was perceived. The rats were trained to bar press at a highly reproducible rate. A single intraperitoneal dose of DEHP (500 mg/kg) markedly inhibited this behavioral performance.

In another experimental design, rats were given free access to a rotating wheel in which they could run ad lib.[2,11] A mechanical counter recorded the revolutions, and control rates of running activity were determined. DEHP

(500 mg/kg ip) virtually eliminated this type of behavioral activity. At this dose of DEHP (500 mg/kg), the rats overtly appear alert; the decrement in behavioral response did not appear to be due to a state of anesthesia or narcosis.

In other experiments, the effect of intravenous DEHP on reticuloendothelial function was determined.[2,11] In these experiments rats were given a test dose of colloidal carbon suspension. The control rate of disappearance of the carbon from the blood was determined. It was observed that DEHP could alter the rate of carbon clearance in either of two directions, depending upon the schedule of administration. Following a single acute dose of DEHP, the clearance rate was significantly decreased; if the same total dose of DEHP was given over four consecutive days, reticuloendothelial function was stimulated and carbon clearance was more rapid. All carbon clearance determinations were made 24 hours after the last dose of DEHP.

These results depict several of the biological alterations that we have observed in our laboratory with DEHP. In addition, in collaboration with DeHaan, we determined that DEHP at a level of 0.4 mg/100 ml in the growth medium was lethal to beating embryonic heart cells in tissue culture.[2] This is the concentration of DEHP attained in human stored blood after 24 to 48 hours of storage.

DeHaan first called our attention to his system when he observed that passage of a serum-containing tissue culture media through a commercially available PVC clinical intravenous drip set (Plexitron R 41) proved lethal to the cells.[12] Although we did establish 0.4 mg of DEHP as being lethal to the tissue culture, we further demonstrated that this level of DEHP was not attained in the media that has passed through the IV drip set. Thus, while we were able to determine a lethal concentration of DEHP for these cultured cells, something else, as yet unidentified, must also be leached from the IV drip set in sufficient concentration to cause cellular death.

We have investigated the possibility of migration of DEHP from Viaflex plastic bags (Travenol PL 146) into simple nutrient solutions such as 5% dextrose, 0.9% saline, or 5% protein hydrolysate. These solutions, after long term storage for periods exceeding one year and under a wide range of ambient temperatures, were found to contain only traces of DEHP.[13] The trace amounts were not different from the analytical blank. A precautionary note should be made, however, concerning the storage of protein-containing solutions in these types of plasticized bags.

CONCLUSION

These data indicate the migration of heretofore unanticipated quantities of DEHP into complex biological solutions such as blood and plasma. The presence of this chemical (as well as other plasticizers) in solutions used for direct intravenous administration to humans calls for reevaluation of the toxicologic impact of these compounds. With the idea of completely avoiding adulteration of the stored product, another alternative would be the development of low-cost, easy-to-fabricate substitutes for the plasticized bags currently being used.

364

References

1. Jaeger RJ, Rubin RJ: Plasticizers from plastic devices: Extraction, metabolism, and accumulation by biological systems. *Science* **170**:460-462, 1970.

2. Jaeger RJ: Studies on the extraction, accumulation, and metabolism of phthalate ester plasticizers from polyvinyl chloride medical devices, thesis. Johns Hopkins University, Baltimore, 1971.

3. Jaeger RJ, Rubin RJ: Extraction, localization, and metabolism of di-2-ethylhexyl phthalate from PVC plastic medical devices. *Environmental Health Perspectives* **1(3)**:95-102, 1973.

4. Jaeger RJ, Rubin RJ: Migration of a phthalate ester plasticizer from polyvinyl chloride blood bags into stored human blood and its localization in human tissues. *New Eng J Med* **287**:1114-1118, 1972.

5. Rubin RJ: Plasticizers in human tissues. Letter to the Editor. *New Eng J Med* **288**:915-916, 1973.

6. Jaeger RJ, Rubin RJ: Di-2-ethylhexyl phthalate, a plasticizer contaminant of platelet concentrates. *Transfusion* **13**:107-108, 1973.

7. Hodge HC: Acute toxicity for rats and mice of 2-ethyl hexanol and 2-ethyl hexyl phthalate. *Proc Soc Exp Biol Med* **53**:20-23, 1943.

8. Food Additives Amendment to the Food, Drug and Cosmetics Act, Subpart E-121.2001, Federal Register (15 October 1968) 33 FR 15281.

9. Schulz CO, Rubin RJ: Distribution, metabolism, and excretion of di-2-ethylhexyl phthalate in the rat. *Environmental Health Perspectives* **1(3)**:123-129, 1971.

10. Valeri CR, Contreras TJ, Feingold H, et al: Accumulation of di-2-ethylhexyl phthalate (DEHP) in whole blood, platelet concentrates, and platelet-poor plasma. I. Effect of DEHP on platelet survival and function. *Environmental Health Perspectives* **1(3)**:103-118, 1973.

11. Rubin RJ, Jaeger RJ: Some pharmacologic and toxicologic effects of di-2-ethylhexyl phthalate (DEHP) and other plasticizers. *Environmental Health Perspectives* **1(3)**:53-59, 1973.

12. Dehaan R: Toxicity of tissue culture media exposed to polyvinyl chloride plastic. *Nature* (New Biology) **231**:85-86, 1971.

13. Rubin RJ: Storage of aqueous solutions for parenteral infusion. Letter to the editor. *Lancet* **1**:965, 1972.

Chapter 13

Chemicals and Particulate Matter

Kenneth E. Avis, D.Sc.

Inadvertent chemical and physical contaminants may be found in total parenteral nutrition solutions. While the toxicology of these contaminants is not clearly established in all instances, their presence is contraindicated. A review of the significance of these contaminants and suggestions for their elimination is presented.

No therapeutic agent administered to patients is free from the risk of injury to at least a few of the recipients. It is administered, however, because the anticipated benefits far exceed the risk of injury. One of our continuing objectives is to seek means to minimize the risk while enhancing the benefits of therapy. Total parenteral nutrition can be provided only directly into the bloodstream. Therefore, considerations for reducing the risk by this intimately direct but highly vulnerable-to-harm route are essential.

The larger the volume of fluid introduced into the bloodstream and the longer the period of administration, the greater the possibility of adverse effects upon the patient. Since parenteral nutrients are administered not in just a few milliliters, but in volumes of several liters a day, and for several days or even several months, the characteristics of the product and parameters associated with safety must be scrutinized with exceptional thoroughness. In addition, since parenteral nutrition is utilized in pediatric care—when the patient is in the very beginning of what is hoped will be a normal length of life—safety characteristics take on different dimensions from those for an adult having a terminal illness.

PARTICULATE MATTER

In 1963[1] and 1964[2] Garvan and Gunner focused attention upon the harmful effects in man and animals that may be produced by the presence of insoluble particles in intravenous solutions (Fig 1, Fig 2).

Others have confirmed their report that particles similar to those found in intravenous solutions could be encountered in the center of granulomas within lung and other vital tissues in man and animals (Fig 3).[3,4]

The report by Jaques and Mariscal in 1951[5] reflected the surge of concern over the safety of intravenous solutions containing such particles, yet earlier studies, such as that of Brewer and Dunning (1947), tended to allay concern.[6] Suspensions of ground glass were injected into the marginal ear vein of rabbits. In one rabbit, 153 injections were administered over a period of nearly one year. Rabbits in the test series appeared to be in perfect health up to the time of sacrifice. Upon autopsy, the glass was found lodged in vital tissues and organs of the animals, but there seemed to be no gross impairment

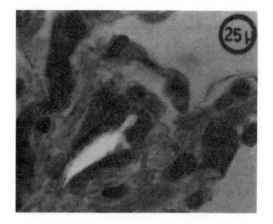

Fig 1. Particles in human lung tissue.

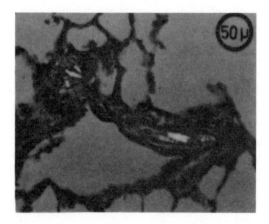

Fig 2. Particles in rabbit lung.

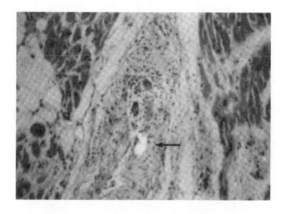

Fig 3. Particles in human heart.

of function. It was concluded that "injection of occasional particles will not give rise to pathology which could be considered dangerous."

Attitudes have changed, and concern is evident everywhere. Much definitive work is needed, however, to clarify a variety of factors. Questions not clearly answered include:

> What kinds of particles and what characteristics cause them to lodge in the capillary wall and generate granulomas? Does the shape, the degree of smoothness or sharpness of edges, the chemical composition, or the surface charge affect the likelihood of the particle lodging in the capillary?
>
> How many circulating insoluble particles are necessary to produce results which will impair the function of vital organs?
>
> What size particles will most likely lodge in the capillaries? Is it reasonable to assume that, as long as the particles are smaller than red blood cells, they will pass through the capillaries without producing an adverse effect?

OCCURRENCE

Particles have been and can still be found in intravenous solutions. The particle counts from solutions distributed in Australia—as reported by Vessey and Kendall in 1966—are summarized in Table 1.[7]

Table 1.—Counts (per ml) for Selected Particle Diameters[7]

Manufacturer	Number of Samples	Particle Diameter			
		2μ mean	3.5μ mean	5μ mean	10μ mean
A1	29	11,760	3,401	1,286	152
A2	16	2,255	586	186	28
B	11	2,212	592	199	26
C	22	185	50	18	8
D	25	1,275	296	97	17
E	9	4,863	1,092	363	35
F	7	245	73	27	10
G	18	241	48	18	9

It is apparent that the control exercised over the manufacture of these solutions affected the particulate content, since the same technology used by manufacturers C, F, and G was available to the others. It is to be noted that the particle counts are for the size indicated and larger and were per milliliter of solution. In this and other studies, it has been found that the number of particles is inversely related to the size.

Processing technology has improved significantly since the Vessey and Kendall report, so that particle counts in intravenous solutions usually are much lower today. This may be seen by comparing the data in Table 1 with that in Table 2, taken from a recent report by Davis and Turco.[8] (Please note that the particle counts in this table are per liter of solution.)

368

Table 2.—Total Particles ($>5\mu$) Per Liter [8]

Manufacturer	Average
A	373
B	98
C	1,490
D	360

Note: Average of 12 samples each of 5 solutions.

No standard exists in the United States as an acceptable limit for particles in intravenous solutions. The Australians have established a limit of not more than 250 particles of 3.5μ and larger per ml of solution (written communication, Department of Health, Commonwealth of Australia). Whether or not such a standard is needed in the United States as a stimulus to the improvement of processing technology is an open question, but the standard in Australia would seem to be behind the current technology.

DETECTION

The detection of particles is most frequently based upon a visual examination of the contents of the container of solution and a decision as to whether or not particles are visible. It is recognized that this method is limited by such factors as: visual acuity, the attention of the inspector, the lighting and the conditions surrounding the inspection, the color and opacity of the product and container wall, and the size limitation of human inspection. Under the best conditions of inspection, particles much smaller than 50μ cannot be seen with the unaided eye. If, as some have suggested, a particle in the size range of 5μ and larger is critical, it might be concluded that human inspection is an exercise in futility. While it is clear that better inspection methods are needed, it is reasonable to assume that, if no particles are observed within the visible range, the particle count at the smaller size ranges should be low (see Table 1).

The **Coulter Counter,** which was used for the data in Table 1, detects smaller particles than a human inspector can and has been widely utilized as an instrument for counting particles.[7] Its operational principle is based on a decrease in electrical conductivity when a particle passes through a capillary between two electrical poles. However, it is a destructive method, because the sample container must be opened to be counted. Other instruments are now available.

Another method widely used is a **membrane filtration technique,** also a destructive technique.[9] A sample of a solution is passed through the membrane filter, and particles present are retained on the surface of the filter. They then are examined and counted by means of a microscope (see Fig 4). This method requires considerable training and experience in microscopy to obtain reproducible results, and it is time-consuming.

NATURE AND SOURCES

It is often possible to identify the nature of at least some of the particles by using the microscopic method of detection, particularly when coupled

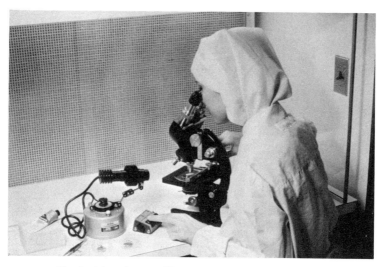

Fig 4. Membrane filter counting equipment.

with staining techniques and the polarizing microscope. Particles most frequently found include cellulose fibers, rubber, chemical particles of various types, glass, and plastic.

Cellulosic or other types of fibers are widely distributed in the environment. They may be on the wall of a "clean" container, in the processing lines of equipment, or in the air at the time of exposure of the solution as it is being prepared for administration. They are generated from clothing, packing material, housekeeping utensils, paper products, and the like. They may enter the product at any time during its history. They should be eliminated during the filtration step of processing, but may be reintroduced at the time of final preparation and administration in the hospital.

Chemical particles may arise from chemical reactions within the product, leaching from rubber closures, residues of contaminants such as detergents, and a variety of other sources. Rubber particles are the result of abrasion of rubber closures or from the fragmentation of the closure as a hypodermic needle or administration set is inserted through the closure. Glass particles normally come from opening a container, such as an ampule, or from glass fragments left in the container at the time of manufacture or during shipment. Plastic particles may be found as a residue from manufacture or as fragments from abrasion of components of the system or tubing.

Potentially, particles may be introduced:

1. During the manufacturing process from a variety of sources;
2. During preparation of the product in the hospital for administration; and
3. During passage through the administration set into the patient.

The first general source of particles and, in part, the third are a responsibility of the manufacturer. The second and third, in part, are the responsibility of the hospital staff.

ELIMINATION

Improvements in processing technology now make it possible to prepare intravenous solutions that have a low particulate content, as shown in Table 2. If proper quality control is exercised in the pharmaceutical plant, the particle level in intravenous solutions can be maintained well below the Australian standard. However, attention must also be given to those smaller volume therapeutic agents which are added to intravenous solutions, such as electrolytes, vitamins, antibiotics, and nutrient concentrates. As may be seen from the data in Table 3, the passage of a solution through an administration set or the addition of an electrolyte, vitamins, or both substantially increased the number of particles in the final mixture. Most of these particles were probably present in the additives, but some may have been introduced through the equipment used to make the addition or through exposure to the environment. If the manipulations are not carried out in a clean environment, the introduction of particulate matter and biological contamination is to be expected.

Table 3.— Total Particles ($>5\mu$) per Liter in D5W of Four Manufacturers Plus an Administration Set and Two Additives [8]

Manufacturer:	A	B	C	D
D_5W	262	40	991	218
D_5W + Set	332	126	1,875	430
D_5W + Set + KCl	506	109	3,402	768
D_5W + Set + Vit	2,748	645	5,130	3,362
D_5W + Set + Vit + KCl	2,958	625	6,380	5,120
D_5W + Set + Vit + KCl + Baxter final filter	21 (80% 5-25μ)	12 (80% 5-25μ)	11	48
D_5W + Set + Vit + KCl + Abbott final filter	14 (80% 5-25μ)	23 (80% 5-25μ)	15	18

The elimination of particulate matter from intravenous solutions, such as those used for total parenteral nutrition, is based upon at least three areas of control:

There must be high manufacturing standards of quality control. The entire preparation of the basic solution and any additives made in the pharmaceutical plant must be based on the best technology available. It is obvious that each of these products must be low in particulate matter if the final nutritional solution is likewise to have a low particulate level.

Manipulations involving the combination of components of the product and addition of other substances must be done by a trained individual utilizing a controlled environment and clean, sterile equipment, preferably by a pharmacist working in a high efficiency particulate air (HEPA) filtered laminar air flow enclosure with adequate assurance that proper technique will be followed (see Fig 5).

Nurses and physicians involved with administration of the product to the patient must maintain strict control of the procedure, thus not reintroducing particulate matter at the time of administration. They also should insist that a high standard of quality be utilized in the procurement of products and that strict control be exercised over the processes utilized in preparing them for use in the patient.

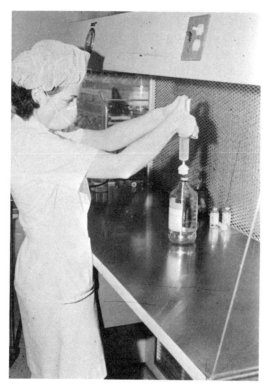

Fig 5. Filtering additive to intravenous solution in horizontal laminar flow enclosure.

Development of the membrane filter probably has contributed most to recent clean solution technology. The closer the filter can be used to the actual point of entry of the solution into the vein of the patient, the greater will be the effectiveness of particle elimination. It is not appropriate, however, to assume that the utilization of a final filter just upstream of the infusion catheter makes it possible to eliminate other quality control procedures. First, not all contaminants can be eliminated by filtration. Pyrogens are an example. Second, the membrane filter functions by screening particulate matter out of the solution as it passes through; thus particulate matter will collect on the surface of the filter and tend to build up a layer that may stop the flow of the liquid. Therefore, if a final filter is to be used, the solution should be cleaned previously, and the final filter used primarily as a safety device.

The membrane filter is a cellulose ester consisting of a very thin, tender sheet. It is easily torn or ruptured if not properly handled and supported in appropriate holders. A back surge of air or fluid through the filter may be sufficient to rupture the membrane. Obviously, a ruptured membrane will not retain particulate matter. Membrane filters are available in a variety of pore sizes, ranging from less than 0.2μ to several microns in pore size. Since the filter functions by sieving, the pore size determines the size particles that will be retained on the surface (see Fig 6, Fig 7). If the filter is to sterilize the solution, an 0.2μ porosity is required. With such a fine-porosity filter, delivery of parenteral nutrition solutions will require a pump to provide the pressure differential needed to effect a reasonable flow rate. If particulate matter elimination is the objective, a 1 to 2μ porosity filter should be adequate, giving substantial flow rate from the hydrostatic pressure resulting from hanging a bottle of solution at the patient's bedside. Clogging of 25-mm filters almost always occurs within 1 to 3 liters of nutritional solution passed through them. This may be due in part to the presence of insoluble particulate matter and in part to the presence of colloidal substances from the amino acids and carbohydrates present in the product. The particulate matter may be of subvisual size.

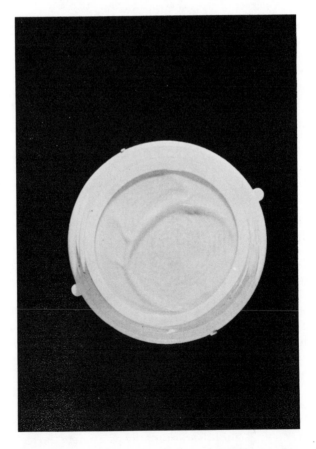

Fig 6. Particulate matter collected on membrane filter from vial of an antibiotic.

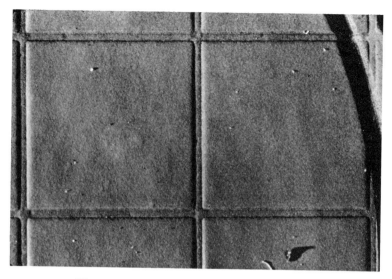

Fig 7. Example of membrane surface.

ENVIRONMENT

The opening of sterile commercial containers, the transfer of the contents of one to another, and the inclusion of various additives, all expose the product to contamination if the environment is not under adequate control. The HEPA filtered laminar air flow enclosure provides a clean environment. However, it is imperative that the filter be installed and maintained so that it is cleaning the air effectively. In addition, it is essential that personnel working in the enclosure are familiar with its limitations and recognize that, unless their movements are properly planned and their technique is confirmed to be aseptic, they can introduce contamination even in a laminar air flow workbench. Recently, it came to my attention that the downstream surface of a HEPA filter in a workbench had apparently been unintentionally splashed with solution. Since it was the custom to turn the blower off at night, adequate time was provided for microorganisms to land on the residue and multiply. Subsequently, when the workbench was used again, microorganisms were blown from the filter directly to the critical working area. The effective use of a laminar flow enclosure is contingent upon a recognition of the limitations in its use.

Since no solution is completely free from particles, and additional particles may be introduced at several points in its history—including preparation for administration at the patient's bedside— a **final filter** should be used. Provided the product has been maintained sterile and the objective is to remove particulate matter, a filter having a porosity of 1 to 2μ should be adequate and would provide a reasonable flow rate.

CHEMICAL PURITY

All chemicals utilized in the preparation of nutritional solutions or added at the time of administration should be of the highest purity obtainable, both physically and chemically. Physical impurities include pieces of wood, cardboard, dust, and insect fragments. Such contaminants are obviously undesirable and are more apt to be found in chemicals of lower quality. Chemical impurities also will be found where quality is lower and they may contribute to toxicities or possibly unexpected chemical reactions with other ingredients in the formulation. Therefore, emphasis should be placed upon quality, not cost, in procurement of ingredients and products.

Solutions for parenteral nutrition are excellent culture media for microorganisms. Therefore, the introduction of only one organism can quickly lead to a serious septic condition. Even if microorganisms should subsequently be eliminated by filtration, the pyrogens produced would not be eliminated. Once present, pyrogens cannot readily be eliminated. Therefore, they must not be introduced. These chemical contaminants also must not be present as impurities in ingredients used to formulate parenteral nutrition solutions.

INCOMPATIBILITY

Precipitation due to chemical reaction will generate particles that are at least as toxic as dirt or lint particles. It is well known that di- or trivalent inorganic cations and anions frequently interact to produce insoluble compounds that will precipitate when conditions are appropriate. Thus, calcium or magnesium ions in the presence of phosphate, sulfate, or carbonate ions—a combination not infrequently found in parenteral nutrition formulas—may interact and precipitate. Insoluble divalent salts of some drugs could be formed in the preparation, also. The amount of precipitate is not always large and may not be readily visible, partly because of the stabilizing properties of amino acids and carbohydrates. However, it may contribute to the plugging of a membrane filter and, if filtered out, will reduce the content of each substance.

The pH often has a pronounced effect upon solubility and the degree of interaction. Additives may significantly alter the pH of the entire nutritional formula. Most vitamin preparations have a low pH, ascorbic acid and thiamin hydrochloride in particular.

CONTAINER COMPONENTS

Glass containers are widely used for parenteral nutrition formulations. However, plastic containers are receiving increasing attention and interest. Rubber closures are necessary to close the openings of glass containers. Therefore, rubber, glass, and plastic container components may be in intimate contact with the product. Leaching of constituents can occur from all three by the action of the solution. The problem is usually greatest with rubber compounds because more additives are normally present.

Both plastic and rubber attract particles, in part because of electrostatic effects. During processing, particles may adhere to the surface of these materials and then be released into the solution during subsequent handling and storage. Both plastic and rubber materials can be abraded with the release of small particles. This is usually a greater factor with rubber compounds, since they are more elastic.

Glass will gradually dissolve in most aqueous solutions, especially when the glass is of the soda lime or soft glass type. Most containers of large-volume parenteral solutions are made of soda lime glass with a resistant surface treatment. Normally this provides a glass which is stable to the attack of nutritional solutions. However, if the container is subjected to abnormal thermal conditions during processing or storage, and if the storage period is quite long, glass flakes may be formed. This would not be expected with normal processing, but the possibility exists.

MISCELLANEOUS CONTAMINANTS

Residues of cleaning agents may be found occasionally in empty containers or equipment incompletely rinsed. If present, the cleaning agent may react with constituents in the formulation.

Surface disinfectants are often used freely on the outside surfaces of containers. All of these agents are toxic to tissue. Should they be inadvertently introduced into the product, toxicity of host tissue may occur and/or chemical reactions may be encountered (eg, alcohol may denature amino acids and reduce their solubility). Therefore, surface disinfectants should be used sparingly and carefully, never leaving pools of the liquid where it may run into the product.

SUMMARY

Particulate matter is a physical contaminant of high incidence which requires the attention of those responsible for the preparation and use of parenteral nutrition solutions. Chemical contaminants are less likely to be introduced in the hospital than in the manufacturing plant; therefore, they present less of a safety hazard at the point of use, provided high quality products are procured.

References

1. Garvan JM, Gunner BW: Intravenous fluids: A solution containing such particles must not be used. *Med J Aust* **2:**140-145, 1963.

2. Garvan JM, Gunner BW: The harmful effects of particles in intravenous solutions. *Med J Aust* **2:**1-6, 1964.

3. Jones AM: Potentially hazardous effects of introducing particulate matter into the vascular system of man and animals, in *Symposium on Safety of Large Volume Parenteral Solutions,* Food and Drug Administration, 1966.

4. Gross MA: The danger of particulate matter in solutions for intravenous use. *Drug Intelligence* **1:**12-13, 1967.

5. Jaques WE, Mariscal GG: A study of the incidence of cottom emboli. *Bull Intern Assoc Med Museums* **32:**63-72, 1951.

6. Brewer JH, Dunning JHF: An *in vitro* and *in vivo* study of glass particles in ampuls. *J Am Pharm Assoc (Sci Ed)* **36:**289-293, 1947.

7. Vessey I, Kendall CE: Determination of particulate matter in intravenous fluids. *Analyst* **91:**273-279, 1966.

8. Davis NM, Turco S: A study of particulate matter in IV infusion fluids. Phase 2. *Am J Hosp Pharm* **28:**621-623, 1971.

9. Trasen B: Membrane filtration technique in analysis for particulate matter. *Bull Parenteral Drug Assoc* **22:**1-8, 1968.

Safety

Colloquium

P. William Curreri, M.D., chairman and editor
Robert H. Henry, M.S., rapporteur

Dr. Curreri: Examination of factors affecting patient morbidity and mortality is an essential preface to development of minimum requirements for safe delivery of parenteral programs. Toward achievement of this goal of safety, our scrutiny of these subjects embraces the following topics:

I. Clinical administration of the currently available hyperosmolar glucose-amino acid solutions
    A. Sepsis
        1. Incidence
        2. Etiology
            a) Intravenous catheter
            b) Depressed host resistance secondary to severe disease
            c) Overuse of systemic antibiotics with opportunistic organism overgrowth
    B. Delivery
        1. Intravenous catheter care
        2. Connective tubing
        3. Filters
        4. Personnel
        5. Inservice education
II. Preparation
    A. Bacteriological quality control
        1. Hospital pharmacy
        2. Manufacturer
    B. Solution constituents
        1. Federal regulation of clinical research

CLINICAL ADMINISTRATION

Sepsis

Dr. Curreri: Sepsis is the major life-threatening complication of parenteral nutrition delivered via the central venous catheter for prolonged periods.

Incidence

Dr. Curreri: Previously reported studies, designed to describe the incidence of septicemia in patients receiving total parenteral hyperosmolar

378

alimentation, have lacked suitable matched controls. For the most part, these have been retrospective studies. Our participants, who represent major medical clinics throughout the United States and Europe, will present data collected prospectively from controlled patient populations.

In every hospital there exists a patient population with terminal disease or minor states of malnutrition in which utilization of parenteral nutrition is *elective*. Few have examined the incidence of sepsis in these patients; but for many reasons one might expect an incidence as high in controls receiving standard diets as is observed in those receiving parenteral alimentation. With the increased utilization of more potent antibiotics, chemotherapeutic drugs, irradiation, and other improved diagnostic and therapeutic modalities, extremely malnourished individuals with extensive disease now survive for longer periods. Frequently they experience recurrent septic complications regardless of the type of alimentation.

If patients receiving total parenteral nutrition do indeed have an increased incidence of sepsis, we are confronted with an even more difficult question: Is the sepsis related to the indwelling catheter (a foreign body in the bloodstream); composition of the solution; methods of manufacture, preparation, and delivery; or all of these?

Our experience indicates that the incidence of sepsis in extremely ill patients with indwelling catheters remains unchanged regardless of the type of solution administered.

If the indwelling central venous catheter becomes contaminated with bacteria or fungi, the source of contamination must be examined. Are these primary infections in which the bacteria gain entrance to the bloodstream through or along the catheter? Are they secondary infections in which microorganisms lodge on the catheter during transient septicemias from a distant septic source in the patient with a gastrointestinal fistula, an infected wound, or a major burn? Such patients have frequent episodes of bacteremia following minor debridement or other minor surgical procedures.

Reflecting on these postulates, I am impelled to ask, specifically: What evidence do we have that incidence of sepsis is increased in an ill, poorly nourished patient receiving total parenteral nutrition as compared to a similar patient with inadequate oral alimentation but without an indwelling venous catheter?

Dr. Ausman: Wei and Hamilton provided parenteral nutrition to approximately 30 children, none of whom had central venous catheters and none of whom got infected. Some patients did have an indwelling catheter inserted peripherally. In the absence of a perfectly controlled study, this is an example of patients in whom no septicemia was observed; but they apparently qualified for parenteral nutrition and were subjected to a slightly different parenteral program than that which requires central venous catheters.

Dr. Border: We have had a high incidence of septicemia in very depleted patients, probably 10% to 20% on ward services in the presence of inadequate catheter management.

In the presence of adequate catheter management and in the presence of vigorous pulmonary management in the severely traumatized patient, we have had essentially no sepsis. I put it that way because the problems of pneumonias are common in depleted patients and in the posttrauma patient. But with vigorous pulmonary management, endotracheal tubes, plasma, positive expiratory pressure breathing, and intelligent use of volume-cycled respiration, our pneumonias have essentially disappeared and, along with them, our septic, bacteremic problems.

Probably a large incidence of hyperosmolar alimentation bacteremia is secondary to sepsis someplace else. Organ sepsis has to be considered organ by organ. The mechanisms of induction of wound sepsis are quite different from those of pneumonic sepsis. Sepsis someplace else, the depleted patient, and inadequate catheter management add up to this high incidence of bacteremia.

If we wait until the patient is so depleted that he is in gross trouble before beginning hyperalimentation, we then have a high incidence of bacteremia. We must start nutrition as soon as we know that the patient has not eaten for one week, if he was previously well nourished; if he was previously malnourished, we must start nutrition as soon as resuscitation is complete. We start early and never let them get depleted. Thus the incidence of catheter sepsis is lowered.

The problem with massive trauma is that the patient is lethargic for a long period of time and will not eat. We begin our intravenous hyperosmolar alimentation as soon as resuscitation is completed. As soon as bowel function returns, we begin progressively to shift to the elemental diet via the nasogastric tube and reduce intravenous alimentation; therefore, the risks of catheter-bottle sepsis decrease. Traumatized patients are at high risk for stress ulcers and massive gastrointestinal bleeding. Nasogastric feedings provide calories as well as increased nutrition to the gastrointestinal tract mucosa.

Dr. Curreri: Let me take some liberty with the figures Dr. Ruberg reported (see p 352). He observed an overall positive culture rate of approximately 12% during parenteral hyperalimentation, with only 4% due to infection via the catheter (ie, either primary infection through the catheter tract or contamination related to the process of putting the catheter into a central vein).

If true, does this imply that the other 8% of these patients would have developed septicemia whether or not they had an indwelling central venous catheter?

Dr. Ruberg: I don't think I can answer that. First, it would be inaccurate to say that 12% of the patients had septicemia. These patients had fever, and, when the catheter was removed, it was found to grow organisms; but not all of these patients had positive blood cultures.

The data suggest that at least a transient bacteremia or fungemia occurred in a significant percentage of the patients. A catheter sitting in the bloodstream forms a perfect focus for the settling of organisms, just as a defective heart valve is a focus where organisms can settle. This is why we will prophylactically put patients with heart valve lesions on antibiotics for minor surgical procedures. In about two thirds of our patients, a definite preexisting source of infection was present before any evidence of catheter contamination appeared.

Dr. Goldmann: I gather you are asking if there is a problem. The best studies have been done with plastic catheters used to deliver conventional intravenous fluids, and there is no doubt that the intravenous system can be responsible for a substantial incidence of septicemia. Some investigators have considered a variety of catheter types, including central venous catheters in the arm, subclavian catheters, angiocaths, and intercaths. The same infection picture holds for all catheter types: The risk of septicemia increases the longer a catheter remains in place. This may be due in part to the fact that numerous infections are caused by contaminated fluids; if the fluid is contaminated, I don't care if you use a scalp vein, it can still cause septicemia.

Dr. Border: You said these series were broken down as to the location of the catheter in the body; but the series I have collected on intravenous catheterization versus septicemia are not broken down as to the anatomic location of the catheter. That is the major defect.

At least one study shows a greater incidence of bacteremia following arm vein catheters than following central venous catheters.

Dr. Goldmann: I should add that some studies utilized an effective surveillance system to distinguish intravenous-related septicemias from septicemias secondary to infection at other sites.

Catheter-associated septicemia has a characteristic clinical picture. The patient is suddenly wracked with a shaking chill and looks terrible. He may spike a temperature to 102°F–105°F and go into shock. Upon withdrawal of the catheter, without any other therapy, the fever disappears, and the patient quickly recovers. This is not always the case; some patients ultimately die with disseminated bacterial endocarditis or fungemia; most IV-associated infections, however, have been cleared rapidly by removing the catheter and the bottle.

Dr. Ruberg: Dr. Goldmann suggests that perhaps the septicemia rates are similar for both central and peripheral venous catheters. The data reported relate to a short duration of peripheral catheterization. Most of the studies show that the catheters or scalp veins were in place between two and four days.

We are talking about very different data in the patients receiving hyperosmolar alimentation. I suggest there is a difference in terms of infection rate with the central venous catheter. The average duration of catheterization in our series of 150 cultured catheters was 16 days. The average time for the appearance of infection was identical (ie, when the contaminated catheters alone were analyzed, these also were in place an average of 16 days). The data suggest that, if the incidence of septicemia and catheter infection is the same in the central and peripheral catheter studies, it certainly is not in the same time sequence. This represents a significant difference.

Dr. Curreri: Also, I suspect there is an increased incidence of transient septicemia, unassociated with indwelling venous catheters, that generally is not recognized. If we obtained a blood culture every hour for 24 hours from a patient who had serious trauma, a serious burn, or a serious neonatal gastrointestinal abnormality, it probably would alarm us to ascertain the number that are positive when no intravenous catheter is in place.

If we put a patient with burns into a Hubbard tank for debridement, we often observe a transient bacteremia, despite the fact that the patient does not appear clinically to have septicemia. The risk of secondary catheter sepsis to a patient with an indwelling catheter under these circumstances is unknown at the present, but would fall close to the 8% estimate of Dr. Ruberg.

Dr. Wilmore: At the US Army Institute of Surgical Research, all intravenous catheters are placed using aseptic technique; but they are removed and reinserted in another infusion site in two to three days. All indwelling catheters, even the centrally placed cannulas, are changed this often. All the catheter tips are cultured upon removal. In 1968 and 1969, we were handling catheters by routine methods: swabbing the site with alcohol, placing the catheter, and changing it every two or three days. In 1970, we initiated a program of daily catheter care: scrubbing the site with Betadion, applying antibiotic ointment and a sterile dressing.

A comparison of the catheter complications associated with catheter care is seen in Table 1. The number of patients with septic thrombophlebitis, diagnosed by biopsy, represents no real change following the program of catheter care. Although there were fewer catheters cultured in 1969 than in 1970, the percentage of positive cultures was about the same.

Table 1.— Effect of Catheter Care on Intravenous Cannulation Complications

	1969 (no catheter care)	1970 (daily catheter care)
Number of admissions	301	325
Patients with thrombophlebitis	52	60
Patients with septic thrombophlebitis	21 (6.97%)	17 (5.25%)
Deaths associated with septic thrombophlebitis	12	15
Number of catheters with positive cultures	31/78	86/237
Percent of catheters with positive cultures	39.7*	36.3

*$(0.50 < p < 0.60)$

This study emphasizes the natural history of the use of antibiotics. Look at the organisms cultured in 1969, when no catheter care was initiated. Compare with the organisms cultured during the use of antibiotic application around the catheter site and see a significant change in recoverable organisms (Table 2). The incidence of *Pseudomonas* decreased, but the incidence of organisms resistant to the antibiotic ointment increased.

Dr. Ruberg: Were all the catheters cultured in 1969?

Dr. Wilmore: No.

Dr. Ruberg: Doesn't this suggest that the catheters cultured were those in individuals where catheter infection was perhaps more suspected, and, for that reason, the culture was done?

Dr. Wilmore: Your criticism is just. However, catheter cultures were taken in a random manner. Several physicians were culturing all of their

Table 2.— Organisms Cultured, 1969-1970

	1969 (no catheter care)	1970 (daily catheter care)
Staphylococcus Positive	8	19
Staphylococcus Negative	4	13
Pseudomonas	14	10*
Providence	13	34
Aerobacter	6	14
Candida	1	12
Serratia		2
E Coli	4	3
Proteus mirabilis	4	4
Bacillus		16†
Mima		1
No Growth	47	151
Total Organisms	103	280

*$X^2 = 12.87$ $p < .001$
†$X^2 = 4.8061$ $p < .05$

catheters through this study. The catheters cultured could not be correlated with the patients with septic thrombophlebitis.

Dr. Curreri: How reliable is culture of the catheter tip, since one has dragged the catheter out through the dirty skin during removal?

Dr. Winters: Valuable, if negative.

Dr. Curreri: Does that not depend on the care with which the catheter was removed? I have seen reports of catheter tip cultures in which every one was positive, but this simply indicates faulty technique. I have not found catheter culture to be valuable in clinical management of the individual patient, although it is occasionally helpful in an epidemiological study of a ward population.

Dr. Goldmann: Investigators who attempted to prepare the skin properly before withdrawing the catheter found a better correlation between cultures of the blood and cultures of the catheter tip than did those investigators who failed to do this preparation. Balagtas, in a study of umbilical catheters in infants (*Pediatrics* **48:**359, 1971), prepared the area carefully before withdrawing the catheter; but, he also cultured the flora of the skin during the time the catheter was in place. He found a correlation, in patients who appeared clinically to have septicemia, between positive blood cultures, organisms on the catheter tip, and the skin flora while the catheter was in place. This implies that it is important which organism is on the skin and what we do to prevent skin and catheter colonization.

Dr. Curreri: To summarize those points in which we have expressed agreement: The indwelling catheter is a pathway of infection in itself. We may disagree on its importance as a primary cause of sepsis, but a reasonable estimate of the incidence would be in the range of 4% to 8% of patients receiving prolonged parenteral nutrition by intravenous catheter.

Etiology

Dr. Curreri: Probably one sees an equal incidence of secondary infection of the catheter from distant septic sites. Certainly, most of the patients with catheter-related septicemia survive. Most are adequately treated by removal of the catheter. The key to avoiding a fatal complication of parenteral nutrition, therefore, is scrupulous and conscientious clinical care.

Reports in the literature suggest that candidiasis is becoming a severe complication of parenteral hyperalimentation. In a review of 12,000 cultures from over 4,000 patients—most of whom were receiving intravenous fluids—it was surprising to find that the incidence of *Candida* in the bloodstream had not significantly increased during the past four years. During this period we utilized parenteral hyperosmolar alimentation much more frequently. Incidences of a number of unusual gram-negative, opportunistic organisms increased, and these were resistant to the antibiotics utilized in our institution. The candidiasis problem may be related also to antibiotic resistance, thus representing the emergence of another opportunistic infection. I have not observed a specific relationship or correlation of fungemia with total parenteral nutrition in our patient population.

Dr. Dudrick: We found two cases of candidiasis among the last 150 patients receiving parenteral hyperosmolar alimentation and one patient with a positive catheter culture for *Candida*.

Let me emphasize that investigators have to collect data. To arrive at a rational conclusion, we have to have numbers. Whether the contamination of the catheter is in removing it, or whether it was contaminated while it was in place, it has been contaminated by something. It was not *de novo* infection; but something contaminated the catheter from the outside or the inside.

Another problem arises when one tries to express the infection rate. A single catheter is left in place for 90 days in one patient, removed at the end of that 90 days, and no catheter bacterial growth is found, no evidence of clinical infection, and a negative blood culture. At the same time another catheter is removed after 24 hours, and something cultured from it. Is that a 50% incidence in catheter infection rate? Is that a fair way to report data? I believe one learns to report data in a manner which describes the conditions under which the data are collected. Otherwise, the data are not meaningful. The investigator who wants to show that hyperosmolar alimentation causes infection or that catheters are harmful attempts this in a manner which cannot be refuted, since the specific conditions of the data collection remain unreported.

Candida is an increasing problem. Most of us lived through the period of staphylococcal epidemics. Pediatricians lived through the era of infectious *Escherichia coli* epidemics. We have lived through *Pseudomonas* superinfection. Now we are living through a period of *Candida* infection. Patients have candidemia who never had intravenous alimentation. The biggest increase in candidemia at our institution occurs following the Wertheim operation in women with carcinoma of the cervix or of the uterus.

Another increased incidence of candidemia is in children who often get thrush, regardless of the method of nutritional therapy. Few adult men have had candidemia. We are dealing with different populations and different clinical problems. All this has to be in the proper perspective for data evaluation.

If a catheter is placed in a baby, the catheter occludes a portion of a vein where it is lodged. There is relatively little, if any, blood flow around the catheter. However, one might reasonably expect the body's immune mechanism to destroy the few organisms introduced at the time of catheter insertion. We create a problem when we overwhelm the host with a bolus of organisms generated in a warm, closed-off, nutrient-supplied area, after which a piece of pus breaks off and metastacizes to the lung or a heart valve.

An adult is different. There *is* a difference between a catheter placed percutaneously into the side of a large vessel like the subclavian and a catheter placed peripherally. In our experience, the subclavian vessel was found to be the best area for catheter insertion. We first tried other areas, starting with the saphenous and the inferior vena cava, proceeding to the cephalic, then to the jugular, finally to the subclavian. We ended up with the percutaneous subclavian catheter because it gave us the lowest infection rate. In one week, with a long-arm catheter in the anticubital space with its tip in the superior vena cava, a 75% positive catheter and blood culture rate will result.

Consider the individual patient when contemplating total parenteral nutrition. Ask, what is the alternative? How many of these patients would die or have an impaired survival rate if we did not feed them? Do we have a choice in any of these areas? We know there are different risks in various patient populations. One ought not to use a catheter in any patient in whom there is no indication for it. When reporting catheter data, one must assess the risks in each patient, examine the alternatives, and present this analysis if the data are to be meaningful.

Dr. Curreri: Development of potent antibiotics against gram-negative organisms (eg, gentamicin and carbenicillin) provides therapeutic weapons to inhibit progression of gram-negative infections in patients with poor nutrition and diminished host resistance. But development of more effective systemic antifungal agents has lagged. Hence, an increased incidence of fungal infections may occur during the next few years, regardless of the route by which nutrients are delivered.

Dr. Duma: Hyperglycemia, both in animals and in humans, may render *Candida* more pathogenic or virulent. This is a concern when patients are receiving high concentrations of glucose.

In searching for candidemia, cultures of the catheter tip may not be as valuable as retrieving blood cultures from the catheter itself. Upon removal, the catheter tip could become contaminated by *Candida* external to the catheter and colonizing surrounding tissues.

Is it important to decide whether or not candidemia or septicemia is primary or secondary? It is important to trace the source, but when an organism lodges on a catheter, it has the potential to produce continual seeding of the bloodstream. It may be academic to consider it secondary.

Delivery

Delivery of hyperosmolar alimentation (HA) fluid requires care and a standardized approach to safeguard the patient.

Catheter care

Dr. Curreri: How often should intravenous catheters be changed? Dr. Wilmore said he inserts a new catheter every 48 hours, while Dr. Ruberg has left indwelling catheters for 90 days. These may represent extreme viewpoints.

How often should the connecting tubing between the bottle and the catheter be changed? It is my experience that if one waits until there is an episode of sepsis to change the catheters, change the tubing, or make other changes, one has waited too long. A small number of these patients will die with septic complications.

Dr. Wilmore: Patients with burns have multiple sources of infection. One of the lethal complications of infection in these individuals is septic thrombophlebitis. This is a form of thrombophlebitis with bacterial invasion within the vein wall. The vein may become suppurative and tender, but the only presenting signs may be those associated with systemic sepsis. Septic thrombophlebitis is best prevented by frequent catheter change; therefore, IV cannulas are removed and reinserted every 48 to 72 hours. Complications from venous catheterization are best treated if the catheter is placed in a peripheral vein. Consequently, many veins of the hands and scalp are used for IV administration. Often in patients with large burns, however, we use subclavian, internal, and external jugular or femoral veins. In these cases, we simply rotate the IV site from side to side, using centrally placed veins.

Dr. Levenson: What is your evidence that you are accomplishing something? I am not saying you are not, but what is your evidence that you are?

Dr. Wilmore: It is in the review of duration of catheterization.

Dr. Levenson: Obviously you cannot correlate it with your review of catheterization in current practice, if you change at 48-hour intervals. I do not find that past experience is evidence.

Dr. Wilmore: A review of the past series shows that increase in catheter infection occurs with increased duration of catheterization.

Dr. Border: The duration of time in which the catheter can safely be left in place depends on the nursing care expended in taking care of it, its anatomical position, and the presence of other sites of sepsis in the patient. In the patients I am studying, we routinely have pulmonary artery, central venous, and arterial catheters in place. They are in place usually for two to four weeks, but we expend several hours each day in taking care of them. Therefore, I do not see an answer to your question in terms of days. The catheter needs to be changed more frequently in a patient with infected burn wounds.

Dr. Curreri: Dr. Wilmore and Dr. Dudrick described patients in whom a *single* central intravenous catheter was maintained for 80 days, proving that with proper care the catheter can be left in place for long periods of time. We should be able to recommend a safe interval for catheter duration in the patient without progressive sepsis (eg, the patient with an enterocutaneous fistula or an omphalocele). Dr. Dudrick, how often do you change your indwelling venous catheters?

Dr. Dudrick: Initially we correlated catheter sepsis with the duration of the indwelling catheter. We have subsequently divided the catheter culture date into periods representing catheter placement duration from 0 to 10, 10 to 20, 20 to 30, and 30 to 40 days. The data show no correlation between the number of days we leave the catheter in place and the incidence of positive catheter cultures. Other physicians have recommended that catheters be pulled routinely at an earlier time, based on an increased rate of sepsis. And didn't Bernard show a positive correlation with time of the number of catheters infected?

I look for clinical signs of septic complications. If a patient had been afebrile for three weeks and suddenly has a temperature of 101°F, which is unexplained, I pull the catheter.

Dr. Wilmore, would you discuss the tables you presented earlier? (See p 381.) Are those results from catheters put in for hyperosmolar alimentation via the subclavian vein route? Or are you including hand catheters and long catheters for CVP monitoring, plus the administration of isotonic solutions? Can you fractionate your data in any way?

Dr. Wilmore: Yes, we can. These were not necessarily nutritional solutions—only a small percentage of them were—but primarily 5% dextrose in water (D_5W) or nornial saline solutions. We were interested in getting information about our bacterial prep around the catheter, because our impression was that our positive catheter cultures correlate best with our positive blood cultures. That is, the organisms that are in the blood, seeding the burn wound and the like, most probably lodge on our catheters, rather than coming in from around the catheter.

Dr. Border: May I object to that? Several times the statement has been made, "lodged on the catheters." What you mean is that you recover an organism from the tip of the catheter after it is dragged through the wound, and you do not know whether that tip is colonized in the vessel or not. It is a semantic problem. We assume we know too much. We are concerned about how commonly bacteremia is associated with fatal outcomes, and that is not saying that it causes the fatal outcome. The patient may be in trouble with multiple organ systems failure. As one symptom of this, he has bacteremia. Alexander's work on *Pseudomonas* showed that if he cleared the *Pseudomonas* with his immune sera the patients went on to die just as they would have otherwise. The *Pseudomonas* was probably just one symptom of this multiple organ system failure.

Dr. Ruberg: Although we recognize the hazards associated with inserting a percutaneous subclavian catheter, it makes sense to treat infection in the simplest way, to totally eliminate what appears to be the source of infection.

We advocate removing a suspect subclavian catheter and reestablishing another central venous route of administration percutaneously.

Dr. Wilmore: One way of preventing catheter complications is simply not to use catheters. We have talked about the development of several solutions that can be administered peripherally, such as fat emulsions and maltose solutions which provide the necessary calories but may be administered by peripheral vein. We are evaluating some of these solutions.

Connective tubing and filters

Dr. Curreri: More dangerous as a potential source of local infection is the tubing that connects the bottle and the catheter.

In reports of septic complications accompanying the administration of total parenteral hyperalimentation, the connecting tubing has been found to be the major source of contamination.

Mr. Ravin: We change tubing every 24 hours. We have found an easy way to accomplish this, utilizing our centralized additive service. A new connective tubing set is provided with every primary bottle ordered for the day. Thus, the nurse does not have to run to a different location to find a connective tubing set.

Dr. Goldmann: Let me give you the background for the CDC recommendation that the infusion apparatus be changed every 24 hours (Goldmann DA, Maki DG, Rhame FS, et al: Guidelines for infection control in intravenous therapy. *Ann Intern Med,* to be published). Members of *Klebsiella* (a genus of the tribe Escherichieae) grow rapidly in D_5W, increasing by more than 5 logs in 24 hours, even when very small inocula are used. *Candida,* incidentally, grows much more slowly in D_5W. Organisms grow differently in total parenteral nutrition fluid. *Candida* grows rapidly in such fluid and by 24 to 48 hours, even with small innocula, will reach a dangerous level. Many bacteria do not reach such numbers within 24 hours. Changing the administration set—bottles and tubing—every 24 hours can greatly reduce the number of organisms to which the patient is exposed if contamination of the IV system should occur. The clinical utility of the 24-hour change was verified during the outbreak of septicemia associated with contaminated Abbott infusion products (Maki DG, Goldmann DA, Rhame FS: Infection control in intravenous therapy. *Ann Intern Med,* to be published).

Dr. Rhoads: Dr. Curreri, could the manufacturers make solutions with the tubing attached?

Dr. Curreri: One of our major objectives is to reduce the handling of infusing equipment to a bare minimum. Dr. Rhoads and Dr. Dudrick (*JAMA* **215:**939, 1971) have developed a prototype of a plastic container in which essentially all of the additives could be combined with the solution in appropriate amounts without violating the packaged solution as it comes from the manufacturing plant (see p 339).

If sterile tubing were attached to such a delivery system, only one connection by nursing personnel would be required. This would be a great advance. But one of the unsolved problems is the development of adequate technique for sterilization of this complete administration set during the manufacturing process.

Dr. Shils: While safety is important, the reason for intravenous feeding is nutritional. My approach is that every patient has nutritional-physiologic problems. These should be reviewed every day with consequent decision on formula composition. Once the patient is stable, little or no change is required; but many of our patients are not physiologically or nutritionally stable for long periods. Since I do not believe that the unit system is flexible enough, I prefer to make the daily solutions in one or two bags on the basis of individual needs. The prepackaged multicompartmental bag would be expensive, complicated, and could not meet all variables in nutrition. Safety can be achieved more simply and inexpensively by closed system transfers of major solutions with additions of small volume nutrients from sterile syringe-type prepackaged solutions as needed.

Mr. Muhlenpoh: At present, it is not possible to process a solution container with an attached connective tubing set and provide the user with sterility assurance. But this can be accomplished by producing solutions and tubing separately with two different means of sterilization. The armed forces have preattached a set to a plastic container.

Dr. Curreri: What are the chances of introducing sterile foreign particles from solutions and additives utilized for total parenteral nutrition? Of what value are in-line filter systems for solution preparation in the pharmacy and for clinical delivery to the patient? Does anyone have either direct or inferential evidence that particulate matter within the solution has produced any morbidity or mortality? The development of foreign body granulomata in the lungs following intravenous dissemination of particulate matter might be expected (see p 365). I am unaware of any data from autopsy material.

Are different techniques required in the treatment of children? Dr. Dudrick, why do you utilize a filter in children and not in adults?

Dr. Dudrick: It is a practical solution to the problems encountered in delivery. The filter was initially utilized in infants to protect the patient from inadvertent contamination of the catheter by nursing personnel during manipulation of the tubing and bottles of solution.

The size of the commercially available in-line filters is an inch in diameter. Using the 0.22μ filter, which is an absolute bacterial filter, acceptable volumes (500 to 700 ml/day) can be delivered—provided the membrane is intact—to infants and small children at the slow flow rates attainable with the filter. Do not utilize the same filter for longer than three days. I always use a constant infusion pump on infants in order to deliver a precise number of microdrops accurately and to maintain positive pressure in the delivery line during Valsalva maneuvers by the infant. Otherwise, blood may be forced up the intravenous connecting tubing to the drip chamber, resulting in a clot in the system with impaired rate of solution delivery.

Using an in-line filter in tandem with a constant infusion pump offers another advantage: The wet filter prevents air passage should the solution in the bottle run dry. This reduces the chances for air embolism. If a filter is used with adults, trouble may be encountered. After infusion of about two liters of solution—regardless of whether or not a constant infusion pump is utilized simultaneously—the filter becomes blocked with particulate matter and the flow rates become unreliable. The filter will also leak, allowing bacteria to grow through a continuum of leaking nutrient solution into the tubing distal to the filter.

We encounter more difficulties with infusion and a higher contamination rate with the filter than without the filter in adults. We have asked the manufacturer to make a larger surface area filter or to put a system together with a prefilter for large particulate matter and a bacterial filter strictly for microorganisms. I am not aware of a controlled study to determine the actual value of in-line filters. Since we have been using the filters in our animal investigations, we have noted fewer septic complications at autopsy.

An in-line filter is not absolutely necessary, and it provides little assurance against contamination in the absence of scrupulous bedside delivery technique. The distal connection between filter and catheter and the skin around the catheter at the puncture site—a major source of infection—create problems. Also, we have observed *Candida* colonized on the proximal side of an 0.22μ filter, while the mycelia were growing through the filter, allowing spores to disseminate intravenously in the patient.

Dr. Curreri: If one can be guaranteed a sterile solution, and if contamination in preparation and delivery is minimized by rigid procedural techniques, one may utilize an in-line filter with larger pore size in order to remove only large particulate matter. Then acceptable flow rates can be attained for high-volume delivery. But in-line filters increase the number of connections. The management of those connections may prove more dangerous than the omission of an in-line filter because of the additional nursing manipulation required.

Dr. Duma: Some in-line filters may not be membrane filters. We do not know, following prolonged daily usage of such filters, what sort of particulate matter may leave the filter. Nor do we know the size of the particles, or what problems the deposition *in vivo* of various materials might produce. Also, we do not know which is more important, small- or large-size particles, or what the clinical significance of each might be. It is possible, depending on the substance of the filter, that certain in-line filters may be more harmful than good from the standpoint of particulate matter.

The mention of *Candida* growing through the filter attests to the fact that filters are not always the final answer. Under hospital conditions we do not know how much damage to pore size occurs (ie, microscopic damage). Data on what various fluids or pressures might do to the filters is not available.

Also, some bacteria in hyperosmolar solutions may lose their cell walls (protoplasts), and these could pass through the filters or multiply in it. There are many questions and problems that have to be considered for which we have no answer at present.

Dr. Curreri: If the filter collects bacteria which subsequently proliferate, endotoxins, exotoxins, and various pyrogens may still reach the patient via the catheter.

Personnel

Dr. Curreri: You have indicated the necessity for a hyperosmolar alimentation team with input from pharmacy, medical, nursing, and specialist members from the dietary division and the department of infectious diseases. In smaller hospitals, this is impractical. Since a specialty team is a prerequisite in administering total parenteral nutrition safely, you advocate localization of such treatment to major medical centers.

How should available personnel be utilized in the preparation and administration of nutritional solutions? How does one monitor the performance of various personnel in the maintenance of sterile technique?

Dr. Dudrick: As an absolute minimum, an interested physician is needed who is willing to work hard 24 hours a day. At our institution, this position is filled by a surgical resident with a minimum of one and a half years of surgical training, who has demonstrated an interest in surgical nutrition and metabolism. He is on call 24 hours a day.

A specialized intravenous TPN nurse sees the patients every day to make sure there are no abnormalities of intake and output or alterations in delivery schedules. She reviews patients with major clinical problems periodically throughout the day. She changes dressings every other day, according to techniques we have published; collects and assembles research data. She contributes to our in-service training program, organizing a course for both the new and the more experienced floor nurses at least four times a year to provide information on current techniques.

The pharmacist is an integral part of the team and we are fortunate in having interested pharmacists to help us insure an acceptable level of quality control. That is the basic team: pharmacist, nurse, and physician.

Dr. Curreri: Is it necessary for every hospital to have this sort of team in order to assure safer delivery of total parenteral nutrition?

Dr. Dudrick: Yes, it is necessary. The nurse with a small patient population does not have to devote full time to parenteral nutrition. I would advise locating the patients geographically in an area, not necessarily an intensive care area, but if possible on one floor or on one ward.

Ideally, the medical responsibility should be limited to a few interested physicians. If every physician in the hospital decides to engage in the administration of total parenteral nutrition, maintenance of strict procedural techniques and collection of meaningful data become nearly impossible.

Other people, with various primary interests, frequently consult with our basic team. These consultants include a psychiatrist, a dietitian, occupational therapists, social workers, and inhalational therapists. Each contributes to optimum total clinical management. Physical therapy is an important part of nutrition. As soon as possible, we undertake a program of passive exercise, gradually progressing to an active exercise program. Such programs affect responses to total parenteral nutrition.

One physician puts in all the catheters. On occasion he might supervise a house officer or a medical student who is learning the technique, but he is the physician responsible. We are offended when somebody puts in a subclavian catheter and then calls us to begin IV, since it prejudices the results we observe in catheter infection rate. We will remove the catheter and insert a new catheter on the other side immediately if we suspect poor technique was used in placing the original catheter. We do not risk accepting another's indiscretions in the technique.

Dr. Curreri: To summarize, the team includes in its basic or smallest element a physician, a nurse who is expert in the maintenance of catheters, and a pharmacist. Then other personnel (eg, physical therapists and dietitians) are utilized more often for data collection and special clinical problems than for day-to-day delivery of total parenteral nutrition.

Dr. Levenson: Can you elaborate on the changing of bottles? Is the doctor responsible for that or is that a nursing responsibility?

Dr. Dudrick: We originally changed bottles ourselves, but now it is a nursing responsibility, and all nurses are instructed in proper techniques.

Dr. Burke: Is it really as necessary to have a team as to have an interested physician responsible for the program?

Dr. Curreri: It is difficult for a physician to provide all the necessary services. Few physicians have enough time or knowledge to be proficient in nursing supervision, nursing education, and pharmaceutical preparations. I would agree with Dr. Dudrick that it takes three interested people: the team nurse who has time to work with nursing and paramedical personnel, the pharmacist who is in an area which you cannot control as a physician or as a nurse, and the physician who must remain responsible for decisions concerning patient care and research programs.

That does not mean that these three individuals devote full time to parenteral nutrition. They are essentially a group responsible for guidance in establishing procedural policies. Nor does it mean excluding other people. It does amount to local hospital regulation of technique in preparation and delivery of these solutions.

Mr. Flack: The pharmacist can provide a surveillance of TPN as he does through the committee on drug surveillance.

Mr. Klotz: The complexity of this therapy demands a team effort. Inexperienced physicians often will alter the composition of the solution or the rate of delivery, even though they are not familiar with the complications of this therapy. Without a team approach and at least one member of the team available 24 hours a day, an inexperienced person will attempt variations in technique without proper consultation; then the incidence of complications will rise.

In-service education

Dr. Curreri: As we agree that there must be a multidisciplinary approach to this type of therapy in very ill patients, we also must examine the team's role in in-house educational programs. The expert nurse must successfully impart her knowledge to the floor nurses before a nurse can accept major responsibility on one of three nursing shifts. Physicians are responsible for the education of residents, students, interns, and other physicians.

Would you comment on your experience with in-service programs for imparting safety information to medical and paramedical personnel, Mr. Ravin?

Mr. Ravin: About a year ago we realized that we had a wide variance of formulations being used in our hospital. The members of the house staff and the attending staff did not have the total picture of what was to be accomplished. As a result of this, one of our physicians, an excellent teacher, was asked to discuss the whole concept of TPN at a house staff conference. He also included practical information which would improve day-to-day clinical management. His discussion was supplemented by a written outline of techniques. This program for the house staff has been successful.

We have also used another approach, the utilization of video taping. We have prepared 15- to 30-minute tapes on venepuncture techniques, on care of the catheters, etc. These are used for nursing orientation and have wide application in training pharmacists.

I urge other hospitals to consider the preparation of educational video tapes. Consistency in teaching is a great advantage. Without the use of video tapes, an important fact may be left out of our educational program.

We ask members of industry to come in and prepare short tapes on their products. We ask the company, "How do you really want your product used?" And we ask them to be explicit and thorough.

Dr. Curreri: Do you use these tapes for practical teaching? Do you videotape a nurse putting together an intravenous system, or an intern or resident putting in a catheter, and then point out the errors in the technique?

Mr. Ravin: We have not done that. We have only tried to show the right way to do it.

Mr. Muhlenpoh: We, as manufacturers, have a responsibility for training personnel who come into contact with our product throughout the hospital. As you have a contract on purchasing these solutions, we have an equal "contract" to train your personnel to use those products correctly. We should explore in-service methods to identify the best methods for carrying out such programs by films, literature, posters, and demonstrations. We solicit physician input of what is meaningful for the purpose of training.

Dr. Duma: May I ask the manufacturers if they would assume the responsibility for such a training program; also would physicians accept and use their programs?

Mr. Muhlenpoh: Each solution manufacturer should answer this question. We developed a motion picture to illustrate the catheterization technique in intravenous alimentation. It was made in cooperation with Dr. Dudrick at the Hospital of the University of Pennsylvania.

We also provided a grant to Dr. Don Francke for his hospital pharmacy journal, *Drug Intelligence*. This grant has allowed a monthly exchange of information on the subject of intravenous solution additives which has been well received by hospital pharmacies. It has provided emphasis on procedures for handling solutions and policies for IV additive programs.

PREPARATION OF SOLUTIONS

Bacteriological Quality Control

Hospital pharmacy

Dr. Curreri: The pharmacist prepares total parenteral nutrition solutions in most hospitals. We have found that close supervision in a central pharmacy results in fewer errors than when additives are mixed by various individuals on the ward.

What kind of quality control is practiced in the pharmacies across the country? Are bottles sampled before additions? How many are using filters when adding additives? How many are sampling the final preparation routinely for bacteriological quality control?

Dr. Burke: We randomly sample the basic formulation HA units at the time of preparation. We do not sample the individual patient formulation routinely when additives are introduced; but we do recover unused formulations, partially used units, and solutions not refrigerated properly, and subject these to bacteriologic survey.

Perhaps as important as culturing solutions, we monitor our aseptic technique by culturing the equipment, tubing, needles, and syringes used in preparing these formulations. This assists us in determining the efficacy of our technique.

Our preparation procedures are written policies and the pharmacist and technician, essentially screening each other, are thus under close supervision. Techniques and procedures are adhered to. To date, we have had no contamination per se in the in-use solutions.

Dr. Brueggeman: We supply in-line filters with all our solutions. The physicians transfer the entire filter unit to a sterile specimen bottle after administration of the fluid. The filters are then examined and cultured in the bacteriology laboratory. In most cases, these filters are sterile. If bacteria are recovered from the filter, the cause must be carefully investigated.

Dr. Avis: I suggest a different type of hospital pharmacy quality control program. In the manufacturing industry, sterility testing is done on a sampling basis. When there is no terminal sterilization involved, another acceptable practice is to run culture media through the process steps to confirm the fact that the process can be carried out without introducing contamination.

This kind of test is much more rigorous than a sample test or culturing a filter. In a hospital pharmacy, this same procedure can be practiced. To test every single batch prepared for an individual patient becomes almost impossible, or at least impractical. If the hospital pharmacy establishes that their technique is a reliable one, and if the same individual carries out the process every time, it should be reproducible. If the technique is rechecked at intervals with the culture media and in actual product tests, quality control would be provided.

Mr. Klotz: As we prepare them in the pharmacy, we periodically set solutions aside for bacteriological and fungal culture. In addition, bottles and filters are periodically recovered from the bedside and cultured. Good in-service education of technicians also is imperative if contact contamination during preparation is to be avoided.

Manufacturer

Dr. Ausman: The USP has been looking at the question of quality control for large-volume parenteral solutions. Never before, to my knowledge, have we examined solution sterility in such detail. The four large-volume parenteral manufacturers have been participating in this cooperative study.

During the examination of quality control from the sterility viewpoint, it has been ascertained that three elements need to be considered: the solution itself, the closure, and the set (the means of administration). Currently, and in the present USP as revised, the solution has only been tested and considered. The closure and the set have equal importance in delivering sterile solutions to the patient.

The solution and the closure are sterilized by steam, and the administration (tubing) set is sterilized by ethylene oxide. There is no variance in these techniques, to our knowledge, among the manufacturers. A few solutions are handled in slightly different ways, but they are not an important part of the volume of solutions produced in this country.

The risk of contamination of solutions sterilized by steam, can be assessed by the formula: $t = D (\log a - \log b)$ where "t" is the length of the sterility cycle, that is the time of sterilization in minutes at 250°F or its equivalent; "D" represents the sensitivity of the organisms to be sterilized by steam sterilization; "a", the ambient load or the quantity of organisms which are present before sterilization occurs; and "b", as you might expect, represents what comes out.

Solving for log b gives the risk factor we all want to know because, as has previously been emphasized, sterility is not absolute. We cannot, in fact, make an absolutely perfect solution every single time. The question is how often do we miss, and then how do we minimize that risk of miss to the point where it is acceptable.

We reviewed the sterilizing cycles that manufacturers use. Most manufacturers, for many of their products, run what is called a four-minute cycle (ie, four minutes or its equivalent at 250°F or 121°C). The "D" value is different for every organism, but the value of 0.21 is never exceeded for any pathologic organism found in a typical medical environment. The values of the organisms ordinarily approach 0.05. The log a value for most manufacturers was nearly the same. The normal value is less than 6,000 organisms per liter going in, but let us say it was 10,000.

We are obliged to solve for log b and the formula now tells us that once in every 10^{16} times one organism will show up in one of the bottles.

That turns out — if you combine total manufacturing in this country — to be one organism every 10 years, an acceptably low risk. That explains why the solution has never been the cause of a significant outbreak of septicemia. The nature of the sterilization cycle is one of overkill.

Manufacturers tend to vary the cycles slightly depending upon the amounts of solution ingredient that are heat-sensitive, but no manufacturer had a cycle with a 250°F equivalent of less than 2.2 minutes.

This formula can be turned around, and we propose to do it. We know what the ambient load is going in, and we know, or we assume an agreement can be reached on acceptable risk factors. We can test for the sensitivity value. Then one knows what cycle must be run.

Let us review the role of sample size in bacteriological quality control of the finished product. To get 90% likelihood of rejecting a lot when it should be rejected (there remains a 10% chance one will miss), one must destructively sample 650 products out of a 1,000 unit lot. The cost of such a program would be prohibitive since there are few bottles left to deliver. Sample size is not the answer to the problem.

Dr. Schaffner: The sample does provide an opportunity, should there be a positive, to identify the organism.

Dr. Ausman: Your point is well made. But bacteriological status is better ascertained by examining the ambient load of bacteria going in than by sampling for organisms coming out. Little is learned because very few bottles are ever contaminated.

We studied the closure also. Tests of the closure and of the administration set, including reexamination of the methods of sterilization, are new. Our engineers believe it is possible to develop risk calculations for both.

Through the methods of manufacture now employed, the likelihood of a sterile solution is immense; the likelihood of a nonsterile solution is extremely remote. A more likely answer to the means of solution contamination could be found in its handling after the manufacturer has delivered it to the hospital.

Mr. Sheffield: The D factor is obviously a function of temperature. We sterilize at 15° or 20° lower than 250°F. What is your D factor at the lower temperature, Dr. Ausman?

Also, I want to comment on your probabilities of acceptance with regard to sampling. Independently, I arbitrarily chose a 10^{-5} value for contamination and ran this through our computers. We came up with a probability of 0.9999 of passing the lot based on 10 samples. When we doubled the sample size to 20, it came out 0.9998, no real difference.

Dr. Ausman: The D factor value referred to organism sensitivity at 250°F. When you sterilize below 250°F, as 90% of the manufacturers do for 90% of their cycles, the cycle time is longer, but it's always possible to calculate an equivalent. Sterilizing at lower temperatures requires a longer sterilization cycle.

Dr. Duma: Dr. Ausman, will you comment on the indicator test strain and also on ethylene oxide sterilization?

Dr. Ausman: Ethylene oxide sterilization is less reliable under normal circumstances than steam, primarily because it is more sensitive to the presence of humidity. Unfortunately, manufacturers of gas sterilization equipment have not been able to develop a device which is sufficiently accurate to detect humidity while sterilization is in progress. We can detect temperature in a product during steam sterilization.

The USP describes the use of a biologic indicator for ethylene oxide sterilization, which has some disadvantages. It requires the manufacturer to willfully bring into his manufacturing site contaminated material. There is always the chance that contaminated material will be lost. The biologic indicator, a soil spore, is used by all manufacturers.

The load is sterilized and is not released until the biologic indicator has cleared and proved to be sterile. Importantly, the labeling specifies only that the fluid pathway of the administration set is sterile.

Dr. Schaffner: You have not mentioned biological indicators in the production of fluid.

Dr. Ausman: There is no need for them as long as we can demonstrate a satisfactory cycle and verify the methods of studying cycle accomplishment by physical measurements. Product temperature, vessel temperature and pressures are far superior to the biological indicator which has the vicissitudes of biology versus the hard science of physics. From a risk analysis viewpoint, it is more advantageous to utilize three more thermometers. Biological indicators are less predictable and less valuable for solution sterilization than for ethylene oxide sterilization of administration sets.

Mr. Sheffield: The equation presented by Dr. Ausman is commonly accepted by industry, but it is valid only if the sterilization container is absolutely closed and remains closed.

The determining factor in the maintenance of sterilization of any single unit then hinges upon the integrity of the closure system. If the probability of leakage at the closure is greater than the probability of kill, then the 10^{-16} probability value which he presented is not valid.

Dr. Ausman: You are right. The probability of contaminating the solution becomes the probability of a leaking closure, and the solution value becomes secondary. This is why everyone is looking at the closure as well as the administration set. For that reason the closure has been taken as a separate entity and is being examined as such.

In addition to the integrity of the closure, one also has to determine the sterilizability of the closure. We have excellent information for that. The sterilizability of all closures now used is the same as the solution itself. The only question is how frequently does the system leak after the cycle has been run. That is being examined to establish a probability.

Mr. Sheffield: I was not thinking about the sterility of the closure itself. I was thinking about the variable pressure circumstances that exist inside the autoclave when you bring the steam pressure down and start adding additional air, and the resultant pressure differential within the unit versus outside the unit. Once you start bringing the nonsterile air back into the autoclave, you could conceivably, with less than an absolute seal, bring the organisms back into the presterilized unit.

Dr. Ausman: Yes. This is examined by engineers when a new closure system is developed. The more complex the closure system becomes, the greater the risk of contamination by the means you have described.

Dr. Schaffner: Recent studies of the microbial environment of manufacturing plants—particularly that portion of the plant where the bottles are stored after sterilization—have shown widespread contamination of the plant with gram-negative bacilli. This was not totally unexpected. The disturbing feature was that some of these organisms have also been found within the metal closure on the top of the bottle, but not on the diaphragm. Is that disturbing?

Dr. Ausman: No. This is the old issue. Each manufacturer defines what is sterile and what is not sterile on his closure. Each manufacturer suggests what should be made sterile before inserting an administration set of his manufacture. If you fail to follow the instructions, the possibility exists that there will be some difficulty. If contamination can occur at the plant site, it can occur in the railroad car, on the way to the hospital, or in the storage areas of the hospital. It is imperative that you know what is warranted to be sterile.

Dr. Schaffner: Do we need a package insert that defines more carefully and precisely how these drugs are to be used?

Dr. Ausman: Unequivocally, yes. We do put package inserts in our product. The FDA requires that anything that carries a New Drug Application (NDA) must have a package insert. I can only plead that more physicians and nurses read the package insert. The FDA exercises care in reviewing what is in the package insert.

Solution Constituents

Dr. Curreri: Since many of us are striving to develop improved nutritional solutions for human use, it would be helpful to know the cost involved in altering the concentration of a single amino acid once a commercially prepared solution has been approved for marketing. What additional testing would be required for federal approval? Would the altered solution have to be subjected to Phases 1, 2, and 3 testing again, or could a manufacturer bypass some of these if only a minor alteration in amino acid concentration were made?

Dr. McDavid: Every time a formula is changed, even if it is an obvious improvement, many of the tests previously completed will have to be repeated. An example of an obvious improvement would be a reduction in the concentration of an ingredient shown to be present in excess. If the development of the product had proceeded as far as Phase 3, then the repetitive work required would be extensive.

Dr. Curreri: But we will want to make changes in these solutions. Investigators will have to find better ways to examine utilization of the nutrients in an animal model in which the results are applicable to human utilization. No one really knows how to do this. We find it difficult, therefore, to specify what product we want the manufacturing firm to develop.

Federal regulation of clinical research

Dr. DeMerre: A change in formulation may bring about the need for two alternatives. If the change is substantial, new experimentation has to be performed, and a new Investigative New Drug (IND) has to be submitted. This would include the need for subjection to Phase 1, Phase 2, and Phase 3 again (see p 450). The pharmacology might have indicated that the product was safe; but effectiveness has to be shown and this will be done through Phases 1, 2, and 3.

If a new drug application is effective and minor changes in the formulation are proposed, it is likely that a supplemental application would be sufficient—provided the changes are of minor magnitude and provided the manufacturing controls remain the same.

Dr. Curreri: What are minor changes and what are major changes? If we have the same qualitative constituent amino acids but change the concentration by no more than a factor of 100%, would this be a minor or major change?

Dr. DeMerre: A 100% change would certainly be a major change. In two cases where this occurred, we called for a supplemental application submission, but we wanted much more. We wanted the experimental data to be updated. This calls for new IND studies, and these cannot be accelerated. If you wanted to lower the concentration of one amino acid and intended to compensate for the decrease in available nitrogen by appropriately increasing the glycine concentration, this would be considered a minor change.

Dr. Curreri: What would be the effect of including one additional amino acid?

Dr. DeMerre: That is a new drug. It is a qualitative as well as a quantitative change in the formulation.

Dr. Curreri: Dr. Munro, you proposed that we investigate the utilization of various formulations of amino acids by gradually increasing the concentration of each amino acid until we saw a rise in the plasma concentration (see p 63).

I presume we could do this intravenously in animals, but would the results be applicable to humans? The cost of intravenous studies in humans would be prohibitive.

Dr. Munro: It is done orally in humans. Simply add tryptophane or valine or other amino acid to the diet, gradually increasing the amount until a break in plasma level of that amino acid occurs. This signals an excess of the amino acid being tested. By all accounts, these studies agree well with known requirements. I do not see any theoretical difficulty in doing the same with parenteral solutions to determine, especially under conditions of disease and injury, what the requirements are in the human subject. It is obvious that these studies will be undertaken when there is reason to believe the patient will benefit.

Dr. Levenson: You can only do that on an individual patient basis when the physician feels that it is critical to the patient's well-being. Current federal regulations would prevent a planned prospective study.

Dr. Duma: Dr. Munro, can you always feel confident that what you give parenterally will give the same results as what you might give orally? An example is iron.

Dr. Munro: We are aware of the transformation of certain amino acids in the gut wall, such as glutamic and aspartic acids. However, most amino acids are absorbed intact. I do not think amino acid absorption is analogous to iron where only 10% is absorbed, and the body is therefore protected against the toxic actions of an excess.

Dr. Levenson: May we ask the FDA another question? In the past, many physicians have administered 10% casein hydrolysate solutions. In current hyperosmolar alimentation solutions, the concentration of hydrolysate or amino acids is roughly half that. Could one double the concentration of amino acids in the current solutions to the same concentrations that have been used in the past?

Dr. DeMerre: You mean you went down from 10% to 5%, and now you would like to return to the 10% level?

If you have an effective NDA for 10%, then through a supplement you went down to 5%, and your NDA is still effective, I cannot see any real objection to returning to the 10% solution. If there is a change in the formulation, the situation is different. In addition, the same container must be used because modification in the container may bring about the necessity for additional investigational studies.

Mr. Muhlenpoh: One of the difficulties in parenteral alimentation is that of "flooding" the patient. Recently manufacturers have attempted to increase the 5% hydrolysate concentrations to 8%, even to 10%. With such concentrations one does not administer as much fluid to the patient while supplying his daily calorie needs.

If an amino acid product is provided in a 5% concentration and is removed to produce a 10% concentration, would this be an NDA supplemental change? Or would it be a manufacturing change?

Dr. DeMerre: This would be a manufacturing change. To go from a lower concentration to a higher concentration means the removal of the aqueous medium. FDA will want to know how the removal is done and under what conditions. This is a change in the manufacturing process and can bring about modifications in the composition. The removal of water may affect the composition of the material. In going from a lower concentration of amino acids to a higher concentration, interreactions may occur among the amino acids. There may be pH changes; in that case, the manufacturing controls have to be disclosed and studied. In contrast, going from a higher concentration to a lower concentration is a matter of dilution and does not pose major problems.

Dr. Munro: Would it be possible to administer the approved solutions parenterally with increasing levels of single amino acids by mouth at the same time to selected patients who retained some oral capacity for absorption? In this way one is testing the levels of oral intake which are sufficient with the intravenous intake to meet requirements. Conclusions about how much extra amino acid the ideal solution would have to contain to meet nutritional requirements could be reached. The intravenous component of the administered amino acids would not have changed.

Dr. Fekl: Optimizing amino acid patterns is only possible by proceeding step by step. This means, in this country, a new IND for every new formula. As an example: When we started to optimize an essential amino acid pattern for adults in Europe, we started with a Rose-pattern. After infusion of this mixture we found that the methionine level in plasma rose. We decreased the methionine concentration in the formula. Other changes in the plasma amino acid pattern were considered in developing new formulations. We always have gone step by step to arrive at a formula which leaves the plasma pattern constantly within normal ranges and results in optimal nitrogen balance.

When I discussed the question of the optimal pattern for newborns with a pediatrician in this country, she said, "We could never do this, because we have to apply for an IND for a distinct amino acid pattern; then we have to get approval for this pattern. We have to show in animal experiments that this pattern works, and I have no animal which I can compare with a human infant. If I find that this pattern is not suitable for the infant, I have to apply for a new IND."

How can we optimize a pattern in a short time without needing a new IND every six months? This is an important question. In Europe, we have the opportunity to start with a reasonable pattern of amino acids and to optimize stepwise. Can we do the same in this country—in infants, for example? How can we proceed in this country in the same successful way, step by step, without requiring 20 years?

Dr. Brueggeman: I would like to ask the FDA opinion on the individual investigator sponsor of an IND versus industry as a sponsor?

Dr. DeMerre: The investigator can be his own sponsor at times. A firm can also be the sponsor and utilize investigators.

Dr. Brueggeman: Is there an abbreviated IND that the investigator is allowed, which is disallowed for industry?

Mr. Sheffield: In the early stages after the Kefauver-Harrison amendments were enacted, which brought about the IND concepts, FDA issued a bulletin of interpretive information. This is what you are referring to, I believe. For bona fide research by individuals—and we are talking basically about university level research—certain requirements were excluded or shortened for IND submission. As far as I know, this is still in force.

Dr. Brueggeman: Can the university investigator who is evaluating a new pattern of amino acids formulate a solution, file an IND, and investigate this in a variety of patients requiring parenteral nutrition?

Mr. Sheffield: Yes, I think so.

Dr. Brueggeman: Without going through all the procedures required of industry?

Mr. Sheffield: I do not think there was ever any exemption from the toxicological information, only from certain aspects of the IND itself. You still had to assure some degree of control over the safety to the patient in your investigation.

Dr. Curreri: The major problem lies in the fact that instead of dealing with a single drug which is covered adequately by law, we are dealing with from 10 to 20 "drugs" in a solution with an almost infinite number of possible combinations of various concentrations of each amino acid.

Mr. Sheffield: Exactly, plus the fact that we are primarily dealing with drugs with which we have had some experience in the past. Whether this fulfills legal requirements becomes a question for our legal people, perhaps.

Dr. Dudrick: Is it conceivable that in the instance of the amino acid formulas, the FDA might define an allowable range of each amino acid concentration instead of an absolute concentration? If so, we might be able to manipulate concentrations within that range in our investigations without having to file a new IND.

Dr. DeMerre: No. A marketed product goes along with a label, and the label has to state exactly what the therapeutic products are. Requests for amino acid changes—what they are and in what concentration—are submitted in writing. Naturally, the text submitted will indicate "plus or minus so much," which is acceptable providing it is a narrow limit.

Dr. McDavid: Dr. Dudrick is referring to a range at the IND level, and you are referring to a range at the NDA level. I think the question was primarily directed to the early IND level, say Phase 2.

Dr. Dudrick: Yes. Then, if we filed an IND for a solution that approached the ideal but proved, after early human investigation, to have a slightly inadequate concentration of one amino acid, we could adjust the concentration of this amino acid without the expense and time required for filing a new IND and restarting toxicity studies from scratch.

Dr. DeMerre: During Phase 1 of the IND stage, modifications can be made and the application amended to change the formulation. When one gets to Phase 2, though, it has to be pretty close to the finished product, which will be the object of the NDA.

Dr. Curreri: But are you still required to repeat the Phase 1 studies if you change the formula significantly at the Phase 2 level?

Dr. DeMerre: It depends on the modification. During Phases 1 and 2, changes may be made and clinical assays may continue, provided the manufacturing remains the same.

Mr. Sheffield: Going back to the premanufactured solution, one of the problems is the relative instability of the aldo group and the alpha amino group in these products. They form complexes which are physiologically inactive. Lack of stability for long-term storage would preclude manufacture and sale through the normal chain of distribution. The instability is accelerated through the live steam sterilization process.

Several years ago reports from Temple University painted a rather poor picture of the stability of a 20% dextrose and protein hydrolysate mixture.

Dr. McDavid: Amino acids react with dextrose. This is one reason we have two separate bottles in the IV Set: the dextrose in one unit and the nitrogen in the other component.

Dr. Carlo: This technical problem is due to the Maillard reaction; the combination of either fructose or glucose with amino acids. This can be avoided by using sorbitol, as is done extensively and satisfactorily in Europe (see p 190).

Let us go back to the regulations controlling modifications in the composition of experimental amino acid solutions. We must remember that the amino acid composition of our diet varies considerably from day to day. The different amino acid patterns in our diet, as Dr. Munro indicated, are altered by passage through the intestinal mucosa first, then through the liver. When we study intravenous preparations, a certain margin for variations should be permitted without facing strict regulations with each change in amino acid concentration.

Dr. Levenson: I want this freedom of movement, too, but I do not think Dr. Carlo's point is relevant. It may be that the variations that are induced continuously by the different food intakes are an important safeguard. However, with total parenteral nutrition, the physician establishes a variation which is going to be given continuously, day in and day out, to an individual without any compensating adjustments from different protein sources. This is a major difference. We do not have enough information to predict the relative toxicity of certain amino acids when given at a constant rate for long periods of time.

Dr. Carlo: But if we look in the European literature, we see that relatively great variations in composition of amino acid solutions have been studied over long periods of time without any problems.

We have evidence that certain formulas, which duplicate egg, egg and potato, casein, or the fibrin amino acid pattern, will vary rather considerably in the relative proportion of their various amino acids. Yet, they all have been used intravenously without toxic reaction. Differences may be observed only in the initial ability of the organism to optimally utilize the nitrogen supplied.

Dr. DeMerre: We cannot utilize toxicity studies or plasma amino acid patterns following oral intake of protein to extrapolate safety factors in a parenteral amino acid solution.

From our standpoint, research performed in foreign countries is usually excellent supporting evidence, but the true evidence comes out of research performed in this country.

Dr. Curreri: It has been my purpose to stimulate discussion of subjects which remain controversial in this relatively new field of therapy. You have been thoughtful and exciting participants. Never before have there been such frank, meaningful exchanges between a large number of clinicians, investigators, paramedical personnel, deputies for industry and representatives of the federal regulatory agencies. We hope this colloquy will provide a stimulus for continued and more extensive cooperative efforts among representatives of these disciplines. This will assist us to meet the challenge of developing better, safer use and administration of this lifesaving therapeutic modality.

Digest of Colloquium

Sepsis in patients receiving total parenteral nutrition is a major life-threatening complication of this therapy.

Incidence and Etiology of Sepsis

The indwelling catheter may, in itself, constitute the pathway by which microorganisms gain entrance to the bloodstream. Colloquium participants agreed that septicemia from other sites of infection, resulting in secondary infection of the catheter, also occurred. The incidence of primary catheter infection was estimated to be between 4% and 8% of patients receiving total parenteral nutrition.

Catheter-associated septicemia has a characteristic clinical picture including shaking chills and elevations of temperature. Upon withdrawal of the catheter the fever promptly disappears in most cases. All investigators agreed that the key to avoiding a fatal septic complication is scrupulous and conscientious daily catheter care.

Candidiasis was also cited as a severe complication of TPN. *Candida* grows rapidly in hypertonic dextrose solutions when the solution is contaminated during pharmacy preparation. As a result of prolonged treatment with antibiotics, patients most frequently requiring total parenteral nutrition may harbor *Candida* in their alimentary or genitourinary tracts. *Candida* superinfection is being reported with increasing frequency in malnourished, elderly females and young children, whether or not they are receiving intravenous nutrients.

In order to reduce the severe complication of persistent septicemia, catheters should be removed promptly at the first clinical sign of sepsis. In patients with a high risk of septicemia (eg, those with thermal injury and trauma), indwelling catheters should be removed and reinserted in new anatomic sites at regular intervals, at least every third day.

Controlled prospective studies to estimate the incidence of sepsis in patients requiring prolonged intravenous catheterization are lacking. Among conditions to be considered in such a study are the regulation of local and systemic antibiotic therapy; catheter size, composition and local care; the severity of patient injury or illness; the composition of the administered nutrient solution; the anatomical location of the indwelling catheter; and the time interval during which the indwelling catheter is left in place.

Delivery

No agreement was reached on the routine clinical use of in-line filters. Several investigators utilized filters with various pore sizes in all patients receiving TPN. Others reserved in-line filters for administration of these solutions to children. Some never use filtering systems.

In-line filters protect against air embolism in children in whom constant infusion pumps are utilized and also prevent backflow of blood into the intravenous line commonly seen in pediatric patients during a Valsalva maneuver.

The use of filters increases the number of joints in the intravenous tubing and requires additional nursing manipulation. As a result, the chances of inadvertent bacterial contamination of the intravenous fluid column are greater. Needed are filters of sufficient surface area to allow the large volume delivery often required in adult patients.

Participants generally agreed with the Communicable Disease Center that all tubing between the solution bottle and the indwelling catheter should be changed every 24 hours.

Personnel

A parenteral alimentation team of medical and paramedical personnel is necessary to maintain proper in-house supervision, educational programs, and quality control. The team should consist minimally of a physician, a pharmacist, and a specially trained nurse. Additional benefits are obtained by including a dietitian, physical therapist, and authority on infectious disease, and other consultants as appropriate.

Pharmacy

Consistent methods to ensure quality control in mixing solutions with additives must be employed in the local hospital pharmacy. Samples of formulated solutions should be retained for culture, or a technique developed for growth media monitoring of the pharmaceutical manipulation.

Manufacturing

Increased protection from bacterial contamination could be obtained if greater emphasis were placed on prepackaging complete solutions, including intake connective tubing and compartmentalized additives. Representatives from the manufacturing industry indicated that sterilization methods permitting the manufacture of such preparations are unavailable.

Package inserts should be furnished with each commercially available TPN unit. Some manufacturers furnish this information, including complete instructions for use, but others do not. Representatives of industry made a plea for more frequent and intensive review of package inserts. The information provided is based on the experience of numerous investigators. Suggestions on safety in the preparation and administration of parenteral nutrients are given.

In-Service Education

Industry participants urge strongly that their hospital representatives be allowed to provide in-service education support. Several examples of current in-house educational techniques were outlined. One of the most interesting utilized house staff clinical conferences to derive data that allowed formulation of a hospital policy outlining acceptable practices for preparation and delivery of solutions. Another effective technique for in-service education employed television tapes of physician, nursing, and pharmaceutical activities for orientation of new personnel. The tapes also provide a critical review of actual per formance. Members of industry were invited to underwrite the cost of additional educational movies or videotapes of their products.

Solutions

Participants from industry indicated that present techniques for assuring sterility of solutions are adequate in meeting the official standards published in the United States Pharmacopoeia (USP). An industry-wide survey revealed that the chance of releasing contaminated solutions was indeed small, on the order of one organism in one of 10^{16} bottles. Thus, they estimated that a single 1-liter bottle would be contaminated over a 10-year period; and they emphasized that test procedures in use may not detect contamination occurring during closure of the solution container.

Food and Drug Administration

The strict requirements of The Food and Drug Administration's New Drug Application (NDA) stimulated a dialogue among investigators, manufacturers, and representatives of the FDA. Any amino acid addition or substantial change in amino acid concentration of a solution in current use would require the costly repetition of toxicological and efficacy studies in animals and humans.

Some confusion remains regarding the requirements for an individual investigator's NDA compared to requirements for investigations sponsored by manufacturing firms (see p 452). It was suggested that more latitude might be allowed individual investigators in pursuing clinical efficacy testing in humans than would be allowed a manufacturer. There is no precedent covering a product with as many active ingredients as are present in a synthetic amino acid solution.

An advisor to the FDA emphasized the regulatory role of this agency in carrying out the laws enacted by Congress, and suggested that the FDA must maintain a rigid position when considering toxicity and efficacy testing of qualified solutions. The more flexible regulations in other lands permit their scientists more rapid progress in testing the efficacy of different amino acid patterns for parenteral nutrition.

Summary

A great variation exists in procedures for quality control in the pharmacy and for delivery and maintenance of parenteral nutrients. A guideline for minimum safety requirements, presently being prepared by various organizations such as the United States Pharmacopoeial Convention, Inc., and the Communicable Disease Center should be a valuable adjunct to the future comparison of institutional performance and practice.

PART THREE

Section Two

Delivery

14 The Problem of Circulatory Access
   John W. Broviac, M.D., and Belding H. Scribner, M.D.
15 Pumps and Filter
   Jay W. Cooke

   Colloquium: Delivery
   Digest of Colloquium
   James A. O'Neill, Jr., M.D., and Charles W. Van Way III, M.D.

SAFETY AND DELIVERY OF SOLUTIONS

Chapter 14

The Problem of Circulatory Access

John W. Broviac, M.D., and Belding H. Scribner, M.D.

Three methods of vascular access for hypertonic infusion have been investigated. Infusion into A-V shunts and fistulas were technically unsatisfactory. The use of a new cuffed atrial Silastic catheter is described that allows safe long-term vascular access for parenteral nutrition.

For the past several years at the University of Washington we have been developing a system known as the artificial gut, which can provide long-term total parenteral nutrition by means of self-infusion at home.[1, 2] During this time we have trained 14 patients who could no longer maintain their health and nutrition with oral intake to mix and infuse their total daily nutritional requirements over a 12- to 14-hour period at night. The pertinent data for these patients are presented in Table 1.

Table 1.—Results in Fourteen Patients Fed Intravenously at Home

Pt.	Age	Original Disease	Weight (kg) (initial)	(final)	Infusions per Week	Duration Months	Degree of Rehab
1*	26	Crohn's disease	32	58-60	5	8	Full
2	47	Crohn's disease	44	56-58	6	6	Partial
3	32	Short bowel syndrome traumatic	69	72-73	6	3	Partial
4†	58	Short bowel syndrome vascular disease	57	60-61	3	4	Full
5	31	S/P total gastrectomy severe dumping syndrome	46	63-65	5	5	Full
6	29	Crohn's disease	41	54-56	5	26‡	Full
7	10	Systemic mast cell disease	19	28-29	7	24‡	Full
8	35	Crohn's disease and fistula formation	40	59-61	5	10	Full
9	42	Radiation bowel disease	43	52-53	5	7	None
10	29	Short bowel syndrome vascular disease	70	85-87	7	11‡	Full
11	61	Multiple bowel fistula	52	57-59	7	6	Full
12	23	Crohn's disease	48	55-57	5	3	Full
13	4	Acrodermatitis enteropathica	10	16-17	7	3‡	Full
14	16	Short bowel syndrome volvulus	57	59-60	6	3‡	Full

*Infused for one month through a femoral A-V shunt.
†Circulatory access via A-V fistula; all others via atrial catheter.
‡Continuing home parenteral nutrition.

All patients were able to gain weight and to maintain their desired weight level by self-administered parenteral nutrition at home. Eleven of the 14 patients were fully rehabilitated; they were able to live a normal life except for the time required for infusion. When no longer forced to rely on oral intake of nutrients, five patients with inflammatory bowel disease had a marked reduction in the frequency and severity of their gastrointestinal symptoms (fever, pain, diarrhea). In addition, most of these patients no longer required treatment with narcotics, corticosteroids, or immunosuppressive drugs. The system also has been used successfully in the management of patients with the short bowel syndrome and appears to offer lifelong nutritional support for those patients not expected to recover small bowel function.

The artificial gut system has proved to be a relatively easy technique for use in the home. It is readily accepted by patients without undue change in their lifestyle. Basically it consists of four parts (Fig 1):

A two-liter bottle in which sterile nutrients can be mixed safely by the patient just prior to infusion;

A small battery operated pump to control the rate of infusion;

A portable stand with a monitoring device to warn the patient that the infusion bottle is nearly empty; and

A method of circulatory access for infusion of concentrated nutrient solutions.

It was apparent from the onset of this program that an essential component of the artificial gut system was a safe method for prolonged circulatory access through which the hypertonic nutrient solutions could be infused. To avoid local vascular endothelial damage and thrombosis, such solutions must be delivered to areas where rapid dilution of solutes occurs. The circulatory access device must not predispose the patient to life-threatening thromboembolic phenomena or air embolus. Above all, it must be bacteriologically safe. Finally, the device itself must not add other risks because of its presence.

In the course of our studies we investigated three basic methods of circulatory access and their modifications: Infusion through a sidearm into a standard external Teflon-Silastic arteriovenous (AV) shunt; infusion into a surgically constructed internal A-V fistula by repeated venipuncture; and infusion via a modified all-Silastic right atrial indwelling catheter. All three permit infusion of solutions into areas of high blood flow for its dilutional effects. The first two are the most frequently utilized modes of circulatory access for repeated hemodialysis. We have observed that blood flow through A-V shunts ranges between 150 to 400 ml/min in patients receiving dialysis, and that through A-V fistulas averages around 600 to 900 ml/min.[3] Similar findings have been noted by D. Sherrard and T. Fleming (unpublished data). Since the maximally tolerated rate of infusion of glucose is not much above 1 gm/kg/hr, a blood flow of 200 ml/min keeps the maximum possible sugar concentration in the venous blood below 1,200 mg/100 ml, which is less than the level sometimes seen in uncontrolled diabetes mellitus. A catheter with the tip in the right atrium empties into a flow equal to the total cardiac output. Theoretically, local vessel irritation, thrombosis, and fibrosis due to hyperosmolar solutions should not occur with any of these methods of circulatory access.

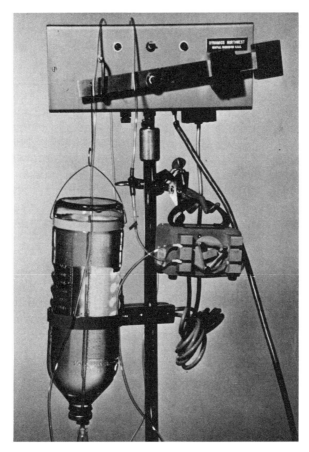

Fig 1. Portable stand with two-liter bottle, small peristaltic pump, and the monitoring device.

EXTERNAL A-V SHUNT

Infusion into external A-V shunts is performed by the addition of a T-connector in its external portion that may be filled with heparin and capped for use on an intermittent basis. Experience with infusion of 50% dextrose in water solution ($D_{50}W$), supplying 3,000 kcal/24 hr into shunts of patients undergoing dialysis had shown it to be without significant complications (eg, increased incidence of infection or thrombosis).[1] The method offers the advantage of delivery of hypertonic solutions at a point where the vessel wall is artificial. However, attempting to apply this technique to patients with severe bowel disease met with failure. First, these patients invariably had tiny fragile veins or veins previously thrombosed by prior intravenous therapy, making insertion of a shunt impossible. Second, shunts once established often clotted despite systemic anticoagulation with coumarin or heparin. Shunts tend to clot rapidly in the nonuremic individual[4] as evidenced by spontaneous thromboses in shunts of patients who have successfully undergone renal transplantation. For these and other reasons this method has been all but abandoned.

However, it still remains a valuable technique for delivery of nutrients to uremic individuals with shunts *in situ*.

INTERNAL A-V FISTULA

Another mode of circulatory access for dialytic treatment is the surgically constructed internal A-V fistula formed in various ways: end-to-end, end-to-side, or side-to-side anastomosis of artery to vein.[5] This route also has been investigated in patients receiving dialysis and found to be exceptionally satisfactory. Infusion is accomplished by repeated venipuncture with a 20-gauge Teflon needle. Although the incidence of local infection is high with indwelling intravenous catheters, little has been published about the use of needles, except to state that infection occurs infrequently, presumably because they are not kept in place for long periods of time.[6] This has been our experience, also.

A-V fistulas promote a hyperdynamic cardiovascular state, manifested by an increase in pulse rate and cardiac output, increased blood volume, and decreased peripheral vascular resistance. In dogs, these changes have been correlated with the size of the fistula[7] and have been found to increase with time.[8] However, with fistula flows of the above magnitude (from 600 to 900 ml/min), the appearance of cardiovascular symptoms or cardiomegaly is extremely rare, even in patients receiving dialysis who are also quite anemic.[3] If symptoms do supervene, it is a simple matter to revise the fistula surgically and reduce the size of the opening between artery and vein.

Thus far, the greatest drawback to use of a fistula has been the difficulty encountered in attempting to construct them in patients with chronic bowel disease. Findings at surgery are similar to that seen during placement of cannulas, namely, a poor venous system. Fistula construction has been attempted 13 times in 9 patients. The results: two successes. Fistulas, once constructed, have been sclerosed by too early or too rapid infusion, especially when the smaller dilated veins were selected for venipuncture. Infusions into the small veins are regularly associated with local inflammation and aching pain, even if extravasation does not occur. Sterile phlebitis also has been seen with infusion at one site for longer than 24 to 36 hours. However, repeated infusions up to 60 gm of dextrose per hour into large veins do not lead to damage. Therefore, it is important when using this mode of access to allow the fistula to mature for several months before use, for until that time the venous system will continue to dilate; and to choose only large veins for sites of infusion.

It may be advisable to construct a single large vessel fistula through which the total fistula blood flow passes. Such a fistula can be constructed by translocation of the saphenous vein to the forearm.[9]

A large-flow fistula can mature with no usable superficial veins available for venipuncture, the greater part of the blood returning via the deeper venous system. This problem can sometimes be corrected by ligating the distal venous branch of the fistula.

In general, fistula usage is restricted to 24 hours per venipuncture site to prevent sterile or bacterial phlebitis. To safely infuse continuously, in our experience, would require changing needle insertion sites every 24 hours at least.

Theoretically, this method is the safest for prolonged parenteral nutrition because it neither requires an indwelling prosthetic device (foreign body and its attendant dangers), nor is the incidence of infection a problem with the use of needles for short-dwell times. Other than the discomfort to the patient from inadvertent extravasation of hypertonic solutions, its only disadvantage is the time required for maturation before usage.

INDWELLING RIGHT ATRIAL CATHETER

Since A-V shunts were not successful for parenteral nutrition in non-uremic patients and A-V fistulas were difficult to establish and required a delay of several weeks between construction and usage, a third method of circulatory access was investigated: an indwelling right atrial catheter. Since its usage was intended for home infusion, it had to be safe yet require minimal professional care. The major problem to overcome was the high incidence of infection associated with indwelling venous catheters in place longer than 48 to 72 hours. In one study, 51% of catheters in place for longer than 48 hours were positive to bacterial culture, with or without associated signs of clinical phlebitis.[10] The magnitude of the problem is evident in that 9% to 43% of hospital septicemias have been shown to be due to indwelling catheters.[11,12] Others have shown the incidence of septicemias occurring with venous catheterization to be between 2.0% to 3.4%.[12-14] This has been reduced to nearly zero but requires in-hospital meticulous care and its attendant costs.[15] Even under these circumstances, the average duration of safe venous catheterization is only 24 days per catheter used.

Bacterial invasion may occur around or through the catheter. The latter is probably quite uncommon as long as sterile solutions, tubing, and administration technique are used. But blood-borne seeding from an infected source elsewhere in the body may lodge in the thrombofibrinous sheath that encases the intravascular segment of most catheters. This makes eradication of the infection difficult unless the catheter is removed.

Invasion occurring along the outside of the catheter is probably the most common, as evidenced by the fact that skin organisms are cultured most frequently, and such infections are often associated with exit site infections.[10,12,13] Organisms may be carried in during the venipuncture if sterile technique of insertion is not followed, or with repeated mechanical movement of the catheter *in situ*. It is equally likely that mechanical irritation may lead to thrombus formation at the site of vessel entry and provide a nidus in which bacteria can multiply. A bacteriologically safe catheter, then, would be one that prevents such infection from occurring.

It has been shown previously that infection could be prevented from developing around hemodialysis cannulas and indwelling peritoneal catheters. This is accomplished by bonding a substance that would promote tissue ingrowth to the outer aspect of the prosthesis in its subcutaneous tunnel.[16,17,18] Dacron felt resulted in the ingrowth and organization of the felt by vascular connective tissue, thus forming an effective mechanical barrier to bacterial invasion, as well as stabilizing the prosthetic access device.[17]

Keeping these principles in mind, an all-Silastic, Dacron-cuffed atrial catheter was developed and investigated in animals and later in patients in whom other modes of circulatory access were unavailable for parenteral nutrition. This catheter (Fig 2) consists of a thin intravascular Silastic segment inserted through a subclavian vein with the tip carefully placed in the right atrium. A thicker reinforced extravascular Silastic segment of the catheter is brought down through a subcutaneous tunnel on the medial aspect of the chest, with the skin exit site low on the chest wall. The Dacron cuff, which is bonded to this segment, is located just below the subclavian insertion, usually in the first intercostal space. Within 10 to 14 days, the cuff is well anchored, thus preventing mechanical dislodgment or bacterial access to the venous system. A tract of granulative tissue forms along the catheter between the cuff and the exit site. This may serve as an additional barrier to infection. At the same time, it permits drainage should sinus tract infection occur. The external end of the catheter contains a fitting that may be capped after a heparin lock is applied. A single heparin lock can maintain patency of these

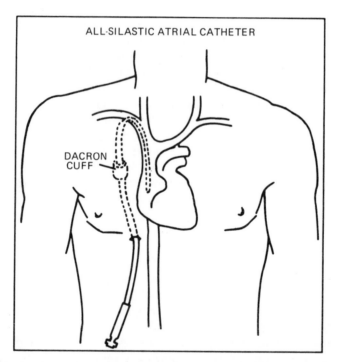

Fig 2. In the schematic above, the tip is situated in midatrial area for adequate dilution of hypertonic solutions; all-Silastic construction avoids mechanical or chemical irritation; Dacron cuff prevents accidental dislodgment and forms a mechanical barrier to bacterial invasion; low skin exit site prevents air embolism with the patient in the upright position; and the external end contains a fitting that may be capped after the catheter is filled with heparin, assuring patency of catheter between infusions.

catheters for at least two weeks, probably indefinitely with periodic replacement. If the catheter is opened with the patient upright, air embolism cannot occur due to positive hydrostatic pressure in the system.

The catheter is inserted percutaneously through a 2- to 3-cm incision beneath the midportion of the clavicle into the subclavian vein using standard sterile technique with local anesthesia and fluoroscopic control. A specially devised split-apart needle is necessary for venipuncture because of the presence of the Dacron cuff. Routine catheter care in the past consisted of daily cleansing of the area with hydrogen peroxide and the application of a sterile dressing. We have avoided the use of antibiotic ointments, because we feel that their usage would predispose our patients to sinus tract infections with either fungi or resistant bacteria. However, recently our patients have been advised to use an iodophor ointment.

Since 1970, 40 such catheters have been inserted into 27 patients to give a total experience of 161 patient months of parenteral nutrition: 108 patient months of unattended home self-infusion by the trained patient and 53 patient months of in-hospital infusion. Twenty-three patients needed only 1 catheter for an average dwell-time of 4.6 months (range 0.5 to 26 months); 3 catheters were used in one patient for an average 3.6 months (0.7 to 5.1); 4 catheters were used in two patients for an average 3.7 months (1.0 to 14.9); and one patient has required 6 catheters for an average 2.5 months (0.9 to 4.0). The average dwell-time for all catheters has been 4.0 months.

Of these 40 catheters, 6 still are in use with an average dwell-time of 7.4 months (1.4 to 26); 7 were removed after an average dwell-time of 2.9 months due to technical difficulties, dislodgement, plugging, or leaking; 21 were no longer needed after an average dwell-time of 3.8 months (0.5 to 22.2) either because the patients died or were able to resume normal oral intake. No deaths were related in any way to the use of the catheter.

Six catheters were removed due to sepsis after an average dwell-time of 2.8 months (1.3 to 5.1). Three episodes of sepsis occurred in 2 out of 14 hospitalized patients at an average rate of 1 for every 1.5 years of patient usage. Of these, two were fungal in origin (Saccharomyces and Candida) and were cured with catheter removal. The other was due to an enterococcus and was cured with catheter removal and a three-week course of antibiotic therapy.

Three episodes of sepsis occurred in 3 of 13 home patients at an average rate of one for every three years of home parenteral nutrition. All three were due to S aureus infection and were cured with catheter removal and a two- to three-week course of antibiotic therapy. Although we have replaced catheters within three afebrile days following catheter removal, we prefer to treat the patient for 7 to 10 days before replacing it. Either way, reinfection with the same organism has not occurred.

During the same period of time, four patients developed catheter exit site infection, two from S epidermidis and two S aureus. Three infections which occurred around catheters that were in place longer than three months were localized to the sinus tract distal to the subcutaneous cuff. They responded within three days to a two-week course of oral antibiotics and did not recur. One infection, present two weeks after catheter insertion, was complicated by sepsis. The catheter was removed. At that time the cuff had not scarred in.

416

This provides evidence that the cuff does prevent infection from occurring around the outside of the catheter once it is well healed in place. Of the six episodes of sepsis that have occurred with this catheter only this one has been associated with an exit site infection. Apparently the others occurred through the catheter because of faulty technique or arose elsewhere in the body, involving the catheter and its fibrin sheath secondarily.

Shown in Figure 3 is the expected rate of sepsis per year of patient treatment when standard subclavian catheters are used with poor but previously common in-hospital techniques,[19] when such catheters are used in hospitals employing sound infection control techniques,[20] and when the cuffed atrial catheter is used with comparable optimum technique. This indirect comparison between the type of central venous catheter used and the degree of care exercised in preventing septicemia has been made by determining the rate of sepsis per year of patient infusion. When TPN catheters are used for withdrawing and infusing blood and measurement of central venous pressure, one can expect a patient receiving intravenous infusion for one year to have seven episodes of catheter-related septicemia.[19] When the infection control recommendations of the Center for Disease Control are followed, this risk is reduced to one episode of sepsis per year of TPN infusion. The use of the cuffed atrial catheter reduces this risk even further.

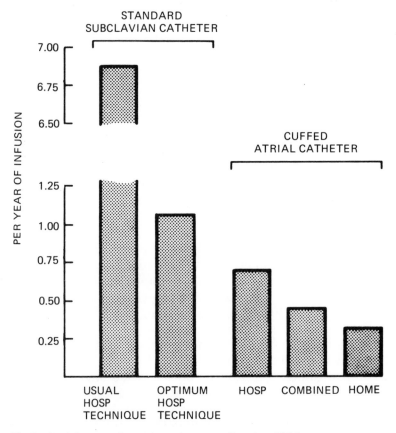

Fig 3. Incidence of septicemia complicating TPN.

We have concluded from our experience with the use of this catheter that it is a relatively safe technique and well worth the slight risk involved when prolonged parenteral nutrition is indicated. Because bacteriemia will lead to seeding of its fibrinous sheath making eradication of the infection difficult, we do not insert the catheter into patients who are currently septic or who are expected to become septic. In these cases the repeated subclavian puncture technique of Wilmore and Dudrick is preferred because of ease of insertion and removal.[15]

Although our research is still in its preliminary or exploratory phase, at this time, a reasonable approach to the management of the patient in need of long-term total or supplemental parenteral nutrition might include the following.

A. For the patient in need of immediate nutrition:

Insert the special right atrial catheter which will permit immediate continuous infusion to promote anabolism.

Construct an A-V fistula if the venous system is well-developed. It takes from two to three months for the veins to fully dilate. At that point, switch to intermittent overnight infusions for maintenance nutrition.

Train the patient for self-infusion in the home using the total artificial gut system.

Continue with use of the catheter if the venous system is poorly formed or badly damaged; it appears to be relatively free of complications. In time, with lack of peripheral IV and with good nutrition, it is possible that the venous system will regenerate enough to sustain a functional fistula.

B. For the patient who needs long-term parenteral nutrition from two months to two years:

Create a functional A-V fistula early, before irreversible damage to the peripheral veins occurs.

Use the fistula at any future date when IV nutrition is necessary.

Train the patient for home infusion if the need arises for long-term parenteral nutrition. From our preliminary data it appears to be safe and avoids the cost of repeated hospitalizations.

References

1. Scribner BH, Cole JJ, Christopher TG, et al: Long-term total parenteral nutrition: The concept of an artificial gut. *JAMA* **212:**457-463, 1970.

418

2. Atkins RC, Vizzo JE, Cole JJ, et al: The artificial gut in hospital and home. Technical improvements. *Trans Am Soc Artif Intern Organs* **16**:260-268, 1970.

3. Johnson G Jr, Blythe WB: Hemodynamic effects of arteriovenous shunts used for hemodialysis. *Ann Surg* **171**:715-723, 1970.

4. Conolly WB, Murphy J, Belzer FO: Intravenous feeding by an arteriovenous shunt. *Surg Forum* **19**:383-384, 1968.

5. Brescia MJ, Cimino JE, Appel K: Chronic hemodialysis using venipuncture and a surgically created arteriovenous fistula. *N Eng J Med* **275**: 1089-1092, 1966.

6. Fekety FR Jr, Thoburn R: Nature and prevention of intravenous catheter infection. *Johns Hopkins Med J* **121**:133-134, 1967.

7. Frank CW, Wang HH, Lammerant J, et al: An experimental study of the immediate hemodynamic adjustments to acute arteriovenous fistulae of various sizes. *J Clin Invest* **34**:722-731, 1955.

8. Schenk WG Jr, Martin JW, Leslie MB, Portin BA: The regional hemodynamics of chronic arteriovenous fistulas. *Surg Gynecol Obstet* **110**: 44-50, 1960.

9. May J, Tiller D, Johnson J, et al: Saphenous-vein arteriovenous fistula in regular dialysis treatment. *N Eng J Med* **280**:770-771, 1969.

10. Druskin MS, Siegel PD: Bacterial contamination of indwelling intravenous polyethylene catheters. *JAMA* **185**:966-968, 1963.

11. Smits H, Freedman LR: Prolonged venous catheterization as a cause of sepsis. *N Eng J Med* **276**:1229-1233, 1967.

12. Bentley DW, Lepper MH: Septicemia related to indwelling venous catheter. *JAMA* **206**:1749-1752, 1968.

13. Collins RN, Braun PA, Zinner SH, et al: Risk of local and systematic infection with polyethylene intravenous catheters. A prospective study of 213 catheterizations. *N Eng J Med* **279**:340-343, 1968.

14. Banks DC, Yates DB, Cawdrey HM, et al: Infection from intravenous catheters. *Lancet* **1**:443-445, 1970.

15. Wilmore DW, Dudrick SJ: Safe long-term venous catheterization. *Arch Surg* **98**:256-258, 1969.

16. McDonald HP Jr, Berber N, Mishva D, et al: Subcutaneous Dacron and Teflon cloth adjuncts for Silastic arteriovenous shunts and peritoneal dialysis catheters. *Trans Am Soc Artif Intern Organs* **14**:176-180, 1968.

17. Striker GE, Tenckhoff HA: A transcutaneous prosthesis for prolonged access to the peritoneal cavity. *Surgery* **69**:70-74, 1971.

18. Tenckhoff H, Schechter H: A bacteriologically safe peritoneal access device. *Trans Am Soc Artif Intern Organs* **14**:181-187, 1968.

19. Curry CR, Quie PG: Fungal septicemia in patients receiving parenteral hyperalimentation. *N Eng J Med* **285**:1221-1225, 1971.

20. Goldmann DA, Maki DG: Infection control in total parenteral nutrition. *JAMA* **223**:1360-1364, 1973.

Chapter 15

Pumps and Filters

Jay W. Cooke

The infusion control (IC) device contributes to precision in administration of parenteral fluids.

An infusion control device provides a controlled, scheduled infusion which is accurate and unaffected by many existing variables. It supplies a metered dose of parenteral fluid to meet the precalculated needs of the patient as determined by the attending physician.[1,2] The device is reliable and relatively simple to operate, and its use does not complicate IV procedure.

The idea of mechanically infusing parenteral fluids emerged in the late 1940s. The syringe pump was developed during the 1950s and the peristaltic pump during the next decade, followed in the 1970s by refinement of the proved peristaltic mechanism.

With the advent of parenteral hyperalimentation procedures, infusion control devices sustained increased interest and further acceptance because they offered advantages over the gravity IV system. To better understand these advantages, we must first examine the nature of the gravity IV system.

THE GRAVITY IV SYSTEM

This method of administration is essentially a manometer, which is dependent on the forces of gravity and is subject to variations of height and pressure. There are many variables which may alter the flow rate during the course of administration:[1]

Height of the IV flask in relation to the patient's infusion site;
Volume of fluid in the IV flask during the course of the infusion;
Uniformity in the size of the drop orifice located in the IV set spear;
Physical properties of the fluid passing through the orifice;
Mechanical properties of the flow control clamp of the IV administration set and its ability to maintain a constant occlusion;
Selection of ancillary devices, such as filters and catheters incorporated into the IV set's fluid pathway, may act as an obstacle to flow; and
Fluctuations in the patient's vascular pressure may occur, varying the amount of resistance against the flow.[2]

Parenteral fluid therapy has placed new and greater demands upon current methods of IV administration. With an infusion control device, fluid volumes and content can be tailored to the patient's needs rather than to the requirements of current IV administration systems. They are designed to create a controlled situation.

APPLICATIONS OF IC DEVICES

Application of infusion control devices exists in situations where the patients require special care.[1] Some examples are: low-birth-weight neonates, fluid-restricted patients, and patients requiring precise administration of parenteral drugs.

Although accepted in caring for the special patient, widespread use of the infusion control device has not occurred and has been resisted to some degree. Yet once patients and hospital staff become familiar with the operation and function of the device, they are reluctant to return to the gravity drip system.

The hospital staff should be trained to use infusion control devices as they are trained in the administration of parenteral fluids by gravity drip. The manufacturers of these devices have recognized the need for in-service training and are willing to provide this assistance.

Advantages

Incorporation of an infusion control device into the parenteral fluid delivery system provides (1) control over the administration of fluids, whether it be at low or high flow rates; (2) a predictable, scheduled infusion, which can be varied with precision at the discretion of the attending staff; and (3) a time-saving factor, since the nursing time spent for frequent readjustment of the gravity drip is no longer required.[1,3] The device is meant to assist the attending staff. Thus, the infusion should be monitored at reasonable intervals. In addition to this, the device continually maintains the flow of parenteral fluid under positive pressure through the administration catheter or needle, thus minimizing the incidence of clotting.[3,4]

Hazards

When a pumping device is used to control IV fluid delivery, the possibility of infusing air is increased since some infusion control devices will continue operating after the bottle has run dry. Use of a microporous membrane filter which is wet (0.22μ or 0.45μ) and is incorporated into the fluid pathway of the IV administration set will act as a mechanical barrier against the infusion of air.[5,6] Other methods are available to monitor the drop rate. When drops cease to fall, an alarm is sounded and the pump is shut off, stopping the infusion. Another method for controlling the infusion of air is using the weight principle to detect a nearly empty fluid flask, thus sounding an alarm and shutting off the device. Finally, plastic IV solution bags can provide safety against the infusion of air, since they utilize a nonvented system which collapses as the solution is administered.

MEMBRANE FILTERS

Membrane filters are available in several pore sizes. The 0.22μ and 0.45μ membrane filters are used most commonly. These filters are useful in removing animate and inanimate material which is larger than the pore of the filter.[6] The 0.45μ filter has received the greatest usage, but it is suggested that the 0.22μ filter be used. It can provide a sterile filtrate, and the 0.45μ filter cannot.[6]

These filters remove particulate matter which may be introduced during the compounding of fluids. Also, they protect against the infusion of precipitates which may result from drug incompatibilities. Thus, microporous membrane filters remove microorganisms, particulate matter, precipitates and protect against the infusion of air.[6] All of these are important when fluids contain many additives.

A 0.22μ filter is recommended for use with an infusion pump, but a filter of this size, which produces a sterile filtrate, may be restrictive to flow in a gravity system. For filters to function properly, it is advisable that all air be removed from the filter case. Difficulties may arise when sufficient quantities of air have descended through the fluid pathway of the administration set into the chamber of the filter, thereby forcing all fluid through the membrane. The situation is termed an "air lock" and stops the flow. In-service training of personnel can aid in minimizing this problem.

TRENDS IN IC DEVICE DEVELOPMENT

Among new ideas for expanding the function of the infusion control device is a possibility for automating the intravenous drug-dosage procedure, a device that will cyclically infuse a parenteral drug and keep the line open continuously. Monitoring a patient's vital signs and the serum levels of the administered drugs is another possibility. Also, closed-loop computerized IV administered systems, utilizing the technology of probes and other sensing devices, may be used to further the advancement of servo-control systems.[1]

With the increasing prominence of infusion-control devices, the design and function will be further refined as time passes and as needs present themselves or are brought to light through the cooperation of engineers and clinicians.[7] Parenteral alimentation will assist in the advancement of these new devices and their success. True advancement in the medical sciences is facilitated through the close cooperation of responsible medical practitioners and concerned patient-oriented companies.

References

1. Wilmore DW: The future of intravenous therapy. *Am J Nurs* **7:** 2334-2338, 1971.

2. Sherman JO, Egan I, Macalad FV: Parenteral hyperalimentation: A useful surgical adjunct. *Surg Clin North Am* **51:**37-47, 1971.

3. Cort DF: Positive infusion control in the treatment of burns in children. *Br J Plast Surg* **23:**395-397, 1970.

4. Atkins RC, Vizzo JE, Cole JJ: The artificial gut in hospital and home: Technical improvements. *Trans Am Soc Artif Intern Organs* **16:**260-266, 1970.

5. Bowman FW, Calhoun MP, White M: Microbiological methods for quality control of membrane filters. *J Pharm Sci* **56:**222-225, 1967.

6. Wilmore DW, Dudrick SJ: An in-line filter for intravenous solutions. *Arch Surg* **99:**462-463, 1969.

7. Ebersman DS: Considerations in the development of total intravenous feedings. *Bull Parenteral Drug Association* **25:**279-286, 1971.

Delivery

Colloquium

James A. O'Neill, Jr., M.D., chairman and editor
Charles W. Van Way III, M.D., rapporteur

Dr. O'Neill: Discussants of the status of various delivery systems gave their evaluation of the techniques and direction for determining what is desirable and what is undesirable. We reviewed, in sequence:

    I. Consideration of sites for catheterization: Peripheral and central venous
    II. Catheter materials
    III. Pumps
    IV. Filters and administrative tubing
    V. Pharmacy procedures
    VI. Responsibilities for safe delivery

CATHETER PLACEMENT

Dr. Hoshal: We have investigated percutaneous supraclavicular sub-clavian catheterization and, as an occasional alternative, the internal jugular approach. Since various types of catheters may have different problems associated with them, we have used Angiocaths almost exclusively. This type of catheter has certain inherent advantages.

The catheter is Teflon. We feel it is the proper length, 5¼ inches. For adults, we use a 14-gauge size which allows rapid flow. The Angiocath has an additional feature of a groove at the connector hub, which permits one to secure the catheter in place with a horizontal mattress stitch around the puncture site. This stitch prevents to-and-fro motion of the catheter, a factor known to be related to wound infection.

The Angiocath needle inserts through the skin easily, but it is eliminated from the system once the catheter is in the vein, since the catheter is on the outside of the needle. This avoids the possibility of the needle shearing off a portion of the catheter and allowing it to embolize, a problem associated with earlier versions of needle-catheter combinations.

Using this catheter and the supraclavicular approach, it takes fewer than ten seconds to place a catheter 95% of the time. We have difficulty in about 4% of our patients; in these it takes two or more attempts to cannulize the subclavian vein. Usually, the problem is related to the angle of insertion and the catheter cannot be threaded into the vein. In 1% of patients another approach must be used, usually into the internal jugular.

Over a three-year period, I have had experiences with 3,000 supraclavicular subclavian catheterizations and about 50 internal jugular catheterizations. The supraclavicular stick has generally been performed on the left side, because I am right-handed and find it easier that way. Ten percent were inserted for hyperalimentation, and 90% were inserted for other reasons, such as central venous pressure monitoring, long-term intravenous antibiotic therapy, or systemic heparinization.

There were three instances of pneumothorax; two of these required tube drainage. The subclavian artery was hit 22 times. We had two transient thoracic duct leaks, which stopped after 48 hours, and two instances of clinically evident subclavian vein thrombosis. "Clinical" is emphasized because of data which indicate that some degree of thrombosis is usually present without obvious clinical signs. One catheter perforated the superior vena cava, resulting in bilateral pleural effusions. We have had eight nonfatal cases of air embolism, not during the catheterization procedure itself, but secondary to disconnection of tubing joints. We have avoided the problem of tubing disconnection by working with industrial engineers to design luer tip extension tubing for our use. We have not had such problems as hemothorax, brachial plexus injury, catheter breakage, embolism, or cardiac perforation.

Occasionally a catheter will not pass into the superior vena cava but will go elsewhere. One catheter entered the inferior thyroid vein; since this patient was receiving TPN, he developed a clinically inflamed thyroid gland. Another patient developed an arteriovenous fistula which occurred about four days after an attempted subclavian catheterization on the right side. This patient had a palpable and audible bruit, and his supraclavicular area and forequarter region had a flushed appearance.

A minimal length of catheter is needed in the vein, inserting only enough so that the catheter enters the superior vena cava. Passing greater lengths into the venous system increases the risk from thrombosis around the catheter. To check catheter tip position, we routinely obtain a chest x-ray after inserting a catheter.

Finally, our program includes a regular schedule of conferences and training sessions to familiarize staff and trainees with methods, techniques, and complications.

Dr. O'Neill: Do you leave these catheters in the same site as long as they appear to be clean, or do you change them to another site once a week?

Dr. Hoshal: They are left in the same location as long as they are needed in all patients, except those with burns. In these, the catheters are changed weekly as a routine.

Dr. O'Neill: May I mention one other problem related to the percutaneous placement of catheters. If one has difficulty advancing a catheter of the type Dr. Hoshal has described and then attempts to replace the needle for a second attempt, a portion of the catheter may be sheared off, and it may embolize. Although he did not encounter such a problem, this has been seen by others and in our institution. In children under four years of age, we generally do not use percutaneous subclavian sticks but have relied on cutdowns, either in the antecubital area or in the neck. This involves either the external or the internal jugular vein or the external facial vein which empties into the internal jugular, allowing use of the internal jugular vein on more than one occasion if necessary. Complications have been encountered with percutaneous subclavian punctures in children under four.

Dr. Broviac: We almost always use the percutaneous subclavian approach for parenteral hyperalimentation in acutely ill patients, but we favor use of a Silastic catheter, which is not stiff and has little tendency to perforate. One can place Silastic catheters in the right atrium without danger of causing mechanical trauma to the vascular system.

Dr. Shils: May I reinforce what Dr. Hoshal said. Hyperalimentation should not be started until the catheter tip location has been established by x-ray.

CATHETER MATERIALS

Dr. Broviac: The catheter with which we have been working is Silastic. The size—smaller than that we were using—is 58/1,000 in in outer diameter and about 29/1,000 in in interior diameter. With the new split-apart needle for insertion, there is only one size available. It is a fine catheter, is radiopaque, and it works well. You can draw blood cultures through it.

Dr. O'Neill: Initially, most of us who become involved in hyperalimentation used polyethylene catheters, available before Teflon; then Portex, available from the British suppliers; and now, more recently, the Silastic catheter which is preferred by the majority.

We have heard that the Teflon catheter is desirable from many points of view. My own preference is for Silastic. I would like to have some consensus on the ideal catheter material.

Dr. Hoshal: My preference is for Silastic, although my experience with it is limited, because it has just come on the market. Silastic is the most flexible material available now, and, at least initially, the tip floats free in the vein so that the infusate is not directed at the vein intima.

The ideal catheter ought to be flexible and easy to insert. It would be best if the needle could be completely eliminated and not connected to the line. It should be possible to insert the catheter without the possibility of the needle shearing it off, and it ought to be easily secured to the skin. There should be no possibility of the catheter becoming disconnected from the hub.

Dr. O'Neill: We need to standardize these materials. When we use Silastic tubing, it is often necessary to construct a hub at the end, using something like an Angiocath to make a satisfactory connection. I suggest that we ask industry to provide us with hubs firmly bound to the catheters, with and without luer locks, so that air embolism may be avoided.

Silastic is ordinarily clear but can be made radiopaque through addition of barium in 5% or 10% concentrations. At the Alder Hay Children's Hospital in England, Silastic catheters of various types, with and without barium and other types of radiopaque substances, were placed in rabbits. No difference was noted in formation of fibrin sheaths around the catheters, but it is our impression that barium impregnation does make these catheters a bit more brittle. I do not believe we have seen any catheters broken off where they were tied into the vein, however.

Dr. Broviac: The only thing that could be more ideal at the present time would be a Silastic catheter that incorporates a heparin bond to prevent formation of a fibrinous sheath. One study has shown that heparin bonded to polyvinyl chloride retarded—but did not eliminate completely—the formation of fibrin sheaths.

Dr. Hoshal: We have used heparin-bonded polyethylene catheters, originally with a modification of Gott's technique. Since fibrin sheaths also form around Silastic, heparin bonding may be of some help there as well. I am not sure that we can ever eliminate some fibrin deposition around the catheter. Where the catheter punctures the vein wall there is going to be some degree of fibrin deposition. How far that will propagate down the catheter is a feature that heparin bonding may alter.

Dr. Rubin: I would like to discuss plasticizers in Silastic and Teflon and ask about using long lengths of such catheter materials as one might use in ambulatory patients. To the best of my knowledge, there are no plasticizers used in Silastic rubber. It is pliable itself.

Fat emulsions may pose certain problems. At the moment, fats are being supplied in glass bottles. If polyvinyl chloride plastic bags are used in the future, fat emulsion might be expected to extract the phthalate plasticizers used in the manufacture of these bags (see p 360).

Mr. Cooke: Dr. O'Neill, could we discuss catheter length? This is a point that would greatly assist the manufacturer of catheters and possibly improve our technique.

Dr. O'Neill: One approach is to make all catheters long and allow the physician to cut off any excess. This takes care of both the pediatric and the adult patient. To catheterize a vein in the antecubital area, one needs a long catheter. Just how far a catheter should be inserted is questionable. Those who prefer to place the tip in the right atrium consider it safe. This may be true to some extent in adults but not necessarily in children, especially the neonate. If we place a catheter in the heart of a neonate who has an anatomic shunt— and many do—it is possible that a bolus of hyperosmolar solution may pass into the coronaries going across such a shunt and produce arrhythmias. We have seen this in two instances. We consider the superior vena cava just above the right atrium the safest position for the catheter tip in infants. In general, we might suggest 14-inch catheters for infants and 30-inch lengths for older individuals.

Dr. Wretlind: In Sweden, and in most of Europe, when we speak about complete intravenous nutrition, we mean intravenous nutrition including fat, carbohydrates, amino acids, and all other nutrients. In most cases, these solutions are given in a peripheral vein. In general, fat and amino acid solutions are given at the same time. The standard solution we use contains 7% amino acids and 10% fructose. As a precaution against thrombophlebitis, we start with fat emulsion, following in a few minutes with the amino acid-carbohydrate solution. The amino acid-carbohydrate solution is finished first, and the fat emulsion runs a little longer. We practically never see thrombophlebitis, but it may be that the intimal cells of the vessel are protected by the fat emulsion.

This needle is left in for about 8 to 12 hours and is then removed. The next day a new setup is used both in adults and infants so that the patient may move about. If patients have problems which require intravenous feedings for longer than two to three weeks, we generally insert a catheter into a major vein.

In infants, 20% fat emulsion is used. Ten percent fat emulsion, now being used in the United States, could serve as well, but it would require a somewhat larger volume. In addition, we used a 10% amino acid and 20% glucose solution earlier, but changed to a mixture of 7% amino acids and 10% glucose. In these two bottles are all the other nutrients, including fat soluble vitamins in the lipid emulsion. In adults the standard amount of fat administered is 12 gm/kg/day and in infants up to 4 gm/kg/day, which means that less carbohydrate is required to supply caloric needs.

Dr. O'Neill: An important aspect of your statement is the potential of getting away from the catheter and its attendant complications.

It has been said that fat and carbohydrate-amino acid solutions may be mixed without difficulty. Now, there must be some admixture at the level of the needle, or at the level of the connection tubing if it is going into a catheter. Do you have any specific data as to whether Intralipid is stable when it mixes with other solutions?

Dr. Wretlind: I do not have data with me, but it has been investigated carefully, and the particle size has been controlled. No instability was noted with the administration methods we currently use. However, we recommend that the two substances should not be mixed in the same bottle; we do not know how long this would be safe.

Dr. Hoshal: The decreased incidence of thrombophlebitis intrigues me. What is the pH of the combined amino acid-glucose solution and fat emulsion at the time of delivery to the vein? We think that acidity is a major factor in thrombophlebitis.

Dr. Wretlind: The pH of the amino acid-carbohydrate solution we use in Sweden is about 5.0, and Intralipid is about 7.5. However, the buffering capacity of Intralipid is practically nil, so the admixture hitting the vein wall would probably be in the range of 5.5.

Dr. O'Neill: We should be careful when we speak about the pH of the solution to stress that we are talking about a local effect on a vein wall. We are not talking about an overall acid-base consideration in a patient. Patients can easily buffer the small acid load these solutions represent (pK vs pH), unless tremendous volumes are given rapidly to small subjects.

Dr. Shils: About seven years ago, Randall and I got the idea of using Scribner-type shunts. The shunts worked well in dogs, but, when they promptly clotted in two nonuremic patients who needed total parenteral nutrition, we gave up. However, Scribner and his group were more persistent and have con-

428

tinued work with some degree of success. About three years ago, we had a patient who had a total small bowel resection; her peripheral veins and almost all of her central veins could no longer be used. In desperation, we thought of an external shunt since no veins were available for an internal shunt. At that time we heard that Scribner had a high-flow shunt and he sent us a Thomas high-flow external shunt for this patient. The Thomas shunt permits such a high flow that heparinization was not required. We used a Millipore filter and a valve which prevented backflow of blood, but which also required a pump because of high resistance (Shils et al, *New Eng J Med*, **283**:341, 1970). The patient then could connect on her side of the Millipore filter, put a sterile closure over it, and be free of the apparatus. We found that we could infuse about 2,000 kilocalories in about 6.5 hours into this patient after she had adapted to the high glucose concentration. This shunt lasted six months, until she developed a staphylococcal infection, and it had to be removed. We then put a low-flow Scribner shunt which required heparinization into her shoulder, and this lasted another six months. That finally had to be removed because of *Candida* infection.

As an emergency measure—or when all suitable arteries and veins for internal AV shunts have been used—external shunts have merit, but internal arteriovenous shunts are preferable.

Dr. Broviac: We have been discouraged with the use of shunts in the patient who has been malnourished for a long period of time, mainly because they clot rapidly and because they become infected readily. Also, we used a Thomas shunt in one patient in whom phlebitis developed, and the shunt clotted off. We allowed it to remain in place and continued intravenous infusions via the right atrial catheter for another four months, at which time the patient was doing well. We decided to remove the shunt at that point. When the shunt was removed, it was grossly infected with *Staphylococcus aureus,* and the patient died within eight hours of fulminant staphylococcal sepsis. This, of course, had infected the fibrinous sheath around the catheter. We have had additional problems with the Thomas shunt in patients receiving dialysis, but I understand that Dr. Thomas has designed a new version which is associated with fewer problems. Investigation of shunts, especially the new high-flow type—even though they may still have the possibility of producing high output cardiac failure—probably should continue in patients who tend to clot Scribner low-flow shunts.

Dr. O'Neill: What happens when high concentrations of glucose are infused in patients with internal shunts?

Dr. Broviac: We have done such infusions in patients treated with dialysis who had well-functioning fistulas (ie, they had one or two veins with a lot of flow through them). In patients with fistulas with enough flow for dilution, we have seen no difficulty with clinical phlebitis or thrombosis of the sub-cutaneous vein. In one patient we even infused 45% sugar at a rate of 3,000 kcal/16 hr without difficulty for some time.

If one can develop a fistula that has available superficial veins to carry an adequate amount of flow, this is probably the ideal mode of circulatory access for a patient who will need it for a long time. This will be especially true if we are able to use fats in this country. Even fistulas with small veins could be used repeatedly.

Dr. Shils: We have been using polyvinyl chloride bags almost exclusively, and we feel we have no worry about plasticizers. Dr. Rubin was kind enough to analyze the contents of some bags that had been stored for some time, and he also analyzed the blood and adipose tissue of patients who, for about a year, had infusions from bags. He reported finding no detectable phthalate plasticizer. However, we put no lipid materials or albumin in these bags.

We also have been concerned about the possibility of an air embolus. We find a pump with an electric drop monitor valuable because it allows us to control infusion rate. It also tends to decrease the frequency of clotting that one gets with gravity drips when they slow down.

PUMPS

Mr. Cooke: The main advantage of a pump is that it is a control device that produces a constant flow. The best pumps work as closed systems to avoid infection.

Dr. Broviac: We like a small, portable Holter pump, a roller pump. It had one small piece of Silastic to which one attached tubing. This was disadvantageous, because frequently the tubing would crack at that point. The new Holter pump tubing has a short prepump segment: a Silastic segment for the pump and a long extension incorporated into it. All one needs is a solution administration set which goes into the short end. The long end is hooked into the patient's catheter. The pump can run for four to six hours on a battery. In the hospital the patient can go to x-ray with it, or to the bathroom at home.

Dr. Shils: How do these pumps protect against air embolism?

Mr. Cooke: The Holter pump is a low-pressure system, and, if one incorporates a Millipore filter of either 0.22μ or 0.45μ, it will act as a mechanical barrier against the infusion of air. The Ivac system utilizes a drop counter; if no drops fall, an alarm sounds, and the pump shuts off. The Sigmamotor 4,000 utilizes the weight method. With this, one hangs the bottle or bag of solution on an arm which weights it. When the container is empty, the scale detects this and an alarm sounds. Of course plastic bags may be the best and easiest method of avoiding infusion of air since bags contain no air and collapse when empty.

Dr. O'Neill: Another advantage of the weight or counterbalance system is that warning is given before the solution runs out. This may help to prevent reactive hypoglycemia.

Accurate regulation systems to produce reliable, constant flow rates are needed for every pump on the market. The ideal has not been achieved for any of them.

Mr. Cooke: You must evaluate pumps on size, portability, function, and cost, and select according to your needs.

What do you feel will be your needs for pumps in the future, how would you employ them, and what would be the requirements of the device?

Dr. O'Neill: We need an inexpensive pump which will allow us to infuse solutions accurately into any age group, which will provide us with a closed system, which will not break down, and which requires little or no maintenance.

Dr. Shils: It should be portable and battery-operated.

Dr. O'Neill: Perhaps we need two types of pumps, one for a patient to carry around with him and another one for heavy-duty use in the hospital. Perhaps we can use pumps in the hospital that will infuse more than one patient at a time.

FILTERS AND ADMINISTRATIVE TUBING

Dr. O'Neill: Let us turn to a consideration of filters. Do we all share the opinion that we should use filters in the pediatric age group and that in the adult age group it probably is not necessary?

Dr. Shils: There are problems with filters beyond the filter. As mentioned earlier, the process of introducing filters into the line is a potential hazard from the point of view of infection. Our policy is to change filters about every four days, but with the whole line from the bottle to the patient.

It would be a further advance if the filter were built in-line, so one could buy the whole unit with the filter in it. This would reduce contamination also.

My experience with the use of filters has been with adults. The filters do clog after four or five days. This does mean that we are removing particulate matter, and the question is whether this particulate matter would be dangerous if it entered the patient. I really do not know. Microprecipitates such as calcium phosphate may comprise a part of the solids.

We have also found that certain materials (eg, Keflin), together with a high concentration of glucose, may precipitate and clog the filter. Our rules are that albumin and antibiotics are infused on the patient side of the filter just to prevent that from happening.

The 0.45μ filter is supposed to take out all bacteria except certain forms of *Pseudomonas*. The 0.22μ filter takes out all bacteria. We have found that the 0.22μ size may require a pump after a day, whereas the 0.45μ filter—which we prefer—will allow gravity drip. It is now available from Travenol as an inexpensive unit encased in plastic. It does not leak and remains sterile.

Dr. O'Neill: We change filters every day but do not know whether it is necessary. Every four days may be perfectly adequate.

Dr. Shils: The filter gets changed every fourth day, but the administration set above the filter is changed twice daily.

Dr. O'Neill: Is there anyone who feels that a filter is not necessary for use in either adults or children?

Dr. Broviac: I do not think it is necessary. We do not use a filter and have not found a high complication rate with our patients.

Dr. O'Neill: Each day, when we change our 0.22μ filter, we send a piece of the diaphragm for culture. Even with this type of surveillance, we obtain positive cultures at times. If we are obtaining positive cultures, presuming we are being reasonably careful, what is happening to those organisms that are not going through a filter at your institution?

Mr. Stone: The need for a filter may be related to the method of preparing the solution. If, in preparation, a solution is filtered through a 0.22μ membrane filter to begin with—a standard means of sterilizing—and bottled under proper conditions, a filter should not be needed.

Dr. Ruberg: The preference for filters in pediatric patients is because the pediatric patient is usually being infused by a pump, and this is an additional protection against air embolus. This is why we use filters in pediatric patients and not in adults.

Dr. O'Neill: To determine the need for filters, hard data on infection rates should be accumulated, with comparative series in both adult and pediatric age groups.

PHARMACY PROCEDURES

Mr. O'Neal: Our pharmacy procedures involve three basic formulas of what we call TPA (Total Parenteral Alimentation) solutions. In the pediatric formula, we use 200 gm of 50% invert sugar and roughly 4 gm of nitrogen from a pure acid solution. In this pediatric formula, we also add electrolytes and vitamins in the pharmacy at the time of compounding the formulation. We standardize these solutions whenever possible. Standardization is imperative from the pharmacy standpoint so that wastage is minimized. However, our physicians may alter the solutions depending upon the patient's electrolyte requirements. We also try to standardize our adult TPA solution, in which we use pure amino acids as a source of nitrogen in the same 4-gm nitrogen concentration. The caloric value is approximately 900 kcal/liter. The pharmacy also adds basic electrolytes that are standard in our hospital. These are 25 mEq of sodium, 40 mEq of potassium, 10 mEq of magnesium; chloride and acetate may vary somewhat. Vitamins are added also.

Our basic formulation technique involves the use of previously sterilized solutions mixed under a laminar air-flow hood through Millipore filtration equipment. We feel that this cleans the solutions of particulate matter at the time that it sterilizes it.

Depending on our patient load, we make a week's supply of these solutions and store them in the refrigerator. We usually take a 5% random sampling at the beginning, in the middle, and at the end of the procedure and do sterility and pyrogen tests. The solutions are quarantined for seven days until our laboratory releases them as being sterile and pyrogen-free.

We have been preparing these solutions successfully for approximately two years and continually monitor their sterility and pyrogenicity. We have no standard method of formulating solutions, and controls vary depending upon the institution. His knowledge of the instability of various admixtures in solution enables the pharmacist to be of assistance to the clinician who requests additions to the bottle.

Dr. Garrett: What is a standard formula? Some use glucose; others use invert sugar. There are others who think that sorbitol and xylitol have a place (see p 190). Even if we could arrive at a standard formula, we would still have to watch for incompatibilities, stability, contamination, and so on. Packaging, shelf life, and stability in shipping would be problems.

Mr. Grant: Even minor changes in formulations involve a two and one-half year lag in the testing required for FDA approval. This is why total formulations have been left to hospital pharmacies.

Mr. O'Neal mentioned that these components are all sterile when he starts to admix them in his sterile system. Do you have some control data to show what comes out after you sterilize it?

Mr. O'Neal: No, we do not do any tests as far as amino acids are concerned. We receive these as an 8% base mixture of essential and nonessential amino acids from the manufacturer.

Dr. McGill: Does anyone have evidence to show that one sugar is better than another, or better than glucose in these formulations? (See p 186.) Why, for example, use invert sugar for pediatric formulations and glucose for adults?

Dr. O'Neill: Evidence indicates that invert sugar is more easily utilized by an immature liver than glucose. This is not necessarily true in the average pediatric patient. It is much more of a consideration in the neonatal group than it is in the older child.

Dr. Garrett: Is it not true that there are more reactions in pediatrics to invert sugar than to glucose? I was surprised that Mr. O'Neal's pediatric formula is invert sugar. I have found that with a solution of invert sugar higher than 5% children may respond with rashes, discomfort, and temperature elevation.

Dr. O'Neill: I have been involved with the use of 10% fructose or invert sugar solutions for at least the past six years. Such reactions, although they do occur, are exceedingly rare. Even with the so-called hyperalimentation solutions, which have a maximum of 10% fructose, reactions of the sort you describe are essentially nonexistent.

Dr. O'Neill: A question that remains unanswered is storage. Should these solutions be made up every 8 hours, every 24 hours, or every two weeks? The only data available about long-term storage (up to a week or two) are the data presented from Vanderbilt.

Mr. O'Neal: Our amino acid mixture remains clear for about two months. We would not want to use a solution stored that long, but, from a physical standpoint, no discoloration occurred in that interval.

Dr. McGill: What does discoloration imply?

Mr. Grant: Probably browning of the sugar. In combination with the amino acids, this apparently is accelerated. It seems to be a factor of concentration. For many years, products in which 5% glucose was combined with 5% casein or fibrin hydrolysate were on the market. These were stable up to two years; but they did not have the other added electrolytes, vitamins, and so forth. We need more data on this point.

Among publications providing information relating to solution and admixture stability, pharmacy manufacturing programs, and other subjects pertinent to our discussion are the *Journal of the American Society of Hospital Pharmacists, Clinical Pharmacy, Drug Intelligence and Clinical Pharmacy,* and *Hospital Pharmacy.* Physicians should become familiar with this information since it is hard to come by otherwise.

RESPONSIBILITIES FOR SAFE DELIVERY

Dr. O'Neill: I would like to consider the broad category of nursing procedures. Is it worthwhile to have a so-called "hyperalimentation team" to standardize protocols? Or, on the other hand, should we all be free agents, whether we are dealing with a university hospital or a private institution? We have pediatricians, internists, surgeons, dermatologists, traumatologists, everyone you can think of, utilizing this method (see p 390). Who should be responsible?

Dr. Hoshal: I work in a community hospital of 550 beds, and there is interest in hyperalimentation among a number of the private staff members, primarily general surgeons. The weight of responsibility falls on the resident staff. As we entered this field we felt the need for some kind of unification.

To accomplish this we developed—through the aid of our pharmacy—what we hoped would be a standard solution with a few necessary variables such as electrolytes. The pharmacy was being besieged by a variety of different orders. The resident staff was unsure how to write orders, and the nurses asked for instruction in the problems involved in administration of the solutions.

We printed a pocket-sized card, on which we gave the constituents of the standard solution, how it meets basic requirements, and the principles and precautions to be followed in administration. The card has been distributed to attending and resident staff physicians and to the nursing staff. Revisions are made periodically. It has been a great help in standardization.

Dr. Kark: What are the data on the rate of infection at St. Joseph's Hospital in Ann Arbor, as opposed to any other hospital nearby with the same kind of people who have a team? If we believe that one has to have meticulous care of the site of injection and everything else, I personally cannot see that, in a big hospital where you have 1,000 beds and a large staff turning over, every individual is going to be careful. In fact, I know that is not so. I wonder if somebody would speak from the team point of view.

Dr. O'Neill: Good comment. I am sure there are no data available, but it makes sense, just as it does in the care of patients with burns. In general, these

434

patients are localized in one area; a few well-trained people can do a better job than if the patients are scattered throughout the hospital.

Dr. McGill: Do you have opportunity for quality control?

Dr. Hoshal: Quality control is supplied through interaction of the hospital pharmacy, the Infectious Disease Committee, an epidemiologist, and myself. We need an IV team which could take the responsibility for catheter care.

Dr. McGill: The new standards for hospital accreditation provide that hospitals will have to identify clearly what their staffs can and cannot do. Some internists may not be allowed to perform this procedure. In response to Dr. Kark's comments, I would think that physicians who have not demonstrated special interest and competence should be prohibited from doing it; perhaps everyone should be prohibited from doing it except those who are part of a group with proved competence and training.

Dr. O'Neill: We all differ depending upon training, background, and practice environment. Emphasis should be placed on evaluation of the individuals who are training these people to go out and utilize the methodology rather than on controlling who should do it and who should not. It may be a function of the hospital executive committee to see who is not using it properly.

Dr. Kark: Do you think this should be done in any community hospital as an occasional procedure? We are approaching a real danger.

Dr. O'Neill: Three or four years ago, the answer would have been that total parenteral nutrition was a research technique, and it should only be utilized in closely controlled research situations. Because of its value, it has been taken out of the research category and applied on a worldwide basis. Its application is ahead of its technical development. It is not possible to say that this cannot be done in a 50-bed hospital in the hills of Tennessee today, because we are training individuals at Vanderbilt who are going to do it there. There may later be hospital controls, but there are none now, and there are essentially no physician controls. We must train these people as well as we can at the moment.

Dr. Kark: I wonder if the patient in the 50-bed hospital in eastern Tennessee who needs this procedure would not be better off if he transferred to Vanderbilt Hospital?

Dr. O'Neill: I think he would, but my opinion has very little to do with it. It is the matter of imposition of controls. Where should patients have cobalt therapy? Where should patients have open heart surgery? Where should patients have neonatal surgery? Where should patients receive hyperosmolar alimentation?

These are questions which will be answered eventually; certainly, they should be recorded in the proceedings of this symposium.

How about records? This also has to do with surveillance—where somebody keeps records on bacteriological control, on the patient's intake and output, weight, and the like? This is also a way to establish standards.

Among other questions: how long is a bottle of solution considered safe after it is opened? Our limit at Vanderbilt is 12 hours.

Dr. Hoshal: Twelve hours is also our limit, once the bottle has been started in an infusion.

Dr. Garrett: Did we not hear that *Candida* can develop a growth pattern within 12 hours, and other bacteria may require about 24 hours? To me, this 12-hour time limit could be lifesaving.

Dr. O'Neill: Our decision was based on this fact. Eight hours might be a more reasonable limit, and it might be more convenient. Nurses change shifts every eight hours, and intake and output records are available every eight hours.

How long do you leave administration sets, filters, and tubing hanging? Our limit is 24 hours.

Dr. Hoshal: We concur that 24 hours is the limit, and we change everything down to the catheter hub daily.

Dr. Sandstead: Additions to the system (eg, central venous pressure manometers) should be designed as closed systems. They should be used only as long as necessary since they are sources of contamination.

Dr. O'Neill: We have heard some differences of opinion about whether filters should be used. Our group changes filters every day and occasionally finds positive cultures. Others do it every four days. Occasionally I will find organisms on the bottle side of the filter after 24 hours, hence I am concerned about leaving it longer than 24 hours.

Dr. McGill: Where do the bugs come from on the bottle side?

Dr. O'Neill: We have not been able to track it down, because the bottle is often empty at the time we change our filter. Presumably, the organisms come from the solutions or administration sets.

How do you feel about drawing blood through the catheters? We avoid any blood drawing from catheters because of the problems of infection and clotting. Furthermore, we have preferred not to give blood or blood products through these catheters, except occasionally in small neonates.

Dr. Hoshal: The procedure should be condemned. Drawing blood through the catheter involves too many possible sources of infection.

Dr. O'Neill: Just before removal of the catheter, it appears to be appropriate to draw a blood culture through it. Most people do this.

How about heparin? Does anybody give heparin routinely? We have not.

Dr. Hoshal: Since the inception of subclavian catheters in our hospital, we have routinely added 10 to 15 mg of heparin to each liter of solution. This was based on a comparative study we did with and without heparin which suggested that fewer clots occurred in catheters when heparin was utilized.

Dr. O'Neill: How many people use insulin routinely in infusions? We have tended not to.

Dr. Hoshal: We use insulin if a patient persistently spills a 4+ urine, and we add the insulin to the bottle. We do not use it prophylactically.

Dr. Kark: We add it to the bottle when necessary.

Dr. Sandstead: Insulin should not be added to the bottle but should be given subcutaneously on a sliding scale if the patient requires it. Each patient is quite different in his response, so one cannot predict how much is required. Most patients, if not diabetic, will wean themselves off insulin within a day or so and then do not require any more insulin.

Dr. O'Neill: Another way to handle the insulin question is to begin a patient on 10% sugar and gradually increase the concentration to 20% over a few days. This is routine in pediatric patients.

Dr. McGill: We have discussed when to initiate parenteral alimentation, but when do we stop? What are the criteria?

Dr. O'Neill: General agreement is that, if a patient can eat and utilize his gastrointestinal tract effectively, that is the best route to use. Sometimes only partial use of the patient's own gut is a big help. If his gastrointestinal tract is not utilizable, either partially or totally, the remainder would have to be made up by means of parenteral support. When the patient's gastrointestinal tract can again take over the job is the time to stop parenteral alimentation. Total parenteral nutrition is a relatively dangerous tool to apply, and we do not use it lightly. We must be careful in the evaluation of patients who may need parenteral nutrition and steer clear of it if a patient can reasonably get by without it. Remember that hyperalimentation is a temporary expedient. The biggest problem is that physicians wait too long to put patients on intravenous hyperalimentation, rather than the opposite.

Digest of Colloquium

Our discussion of delivery had the dual purpose of summarizing currently utilized methods, materials, and techniques for the administration of various types of nutritional solutions and reaching a consensus regarding the best available delivery systems and components.

ADMINISTRATION SITES

Peripheral venous sites may be used for the administration of fat solutions combined with amino acids and 10% glucose. Central venous catheterization is required for the administration of hyperosmolar solutions. Sites discussed include the jugular system, anterior cervical, cephalic, and subclavian systems. Either the subclavicular or supraclavicular approach to the subclavin vein is applicable to most adults.

Percutaneous methods of placement in the subclavin venous system are desirable in the adult, but these methods are probably not applicable in patients below the age of four years because of lack of safety. In young patients, cutdown placement is necessary. When inserted via a cutdown, catheters should be brought out a separate stab wound distant from the incision site itself in order to decrease the potential of infection. Catheters should be firmly sutured so that movement is minimized. X-ray confirmation of catheter position prior to utilization for parenteral alimentation is essential.

Complications include extravasation of solutions into the thorax and mediastinum, pneumothorax, venous thrombosis and embolism, perforation of the vein, thoracic duct leaks, right atrial perforation, arrhythmias due to intracardiac shunts, catheter embolization, and the almost routine formation of fibrin sheaths around catheters which have the capability of either embolizing or serving as sources for bacterial or fungal growth. Appropriate training of personnel is vital in order to minimize these problems which are related, at least in part, to misapplication of methodology.

CATHETERS

Various types of catheters include polyethylene, polyvinyl chloride, Portex, Teflon, and Silastic. It was agreed that Silastic (preferably with barium impregnation) is an ideal material, although Teflon and polyethylene are used widely. Silastic is extremely pliable with less tendency to perforate the heart or venous structures. It may also have a lessened tendency to initiate thrombosis.

Fibrin sheaths may form around the catheter with all types of materials, although a little less often with Silastic. These fibrin sheaths may be fixed to the vein wall or, disturbingly, often float free in the vein with the potential of either partial or total embolization. Observations in a few patients indicated that the amount of fibrinous sheathing was less when heparin bonding was utilized. But no animal data—essential on this point—were available.

Silastic tubing is not routinely supplied with appropriate adapter heads for intravenous tubing. Also, barium impregnation of silastic tubing to make it radiopaque is expensive. It is not known at present just what the plasticizer release or other physiocochemical problems might be with Silastic, but presumably the risk would be low or nonexistent.

One technique, developed from extensive experience with the utilization of fat solutions in Scandinavia, included simultaneous infusion of an admixture of glucose and amino acids with Intralipid through a Y-tube situated close to the hub of a small needle appropriate for insertion into peripheral veins. The distinct advantage of this technique is that it avoids the necessity for any form of central venous catheterization with its attendant complications.

The system offers a further advantage, the ability to infuse over a period of 5 to 6 hours during the day, leaving the patient at least 12 hours free and unencumbered. Problems with the stability of fat particles have not been encountered with this type of dual infusion which also affords, apparently, a decreased incidence of thrombophlebitis when fat solutions are utilized.

In considering whether blood should be drawn or administered through the catheter, the consensus was that blood should not be drawn through the catheter except for culture at the time of catheter removal. Blood and blood products should not be administered through the catheter unless necessary, as in the neonate.

Although it was agreed that heparin should not be used routinely, results of one comparative study suggested that fewer clots occurred in catheters when heparin was utilized. Heparin bonding might be useful in the future.

Should insulin be used routinely in infusions to control hyperglycemia or for the possible advantage of improving amino acid utilization? Insulin is not used routinely at present except to control episodic hyperglycemia.

SHUNTS

Participants described experiences with external shunting devices of the Thomas high- and low-flow varieties and of the Scribner variety. Many problems are associated with use of the high-flow shunt. External shunts should be reserved for those patients who either have no readily available central veins or who require long-term administration of hyperalimentation solutions. Internal shunts may be useful and are probably the safest for the long-term patient from the standpoint of avoiding infection; but it takes about two months for an internal shunt to be established, and thrombosis can be a problem, especially when the shunt is constructed late in the patient's hospital course. The consensus was that in adult patients percutaneous catheterization of the subclavin vein is one of the most useful routes for fluid administration. When veins are not sufficiently available, shunts are an additional expedient which may be beneficial in selected instances.

PUMPS

In a comparative review of the various types of administration pumps, these facts were highlighted:

Constant infusion by pump may help to reduce incidence of thrombosis.

The Ivac system is one of the most reliable with respect to long-term use and one of the safest with respect to avoidance of air embolism because of the photoelectric drop control mechanism.

The Holter system can be run on battery power and is small enough to be portable, both of which are desirable qualities.

The counterbalance system is a control mechanism which prevents air embolism and also avoids the termination of infusions too rapidly, which might expose the patient to the potential danger of reactive hypoglycemia. With this method, the weight of the bottle of infusate provides feedback to warn when the solution is falling to a critical level.

Despite the concern about air embolism with pump utilization, the majority of instances of air embolism associated with pumps have come from disconnection of administration tubing allowing the passive passage of air into the system.

We need an inexpensive pump which is reliable and which uses a closed system, preferably of the peristaltic type, which would allow accurate, constant administration of fluids without the possibility of air embolism.

Further areas for research include improvement of administration control systems and miniaturization of equipment.

FILTERS

If solutions are prepared appropriately in the pharmacy, utilizing filters in formulation, it may not be necessary to use them during the time of administration. Use of filters in infants and children is desirable because of frequent alterations in the composition of solutions and the consequent hazard of infection.

If filters are monitored daily, bacterial and fungal organisms can often be found on the infusion side of the filter. The relationship of this to sepsis is not clear.

Millipore filters of the 0.22μ or 0.45μ size will effectively prevent air embolism. This is a distinct advantage in the pediatric age group where anatomic or physiologic shunts may allow the passage of even small bubbles of air into the coronary or intracranial vascular systems. The 0.45μ filter will remove paticulate material and bacteria, except for *Pseudomonas*. The 0.22μ filter will remove essentially all bacterial and fungal organisms in addition to particulate matter, and this would appear to pose a distinct advantage. The 0.22μ filter requires the use of an infusion pump.

PHARMACY PROCEDURES

A detailed description of how solutions are prepared in the Vanderbilt University Medical Center pharmacy was given. Presterilized solutions of distilled water, amino acids, glucose, electrolytes, and vitamins are mixed and passed through a vacuum-controlled Millipore filter. Appropriate surveillance is carried out for bacteriologic control and for identification of pyrogens.

The solutions are then quarantined for a period of seven days, and utilized after storage at 4°C for periods of up to two weeks, the average being one week. This is in contradistinction to standard practice in many other centers, where solutions are used within a one- or two-day period because of apparent bacteriologic overgrowth.

In another method of formulation, amino acids and glucose are mixed adding electrolytes, vitamins, and other constituents later. Other pharmacies use other techniques. Which is the best method? There is no information at the present time. All agree that solutions should be prepared and mixed under a laminar air-flow hood.

Each hospital should have a group primarily responsible for the education of those who apply parenteral feeding. Virtually every medical specialist will apply this method at some time or other, and he should be educated.

Others feel that parenteral feeding should be administered only by a certified group of experts.

No standard records are being kept in hospitals. There have been relatively few guidelines as to what needs to be monitored, and how often this should be done.

AREAS FOR STUDY

The most impressive need at present is thorough clinical evaluation of techniques based on firmly controlled background data. Until all of these data are brought in and compared, it will not be possible to achieve true standardization of procedures and techniques.

Local tolerance to thrombophlebitis is an important consideration. We tend to forget that hyperosmolarity is not the only factor.

The improved local tolerance of combined infusion of Intralipid and protein hydrolysates was related to the fact that use of Swedish Aminosol is followed with approximately an 80% incidence of venous irritation; when the solution is diluted venous tolerance improves automatically.

The pH, the buffer capacity, and the presence or absence of irritating impurities in these solutions are to be considered. In the protein hydrolysates, we know that the pH is around 5.2; we know they contain decomposition products which are poorly defined, and that these may have irritant properties. Some carbohydrates are more irritating than the corresponding sugar alcohols. Also, when glucose is sterilized, caramelization with formation of acidic material occurs. These acidic materials are potential irritants. Tolerance may be improved by purity in composition.

PART FOUR

16 FDA Regulatory Practices and Philosophy
Leon J. DeMerre, Ph.D.

FDA REGULATORY
PRACTICES AND
PHILOSOPHY

Chapter 16

FDA Regulatory Practices and Philosophy

Leon J. DeMerre, Ph.D.†

Total parenteral nutrition is governed by the Code of Federal Regulations. The Food and Drug Administration approves the marketing of parenteral nutrition drugs after intensive review of the manufacturing processes, the source and composition of materials used for the drug containers, animal, stability, and clinical studies. These stringent requirements help maintain adequate consumer protection.

Regulatory practices governing the manufacture, quality control, labeling, and marketing of solutions used in total parenteral nutrition are those that must be adhered to for all drugs approved by the Food and Drug Administration (FDA). Exhaustive precautions are taken for production of such materials.

FOOD AND DRUG ADMINISTRATION: FUNCTIONS

Enumeration of salient points related to establishment of the Food and Drug Administration as a bona fide regulatory body provides a key to its functions:

• In 1848 Congress passed the Import Drugs Act to prevent the importation of adulterated drugs. This was the first federal statute to insure the quality of drugs. It was passed when quinine used by American troops in Mexico to treat malaria was found to be adulterated. By this act of Congress, the federal government entered the drug field.

• In 1902, the Public Health Service (PHS) Act was passed regulating biologics and trivalent arsenicals, currently controlled by the Division of Biologics Standards (DBS), National Institutes of Health (NIH).

• In 1906, the original Pure Food and Drug Act passed Congress and was signed by President Theodore Roosevelt. In this happening the *regulatory* functions of the Food and Drug Administration originated. The act regulated interstate commerce in misbranded and adulterated foods, drinks, and drugs only in terms of "purity" of these products.

• A major step was taken when the Federal Food, Drug, and Cosmetic Act of 1938 was enacted. This followed the "sulfonilamide incident" in which more than 100 patients died because the drug was dissolved in a poisonous solvent and marketed without proper toxicity testing. The 1938 law required the manufacturer of a new drug to test it for safety before marketing it.

†Dr. DeMerre died March 21, 1974.

• The Kefauver-Harris Amendments of 1962 were an additional major step aimed at consumer protection. Influenced by the discovery that thalidomide, a mild sedative, when given to pregnant women caused limb defects in the fetus in a number of cases, these amendments were passed to assure a greater degree of safety and to strengthen new drug clearance procedures. For the first time, drug manufacturers were required to prove to the FDA the effectiveness of their products before marketing them.

The current National Formulary (NF) contains 91 monographs and the United States Pharmacopaeia (USP) 165 monographs in the category of "Injections," an indication of the importance of this therapeutic type of administration.

REQUIREMENTS AND CLEARANCE PROCEDURES

Manufacturers of large-volume parenterals and nutrient replenisher solutions must meet specific requirements and clearance procedures. Narrowing to essentials, we will consider protein hydrolysates and amino acid mixtures for parenteral administration. It is recognized, however, that various additives are commonly administered with these parenteral nutrient solutions (eg, B-complex vitamins are frequently added to postoperative infusions). Injectable amino acid mixtures may be used in combination with the easily metabolized energy ingredient dextrose. When plastic containers are used, the FDA requires a warning that additives may not be compatible with the solution, the container, and/or the administration set.

Prior to marketing a *nutrient replenisher solution,* the manufacturer must be in compliance with a number of requirements. Once again, protein hydrolysates and amino acids will be taken as paradigms for their acceptance as raw materials. Although "Protein Hydrolysate Injection" is listed in the USP, the FDA cannot accept a mere commitment that the raw product used complies with the compendial requirements; the reason is that a pure chemical entity is not obtained. The only major requirement in the USP concerning the composition of this injection is that no less than 50% of the total nitrogen present be in the form of gamma-amino nitrogen. Because of the widely different nature of the proteins from which the amino acids and peptides are derived—differences in polymeric chain length, cross linkages, amino acid components and their sequence in the chain—identification of the source of the raw material must include:

The nature of the raw material from which the hydrolysate is derived (eg, casein, yeast, soy proteins);

The type of hydrolysis to which the raw proteinaceous material has been subjected to reach the peptide and amino acid states (acid and enzymatic methods are the most common);

Assurance that the USP monograph requirements are fulfilled.

PREPARATION OF AMINO ACIDS

Methods of preparation of amino acids are typical for the analysis and justification of our requests. We shall take them as concrete examples. Three methods can be, and are, utilized for their preparation. Used on a selective basis, they are: separation from protein hydrolysates, bacterial fermentation, and organic synthesis.

A review of these modes of production may show the intricacies involved in obtaining the new drug substances. Some amino acids are obtained more easily by one method than by another. This does not preclude some overlapping, however.

Separation From Protein Hydrolysates

The following amino acids are generally obtained by separation from soybean protein hydrolysates.

L-leucine
L-phenylalanine
L-arginine
L-histidine
L-serine

The method—which must be submitted in detail by the manufacturer to the Bureau of Drugs—consists of drying and dehulling the beans, extracting the oil in an organic solvent (n-hexane is preferred), hydrolyzing the defatted proteins with hydrochloric acid under pressure, separating the amino acids under well-defined conditions by means of ion-exchange resins, and elution at the required pH. The last step is followed by as many recrystallizations as are necessary to obtain pure compounds.

The description of this method may not be submitted by the manufacturer in a theoretical manner. The type, size, and nature of the equipment used must be stated. Recommendations are that the yields of the in-step pivotal compounds be given as well as the yield of the finished pure product. Now, a word of justification for these requests: Impurities may be entrained from the metal of the vessels or, as may be the case, from their plastic linings, where the hydrolysis and purification are performed. The reagents used in the process and their specifications must be known in order that impurities, if present, can be traced to their source. Also, yields are of great importance. Low yields indicate, in general, an incomplete reaction entailing the necessity for total elimination of by-products.

Bacterial Fermentation

The following amino acids are usually produced by bacterial fermentation:

L-proline
L-leucine (also from hydrolysates)
L-threonine
L-valine
L-alanine

In this case the essential requirements comprise the exact composition of the fermenting broths, the origin of the stock cultures, and taxonomy of the organisms (genus, family, complete determinative identity).

For example, L-valine is obtained by the action of *Brevibacterium lactofermentum* under certain conditions of temperature and pH when grown in a medium which is essentially a beef extract broth with adequate salinity. The cultures must be pure. During the fermentation process, repeated checks must be made to show that mutations have not occurred. The purification process is of the greatest importance since most bacteria will produce pyrogenic substances which must be totally eliminated.

Organic Synthesis

The preferred path for the preparation of some amino acids is a true organic synthesis. The following amino acids belong to this category:

DL-methionine
L-tryptophan
glycine (aminoacetic acid)
alanine

The most commonly used technique is the Strecker reaction or cyanohydrin synthesis, schematized for alanine, as follows:

$$CH_3CHO \xrightarrow{NH_3, HCN} CH_3CHNH_2 \xrightarrow{2H_2O} CH_3CHNH_2$$

acetaldehyde　　　　　aminonitrile (—CN)　　　alanine (—COOH)

Note that hydrogen cyanide has a major role in this synthesis. Consequently, amino acids obtained by this route must be carefully tested for the possible presence of cyanide residue.

ACCEPTANCE SPECIFICATIONS

The following rules are applied to the delivery and acceptance specifications which regulate raw materials. Raw materials which will be a part of the finished drug, either as such or in combination, or that will be intermediates for the finished preparation, are the object of strict controls. These comprise a list of specifications provided by the supplier or suppliers of the ingredients. Each batch, upon delivery, must be accompanied by a certificate indicating that the tests substantiating the specifications have been performed.

The acceptance tests for raw materials made by the manufacturer of the finished drug may be either a repeat of all parameters stated in the specifications or may be limited in some cases to the more sensitive assays in the series. These are proposed by the manufacturer and will be judged adequate or inadequate by the FDA chemistry specialist. It should be added that no *ex cathedra* decisions are ever made in this regard but that a conclusion is reached on a rational basis, usually after agreement between FDA and the applicant.

For compounds which are not official compendial items, the firms are requested to verify the degree of purity of their products by a series of tests which will guarantee their integrity beyond any doubt.

For USP or NF compounds which are supplied as such and for which a certificate is provided attesting to their conformance with the compendial monographs, a repeat of all parameters listed is generally not required. But aminoacetic acid (glycine) and methionine are two amino acids which appear in the National Formulary (NF XIII); in these cases—although there is actually no written rule—the reviewing chemist usually will be satisfied with the identification assays for acceptance.

Drug master file If the manufacturer of the finished drug (eg, a mixture of amino acids) is not the maker of the individual amino acids, a complete description of the methods used for their preparation is requested from the suppliers. If the supplier chooses to furnish the detailed information to his customer, this will be included in the application. However—and this is more often the case—the supplier feels that his trade secrets should not be divulged to his client. In that instance, he may submit every detail of the preparation, whether it be an extraction or a synthesis, to the Food and Drug Administration. This is done in the form of a Drug Master File, with authorization given to the FDA to consult it on behalf of the application. The information should be given in terms of a typical batch and must include all steps of the preparation, the controls effected at each step, and the purification process. The equipment and its nature must be provided: The types of vessels used (stainless steel, plastic-coated interior), the type and nature of the stirrers, the type and nature of the tubing, and all other details concerning the production of a batch.

The information thus submitted is confidential and is protected in the Code of Federal Regulations, paragraph 130.32. More precisely, and I quote: "(b) Section 301 (j) of the Act makes it an offense to divulge to unauthorized persons any information acquired from a new drug application concerning any method or process that is a trade secret." This statement applies equally to New Drug Applications (NDA) and Drug Master Files.

Submission of a Drug Master File by a supplier is a commitment that all phases of the manufacturing process therein described are being followed to the letter. In this regard, FDA has additional regulatory power, as the Agency may, and usually does, request a plant inspection. The federal inspector follows all the steps of the preparation or preparations under consideration and reports to the reviewing FDA division the status of the manufacturing processes. Deviations from good manufacturing practices, if any, are reported.

Rather frequently raw materials are manufactured abroad, and this is the case for amino acids. The foreign manufacturer must, in addition to the submission of a Drug Master File, agree to have his plant inspected. The formulation of the dosage form (ie, the finished product and its manufacturing) are the object of a thorough FDA scrutiny.

Taking again as an example the concrete case of a nutrient parenteral solution of amino acids, the following requirements must be met:

All components must be listed, and assurance must be given that the amino acids have been subjected to all required acceptance tests.

The composition is then stated; it may be given in terms of percent, in terms of quantities per dosage form unit, but it is

448

particularly helpful when a submission of the quantities used is given for a typical batch.

Not only must the various amino acids meet all specifications, but the solution must be prepared with pretested "Water for Injection, USP."

The facilities and the qualifications of the personnel responsible for directing the manufacture and control of the drug should be adequately described with areas of activity clearly depicted: general processing area, aseptic filling area, inspection area, storage area. The description of the manufacturing and processing, including details of the aseptic filling operations, must be given in detail. The preparatory procedures employed for the packaging components must be provided. Should ethylene oxide sterilization be employed, adequate evidence must be given for the complete removal of any residual gas from the packaging components.

The laboratory controls call for acceptance specifications and testing methods employed to assure that the pharmaceutical dosage form has the identity, strength, quality, and safety required.

Analytical methods used for the finished product must be described in detail. In the case of amino acid solutions, automatic analyzers have now been constructed that will give with great accuracy the quantitative composition of the finished product. However, a knowledge of the composition is not sufficient. A number of tests must be made prior to the release of a parenteral solution. Among them are absorption curves for the active ingredients. These will detect impurities. Other tests are required for color, clarity, presence of particulate matter, pH, sterility, and pyrogenicity.

The following rule is generally adopted with regard to methods: If a method is in use for the compound to be analyzed, and this method may be found in an official compendium, it is deemed acceptable, provided no demonstrated interference exists because of other ingredients (eg, dextrose in the presence of amino acids). Methods not officially accepted must be validated. The procedure is as follows:

Samples of the finished drug, as well as other samples required by NDA Form 356-H, must be forwarded to the Bureau of Drugs.

The samples must be accompanied by an analysis of their particular batch number.

The methods are then forwarded along with the samples to the FDA laboratories to determine their suitability to serve as FDA regulatory methods.

Stability studies are directly linked to the laboratory controls and are the determining factor in the establishment of an expiration date. Stability studies for any drug must be performed in the container and/or package that will be marketed.

Traditionally, large volume parenterals have been packaged in glass bottles fitted with an ampule-type rubber stopper and a breather-tube to permit displacement of the solution with air as it flows out of the inverted bottle. This package is sold in conjunction with an administration set basically consisting of a length of rubber or plastic tubing with needle adapters at each end. The applicant must show evidence that the container is Type I or Type II glass and meets the USP requirements for resistance to interaction with the solution and that the tubing has been tested for leachables. (This requirement will be discussed further.)

Development of plastic bags for use with parenteral solutions has provided the consumer with a container having a great many advantages, such as reduction in weight, reduction in breakage, elimination of the breather-tube, more compact storage.

It has, however, presented the manufacturer, and of course the regulatory agency, with a series of new problems.

The most widely used plastic bag is fabricated from sheets of plastic film made from polyvinyl chloride (PVC) resin. To achieve the desirable characteristics of this film (soft, pliable, heat-resistant), it is compounded with the addition of various plasticizers, stabilizers, antioxidants, and coloring compounds. Unfortunately, many of these additives are leached from the film in contact with the solution with which they are packaged. The USP has designed a series of test solutions (sodium chloride, sodium chloride in alcohol, polyethylene glycol 400, vegetable oil).

The solutions after extraction are injected into test animals and checked for toxic reactions. Frequently it is requested that an additional test solution be used, the actual drug solution which will be packaged with the film. Physicochemical tests on the container are also required, such as transparency, flexibility, tensile strength, thermal stability, elasticity, nonvolatile residues, heavy metals. Another unfortunate characteristic of the PVC film is its ability to "breathe." Vapor transmission through the film must therefore be determined. The amount of solution lost by this "breathing" action can be an important factor over a period of months in storage, resulting in a concentration of the solution in the bag and providing a potential pathway for microbial contamination.

Most manufacturers have solved this problem by packing the bags in individual high-density polyethylene envelopes or multiple bag packing in metal cans. The administration sets are still of the same basic design, except that they are now prepared from plastic tubing. The sets are generally packed separately and are gas-sterilized.

As mentioned earlier, the shelf-life testing must be performed on the drug in its finished form. In this regard, adequate information should be supplied with respect to the characteristics and age-testing of the proposed container, closure or other component parts of the drug package with the intended formulation to ascertain their compatibility and suitability. Long-term data are required. Short-term and accelerated aging results are good supporting evidence, but cannot be substituted for long-term aging under normal storage conditions. In designing stability studies, some of the factors which must be investigated and evaluated should include but are not limited to: quantitation of active ingredients, temperature, volume of contents, pH, possible oxidation, integrity of preservatives if applicable, trace metals, compatibility of container and contents, preservation of sterility, resistance to light, discoloration, particulate matter.

The compatibility of container and contents is of the utmost importance where large volume parenterals are concerned. Interest has increased in this particular factor because of the growing use of plastics for the packaging of drugs of this type. Stability testing in the case of nutrition parenterals housed in plastic containers is particularly exhaustive. In addition to the series of tests mentioned above, assays must show that, over the storage period corresponding to the expiration time, leachables from the container into the solution have remained stationary. This is the reason the exact composition of the plastic and the history of its fabrication must be known in detail at the Bureau of Drugs level.

SAFETY AND EFFICACY STUDIES

The safety and efficacy of parenteral nutrients must be adequately demonstrated. This is done, first of all, by suitable acute, subacute, and chronic toxicity studies in one or more species of animals. However, in the case of a common essential nutrient like glucose, safety and efficacy would be acceptable on a historical basis. For more complex nutrients, like fat emulsions, protein hydrolysates and amino acid mixtures, detailed testing is required. In particular, the toxicity studies should rule out such adverse effects as teratogenicity and ophthalmic pathology in animals. This does not, of course, preclude such effects in humans, but it does provide a basis for proceeding to clinical trials. Efficacy is a somewhat controversial matter with the more complex nutrients. In animals, efficacy may be studied by serial determination of body weight, nitrogen balance determinations, and observation of the general state of the animal during prolonged periods of infusion. Various human clinical states of malnutrition may be simulated, with or without surgery.

Clinical trials On the basis of acceptable toxicity studies on animals and evidence of efficacy, clinical trials may then be undertaken. These are divided into progressive phases.

Phase 1 studies involve infusion of the nutrient into human volunteers. In this phase, the main interest consists in confirming the safety of the product (eg, ophthalmic pathology should be ruled out). Detailed pharmacologic studies are also indicated in this phase to establish the metabolism and fate of the nutrient if possible. More detailed blood and urine determinations can be done with normal volunteers than would be possible with actual clinical patients.

If the safety of the particular nutrient is confirmed, clinical trials then proceed to **Phase 2,** which involves testing in a relatively small number of patients. The main interest now is in demonstrating efficacy in the actual clinical situation for which the nutrient is intended. But considerations of safety are always of the utmost importance. Thus, in Phase 2, it would be important to obtain some estimate of the incidence of adverse reactions to be expected in large-scale Phase 3 trials (eg, fat emulsions have been associated with a high incidence of severe febrile reactions).

Phase 3 trials involve large numbers of clinical patients. It is in this phase that the degree of efficacy of the product is firmly established. For parenteral products that are to be used in pediatric patients, specific clinical studies in the pediatric age range are required, preferably in the "retrograde" pattern. The incidence of various adverse reactions is determined in the actual clinical situation. Some clinicians feel that the complex nutrients are of benefit only in severe nutritional deficiency, and that the ordinary surgical or medical patient has no need for this therapy.

LABELING REQUIREMENTS

Since nutrition parenterals are prescription drugs, they are subject to the general requirements for such drugs.

The label on the primary container—the primary label—must bear:

The proper name of the product which is the common or usual name. (A trade name may be used but it must be defined.)

The volume of the contents of a unit and the potency of the drug. (In the case of nutrition parenterals, the label must express the quantity of each therapeutically active ingredient.)

The dose and route of administration recommended, or reference to such directions in an enclosed circular.

The legend: "CAUTION: Federal law prohibits dispensing without prescription."

Name and address of the manufacturer or distributor.

Lot number.

Expiration date.

The package insert which is part of the labeling must be in conformance with the following format and order:

1. Description
2. Actions
3. Indications
4. Contraindications
5. Warnings
6. Precautions
7. Adverse reactions
8. Dosage and Administration
9. Overdosage (where applicable)
10. How supplied

Animal pharmacology and toxicology, clinical studies, references, if any (limited to a minimum), are optional. If used, they should be placed after the required information.

The essential information to be found in the insert is derived from the clinical studies and experience of the drug house. Advertising material must strictly adhere to the information contained in the package insert.

POSTAPPROVAL OF NDA

After an NDA has fulfilled all of the requirements that were discussed and has been approved for marketing, Federal Regulations require the agency to continue surveillance of the drug by the application of two procedures. This constitutes the postapproval of the New Drug Application.

The Code of Federal Regulations (21 CFR 130.13) provides for the holder of the New Drug Application to establish and maintain records and make reports at regular intervals concerning:

Clinical experience with the drug, either by the applicant, reported to him by persons using the drug, or published in the scientific literature;

Animal experience, studies, investigations or tests conducted by or reported to him;

Experience, investigations, studies, or tests involving the chemical or physical properties of the drug;

Copies of all mailing pieces and other labeling used in promoting the drug;

Information concerning the quantity of the drug distributed so that the Bureau of Drugs can estimate the incidence of adverse effects reported as being associated with the drug;

Information concerning any change from the conditions described in the original application. (This point is further elaborated in Part 130.9, which describes the supplemental application procedure.)

In general, any change in the original application requires the filing and approval of a supplemental application before the change may be made. This includes changes in labeling, addition of claims, revision of manufacturing or control procedures, change in manufacturing facilities, or provision for an outside firm to participate in any phase of the preparation, packaging, or distribution of the drug. There are certain exceptions to this general rule. The following changes may be made without filing a supplemental application if the change is reported to the agency in the next periodic report or within 60 days, whichever comes first:

A different container size for solid oral dosage forms

Change in personnel

Change in equipment that does not alter the method of manufacture

Change in commercial batch size

Change to more stringent specifications

Inclusion of *additional* specifications

Alteration of specifications for inactive ingredients in order to conform to revised compendia

Introduction of a product identification coding system

Addition of an expiration date to the labeling along with stability data in support of the dating

Change from paper labels to direct printing on glass containers

Another exception to the rule requiring prior approval of supplements lists changes which require filing of a supplemental application, but which may be made immediately effective. These are:

Addition to the labeling of additional warnings, contraindications, adverse reactions, and precautions

Deletion from the labeling of false, misleading, or unsupported indications for use of the drug

Changes in the methods of manufacture or control that give increased assurance of identity, strength, quality, and purity of the drug

All other changes require submission of a supplemental application that is documented and well organized. Only those areas in the original application that are the subjects of the change need to be submitted. All parts of the original application that are not mentioned in the supplement remain unchanged by reference. Each New Drug Application must be self-supporting.

APPENDIX A

VITAMIN
PREPARATIONS
FOR PARENTERAL USE

Vitamin Preparations for Parenteral Use

A Statement of the
Nutrition Advisory Group on Total Parenteral Nutrition
Department of Foods and Nutrition
American Medical Association

In the Federal Register (vol 37, No. 241, Thursday, December 14, 1972, p 26626, XI. PARENTERAL MULTIVITAMIN PRODUCTS) parenteral multivitamins are listed which " . . . have been declared 'ineffective' as currently formulated in a FEDERAL REGISTER statement dated February 27, 1972. Because of the critical medical importance of parenteral multivitamins in preventing or treating hypovitaminosis in certain disease states or postoperative conditions, the lack of any alternative drugs for this purpose, and the fact that the only issue involved is the precise formulation that is appropriate for these products, these products should remain on the market until appropriate reformulation can be agreed upon by experts."

The Nutrition Advisory Group on Total Parenteral Nutrition of the Department of Foods and Nutrition of the AMA has adopted the following statement with respect to tentative formulations for parenteral multivitamin preparations. This statement is brought to the attention of the Food and Drug Administration (FDA) for its consideration in deciding upon the adoption of an effective and safe dosage.

1. The Nutrition Advisory Group is in full agreement with the need for reformulation of parenteral multivitamins since it considers present preparations inadequate in their omission of certain essential nutrients, too variable in dosages, unphysiologic, and potentially toxic in content of one or more components and failing to take into account differences between pediatric and adult maintenance and therapeutic requirements.

2. At the same time the Nutrition Advisory Group supports the FDA decision to permit present commercial preparations to remain on the market in order to meet the requirement for parenteral vitamins until more suitable formulations are available.

3. Proposals for specific reformulations which may supplant present preparations are made with the understanding that there are unsolved nutritional problems involved in potential long-term use of the various essential nutrients. These problem areas include:

a) The present state of medical knowledge about the requirements of each of the vitamins is meager when they are given by the intravenous route in conjunction with routine or high caloric intravenous fluids. The lack of information in this area is compounded by differences in requirements for individuals of different ages and with varying disease states.

458

b) The human requirements for certain nutrients will probably vary appreciably as the composition of the overall parenteral nutritional formula varies (eg, thiamin requirements will rise as carbohydrate contributions to total calories increase, whereas tocopherol requirement will probably decrease).

c) Biotin which may not be necessary in the ordinary diet of normal individuals may be essential in the formulation when the intestinal tract is not utilized or where the normal intestinal flora are markedly altered by disease, drug treatment or, bowel resection.

4. New formulations (Table 1) are suggested for consideration with the following precautions and provisos:

a) There shall be two formulations for intravenous multivitamins; one is for children above the age of ten and for adults (designated as "adult" formulation); the other is for infants and children less than ten years of age (designated as "pediatric" formulation).

Table 1.— Working Draft of Suggested Composition for Intravenous Multivitamin Preparation for Daily Maintenance of Adequate Vitamin Status*

| | | Formulations | |
| | | Pediatric (from infancy to 10 years) | Adult (11 years and older) |
Vitamin	Units		
A	I.U.	2,500 †	4,000
D	I.U.	400 †	400
E	I.U.	7 †	15 †
Thiamin	mg	1.2	3.0
Riboflavin	mg	1.4	3.6
Niacin	mg	17	40
B_6	mg	1	4
Pantothenic acid	mg	6	15
Folacin	µg	140	800
Ascorbic acid	mg	100	90
B_{12}	µg	0.7	6
Biotin	µg	20	60

*See paragraphs 6d and 7b concerning volume and physical character.
†In stable water-dispersible form.

b) In the recommended dosages these formulations are for use as a daily maintenance dosage for patients on total parenteral nutrition or for other routine administration where the intravenous route is required.

c) Where there is actual or presumed evidence for *multiple* vitamin deficiency or *markedly increased* requirements, short-term multiple dosage (up to three-fold) may be advisable for two or more days before return to the usual daily dosage.

d) Where actual or presumed evidence for deficiency of a single vitamin occurs, supplementation with the specific vitamin concerned may be necessary in addition to the daily multivitamin dosage. For this purpose there shall be available injectable preparations of each of the vitamins in pure form for clinical use.

e) Because of the possibility of increased excretion of water-soluble vitamins when the multivitamin preparation is given rapidly, it is recommended that instruction be given advising that the daily dosage be administered over a number of hours as part of the intravenous feeding schedule rather than by rapid injection.

5. The formulations are based on the following general propositions:

a) Multivitamin preparations—rather than individual vitamins—should be made available and utilized on a routine basis because there is a need for the broad spectrum of vitamins in meeting demands for new tissue in growing children and in rehabilitating undernourished adults; these are the types of patients requiring prolonged intravenous feeding. Furthermore, single vitamin deficiencies are the exception rather than the rule in the United States.

b) There are few specific or pathognomonic signs of early vitamin deficiency which permit objective decision by the physician for specific vitamin therapy.

c) Use of specific vitamins or an incomplete multivitamin formulation on a repetitive basis required in prolonged parenteral feeding creates a likelihood for accidental prolonged omission of one or more vitamins and development of deficiency. Availability of and provision of a complete formulation will prevent such an occurrence.

d) Few laboratories have the capability of providing rapid, accurate information to physicians with respect to specific vitamin depletion; hence, the physician is often on safer ground by providing a multivitamin preparation. Nevertheless, the use of specific laboratory tests for the assessment of nutritional status is strongly recommended prior to the initiation of long-term parenteral therapy and as an adjunct in monitoring the effectiveness of such therapy.

e) Fat-soluble vitamins are not excreted in the urine as are water-soluble vitamins; they tend to have an appreciably longer half-life than do water-soluble vitamins. For this reason there is more likelihood of overdosage with the fat-soluble vitamins and less chance of acute depletion occurring as compared to water-soluble vitamins. Therefore, relatively smaller amounts of fat-soluble vitamins are given with respect to the Recommended Dietary Allowances (RDA) than are given of the water-soluble vitamins.

f) The RDA provide safety factors in stated amounts of each of the vitamins (ie, they are *not* minimum values but rather amounts designed to maintain the average American in good vitamin nutrition). Furthermore, the amounts given in the RDA provide for oral intakes with some losses related to incomplete digestion and absorption for some of the vitamins. However, absorption from the intestinal tract may often result in more efficient utilization than that obtained with intravenous administrations; when water-soluble vitamins are administered too rapidly intravenously, levels may transiently exceed renal thresholds with resultant increased losses. While more data on such losses in clinical situations are required, it seems prudent to provide amounts of water-soluble vitamins in modest excess of the RDA.

g) Amounts in excess of RDA are also provided for water-soluble vitamins as a safety factor in meeting increased needs secondary to hypermetabolic states, trauma, previous inadequate intake, and the needs of new tissue replacement. Again, there are few hard scientific data to provide accurate guides. Clinical experience and data obtained in trials of these formulations will allow verification or modification of dosage levels for future use. The recommended dosages would seem adequate at this time.

h) The proposed formulations do not provide for ranges of values for each nutrient. A single value for each vitamin in each formulation appears desirable. Tolerances about the proposed figures shall be based on acceptable stability standards.

6. Pediatric formulation

a) The figures in the pediatric intravenous formulation are based on data provided in Table 2. The approximate mean RDA value per kg of body weight for infants up to one year of age has been calculated for each vitamin from the range of RDA values for this age group. These figures have been compared with the RDA range for children 1 to 10 years of age. Table 2 also includes, for comparison, the minimal vitamin levels for infants per 100 kcal of formula (roughly equivalent to 1 kg of body weight) proposed by the American Academy of Pediatrics (AAP) Committee on Nutrition. It will be noted that the mean RDA values are higher than the AAP figures for vitamins D, E, thiamin, niacin, folacin, approximately equal for A, riboflavin, and B_6 and lower for ascorbic acid and vitamin B_{12}.

b) Adequate provision from five to ten years of age appears to be met by:

1) Providing approximately ten times the mean RDA per kg for vitamins A and E in the *total* formulation.

2) Providing vitamin D at slightly more than seven times the mean RDA per kg for a total of 400 units in the total formulation. Since a major role of this vitamin involves calcium transport across the intestinal mucosa and since calcium and phosphate are given as part of the total parenteral regimen for children, this amount appears adequate.

3) Providing approximately 20 times the mean RDA per kg for each of the water-soluble vitamins in the total formulation. For pantothenate and biotin, where no RDA standards have been established, the figures used are 20 times the content present in the volume of human milk providing 100 kilo-calories.

c) Vitamin requirements for children should be met by the following recommended schedule:

1) 10% of the total formulation provided is given daily per kg body weight to a maximum at 10 kg.

2) Above this weight up to age 10 years, the total formulation is given daily unless there is evidence for increased or decreased need based on clinical or laboratory data.

d) It will be noted that no recommendation is made concerning the volume, character, or container(s) to be utilized for the total formulation. Expert advice of vitamin technologists should be obtained in developing stable and efficacious preparations.

e) However, it appears desirable to have a final volume on a simple decimal scale (ie, 10 ml) to simplify dosage calculation and administration.

7. Adult formulation

a) The figures for the adult formulation are based on the RDA recom-

Table 2.—Working Draft of Pediatric Vitamin Standards (RDA* & AAP†) in Comparison with Proposed Pediatric Formulation for Intravenous Multivitamins

Vitamin	Units	Infants RDA Range per kg	Infants RDA Mean	Infants AAP Per 100 kcal	Children RDA Range: 1-10 yrs.	Children Content in Total Formulation
A	I.U.	222-233	227	250	2,000-3,300	2,500
D	I.U.	44-66	55	40	400	400
E	I.U.	0.55-0.66	0.6	0.3	7-10	7
Thiamin	mg	0.05-0.055	0.053	0.025	0.7-1.2	1.2
Riboflavin	mg	0.07	0.07	0.06	0.8-1.2	1.4
Niacin	mg	0.8-0.9	0.85	0.25	9-16	17
B_6	mg	0.04-0.05	0.045	0.035	0.6-1.2	1
Pantothenic acid	mg	0.3‡	0.3	0.3	5-10	6
Folacin	µg	6-8	7	4	100-300	140
B_{12}	µg	0.03-0.04	0.035	0.15	1-2	0.7
Biotin	µg	1†	1	-	?	20
Ascorbic acid	mg	4-6	5	8	40	100

*RDA (1974).

†AAP—American Academy of Pediatrics, Committee on Nutrition: Minimum vitamin levels per 100 kcal of formula (Pediatrics, **40**:916-922, 1967—Table 1).

‡Based on content of human milk per 100 kcal.

mendation for individuals of both sexes in the age range 11 to 51 + years. The range of figures for such individuals is given in Table 3 in comparison with the recommended formulation. The following position has been taken with regard to specific vitamins:

1) Vitamin A is proposed at 4,000 IU since the RDA for this vitamin assumes that a significant amount of carotene is consumed; the latter is less well absorbed than vitamin A.

2) Vitamin E at 15 IU is taken arbitrarily as an average figure. This is probably unnecessarily high for high glucose infusions. Further data are needed for adequacy when polyunsaturated fats become accepted for IV administration.

3) All of the water-soluble vitamins are recommended in amounts which are twice the highest RDA figures for this broad age group. Certain vitamins such as ascorbic acid may be required in larger amounts under conditions of severe stress, such as major burns and trauma. These should be given in additional amounts as indicated. No data are available for biotin requirements; the figure of 60µg is based on preliminary data with adults on prolonged parenteral feeding which indicate that the amount is associated with normal blood levels. Other vitamins are probably present in excess of need for most patients; however, until more data are available, these figures are recommended.

Table 3.— Working Draft of Suggested Composition for Adult Intravenous Multivitamin Preparation for Daily Maintenance of Adequate Vitamin Status and Comparison with RDA (1974)

Vitamin	Units	Daily Adult Dosage	RDA Adult Range‡
A	I.U.	4,000*	4,000-5,000§
D	I.U.	400*	400
E	I.U.	15*	12-15
Thiamin	mg	3.0	1.0-1.5
Riboflavin	mg	3.6	1.1-1.8
Niacin	mg	40	12-20
B$_6$	mg	4	1.6-2.0
Pantothenic acid	mg	15	5-10†
Folacin	µg	800	400ø
B$_{12}$	µg	6	3.0
Biotin	µg	60	150-300†
Ascorbic acid	mg	90	45

*In stable water-dispersible form.
†RDA not established; amounts considered to be adequate in usual dietary intake.
‡Ranges for ages 11-51+ both sexes; does not include requirements for pregnancy or lactation.
§Assumes 50% of intake as carotene which is less available than the vitamin.
øFolacin refers to dietary sources as determined by *Lactobacillus casei* assay.

b) The comments made in paragraph 6d hold here with respect to volume and physical characteristics of the preparation. Unlike the pediatric formulation, the adult preparation should be given as a single volume on a daily basis unless clinical and laboratory data indicate otherwise.

8. Since the requirement for biotin in man under circumstances requiring intravenous administration is unknown, its incorporation into a multivitamin preparation is deemed advisable until more specific information permits its exclusion or a modification of its dosage.

9. Vitamin K is necessary for man but is not included in this formulation in order to permit flexibility for administration of coumadin-type anticoagulants. For patients not receiving such anticoagulants where maintenance of normal prothrombin is desirable, Vitamin K in parenteral form is recommended in moderate dosage (2 to 4 mg) once weekly for adults and older children and approximately one-tenth of these amounts once weekly for infants.

10. The Nutrition Advisory Group believes that these formulations are more useful and more advisable for maintenance than any one or combination of parenteral preparations available today. However, it states without reservation its unanimous opinion that the present state of knowledge of parenteral vitamin requirements and technical formulation is far from complete. It recommends:

a) That technical information be obtained from those with experience in vitamin formulation and stability.

b) That the final formulation be tested in experimental animals and then in patients under clinical conditions with suitable measurements to insure:

1) Efficacy.

2) Freedom from side effects related to agents which may be necessary for stability and solubility.

3) Retention of potency in water dispersion in plastic and other containers and under other conditions of clinical usage which may bring it into contact with any one of the number of additives and nutrients ordinarily used in parenteral nutrition. The Nutrition Advisory Group will present, in a separate statement, its recommendations for the testing of the proposed formulations to insure that they meet these criteria.

11. a) In addition to the multivitamin intravenous formulations specified above, there is need for a formulation of *water soluble vitamins for intramuscular use*. This preparation is designed for those patients who are not receiving intravenous fluids and who meet the following clinical criteria:

1) Intake or absorption is inadequate and oral intake of vitamins must be supplemented by the intramuscular route.

2) There is known or suspected depletion of multiple water-soluble vitamins and immediate treatment by the intramuscular route is advisable.

b) The vitamin composition of the intramuscular formulation should be that of the adult intravenous multivitamin preparation *without* the fat-soluble vitamins A, D, E, and K (Table 4). The fat-soluble vitamins A, D, and K are available in high potency purified form for intramuscular injection when needed.

c) The specific formulation shall be in small volume, *suitable, safe, and efficacious* when given by the intramuscular route.

d) The same formulations shall be used for children in partial dosage on a weight and age basis.

e) Clinical testing of this formulation shall be conducted prior to its approval for unrestricted clinical use.

Preliminary evidence suggests that some vitamins may be unstable when in solution with other nutrients under certain conditions. For these and other reasons the reformulations should be accepted for use only after there

**Table 4.— Working Draft of Suggested Composition for
Water-Soluble Vitamins for Intramuscular Injection***

Vitamin	Units	Amount
Thiamin	mg	3.0
Riboflavin	mg	3.6
Niacin	mg	40
B_6	mg	4
Pantothenic acid	mg	15
Folacin	μg	800
Ascorbic acid	mg	90
B_{12}	μg	6
Biotin	μg	60

*Daily maintenance when not included in parenteral solutions, see paragraph 11.

has been adequate testing for toxicity, stability and compatibility (see paragraph 10). This procedure should then be followed by clinical testing in order to insure that adequate serum and urine levels are maintained in a variety of patients.

APPENDIX B

RECOMMENDED
DAILY DIETARY
ALLOWANCES

Food and Nutrition Board, National Academy of Sciences-National Research Council
Recommended Daily Dietary Allowances,* Revised 1974
(Designed for the maintenance of good nutrition of practically all healthy people in the USA)

	Age	Weight		Height		Energy	Protein	Vitamin A Activity		Vita- min D	Vita- min E Activity ‖
	(years)	(kg)	(lbs)	(cm)	(in)	(kcal)†	(g)	(RE)‡	(IU)	(IU)	(IU)
Infants	0.0-0.5	6	14	60	24	kg x 117	kg x 2.2	420§	1,400	400	4
	0.5-1.0	9	20	71	28	kg x 108	kg x 2.0	400	2,000	400	5
Children	1-3	13	28	86	34	1,300	23	400	2,000	400	7
	4-6	20	44	110	44	1,800	30	500	2,500	400	9
	7-10	30	66	135	54	2,400	36	700	3,300	400	10
Males	11-14	44	97	158	63	2,800	44	1,000	5,000	400	12
	15-18	61	134	172	69	3,000	54	1,000	5,000	400	15
	19-22	67	147	172	69	3,000	54	1,000	5,000	400	15
	23-50	70	154	172	69	2,700	56	1,000	5,000		15
	51+	70	154	172	69	2,400	56	1,000	5,000		15
Females	11-14	44	97	155	62	2,400	44	800	4,000	400	12
	15-18	54	119	162	65	2,100	48	800	4,000	400	12
	19-22	58	128	162	65	2,100	46	800	4,000	400	12
	23-50	58	128	162	65	2,000	46	800	4,000		12
	51+	58	128	162	65	1,800	46	800	4,000		12
Pregnant						+300	+30	1,000	5,000	400	15
Lactating						+500	+20	1,200	6,000	400	15

* The allowances are intended to provide for individual variations among most normal persons as they live in the United States under usual environmental stresses. Diets should be based on a variety of common foods in order to provide other nutrients for which human requirements have been less well defined.

† Kilojoules (kJ) = 4.2 × kcal

‡ Retinol equivalents

§ Assumed to be all as retinol in milk during the first six months of life. All subsequent intakes are assumed to be one-half as retinol and one-half as β-carotene when calculated from international units. As retinol equivalents, three-fourths are as retinol and one-fourth as β-carotene.

	Water-Soluble Vitamins						Minerals					
Ascorbic Acid (mg)	Folacin** (µg)	Niacin†† (mg)	Riboflavin (mg)	Thiamin (mg)	Vitamin B$_6$ (mg)	Vitamin B$_{12}$ (µg)	Calcium (mg)	Phosphorus (mg)	Iodine (µg)	Iron (mg)	Magnesium (mg)	Zinc (mg)
35	50	5	0.4	0.3	0.3	0.3	360	240	35	10	60	3
35	50	8	0.6	0.5	0.4	0.3	540	400	45	15	70	5
40	100	9	0.8	0.7	0.6	1.0	800	800	60	15	150	10
40	200	12	1.1	0.9	0.9	1.5	800	800	80	10	200	10
40	300	16	1.2	1.2	1.2	2.0	800	800	110	10	250	10
45	400	18	1.5	1.4	1.6	3.0	1,200	1,200	130	18	350	15
45	400	20	1.8	1.5	2.0	3.0	1,200	1,200	150	18	400	15
45	400	20	1.8	1.5	2.0	3.0	800	800	140	10	350	15
45	400	18	1.6	1.4	2.0	3.0	800	800	130	10	350	15
45	400	16	1.5	1.2	2.0	3.0	800	800	110	10	350	15
45	400	16	1.3	1.2	1.6	3.0	1,200	1,200	115	18	300	15
45	400	14	1.4	1.1	2.0	3.0	1,200	1,200	115	18	300	15
45	400	14	1.4	1.1	2.0	3.0	800	800	100	18	300	15
45	400	13	1.2	1.0	2.0	3.0	800	800	100	18	300	15
45	400	12	1.1	1.0	2.0	3.0	800	800	80	10	300	15
60	800	+2	+0.3	+0.3	2.5	4.0	1,200	1,200	125	18+ ‡‡	450	20
80	600	+4	+0.5	+0.3	2.5	4.0	1,200	1,200	150	18	450	25

‖ Total vitamin E activity, estimated to be 80 percent as α-tocopherol and 20 percent other tocopherols.

**The folacin allowances refer to dietary sources as determined by *Lactobacillus casei* assay. Pure forms of folacin may be effective in doses less than one-fourth of the RDA.

††Although allowances are expressed as niacin, it is recognized that on the average 1 mg of niacin is derived from each 60 mg of dietary tryptophan.

‡‡This increased requirement cannot be met by ordinary diets; therefore, the use of supplemental iron is recommended.

APPENDIX C

PARTICIPANTS

Authors

Kenneth E. Avis
College of Pharmacy
University of Tennessee
  Medical Units
Memphis, Tennessee

John W. Broviac
Division of Nephrology
University of Washington
School of Medicine
Seattle, Washington

W. Arthur Burke
Wilmington Medical Center
Wilmington, Delaware

George F. Cahill, Jr.
Elliott P. Joslin
  Research Laboratory
Harvard Medical School
Boston, Massachusetts

Jay W. Cooke
Sicklerville, New Jersey
(Formerly with
  Extracorporeal Medical
  Specialties, Inc.)

Leon J. DeMerre
Division of Research
  and Classification
Food and Drug
  Administration
Rockville, Maryland

Stanley J. Dudrick
Department of Surgery
University of Texas
  Medical School at Houston
Houston, Texas

Donald A. Goldmann
Department of Medicine
Massachusetts
  General Hospital
Boston, Massachusetts
(Formerly with
  Hospital Infection Section
  Center for Disease Control
  Atlanta, Georgia)

Harry L. Greene
Department of Pediatrics
Vanderbilt University
  School of Medicine
Nashville, Tennessee

Rudolph J. Jaeger
Kresge Center for
  Environmental Health
Harvard School of
  Public Health
Boston, Massachusetts

John M. Kinney
Department of Surgery
College of Physicians &
  Surgeons of
  Columbia University
New York, New York

Dennis G. Maki
Department of Medicine
Massachusetts
  General Hospital
Boston, Massachusetts

H. C. Meng
Department of Physiology
Vanderbilt University
  School of Medicine
Nashville, Tennessee

Hamish N. Munro
Department of Nutrition and
    Food Science
Massachusetts Institute
    of Technology
Cambridge, Massachusetts

Robert L. Ruberg
Department of Surgery
Hospital of the
    University of Pennsylvania
Philadelphia, Pennsylvania

Robert J. Rubin
School of Hygiene and
    Public Health
Johns Hopkins University
Baltimore, Maryland

William Schaffner
Division of
    Infectious Diseases
Vanderbilt University
    School of Medicine
Nashville, Tennessee

Belding H. Scribner
Department of Medicine
University of Washington
    School of Medicine
Seattle, Washington

Maurice E. Shils
Memorial Hospital for
    Cancer and Allied Diseases
Cornell University
    Medical College
New York, New York

Chairmen and Rapporteurs

William P. Curreri
Department of Surgery
SW Medical School
University of Texas
Dallas, Texas

Hans Fisher
Cook College
Rutgers University
New Brunswick, New Jersey

Robert H. Henry
The United States
    Pharmacopeial
    Convention, Inc.
Rockville, Maryland

Stanley M. Levenson
Albert Einstein College
    of Medicine
Yeshiva University
Bronx, New York

James A. O'Neill, Jr.
Division of Pediatric Surgery
Vanderbilt University
    School of Medicine
Nashville, Tennessee

Harold H. Sandstead
Human Nutrition Laboratory
    North Central Region
US Department
    of Agriculture
Grand Forks, North Dakota

William Schumer
Abraham Lincoln School
    of Medicine
University of Illinois
    College of Medicine
Chicago, Illinois

Theodore B. Van Itallie
Department of Medicine
College of Physicians &
    Surgeons of
    Columbia University
New York, New York

Charles W. Van Way III
Department of Surgery
Ireland Army Hospital
Fort Knox, Kentucky

Douglas W. Wilmore
US Army Institute of
    Surgical Research
Brooke Army Medical Center
Fort Sam Houston, Texas

Robert W. Winters
Department of Pediatrics
College of Physicians &
    Surgeons of
    Columbia University
New York, New York

Arvid Wretlind
Karolinska Institutet
Stockholm, Sweden

Other Participants

Daniel Abrego
Department of Surgery
Meharry Medical College
Nashville, Tennessee

R. Ali
Pharmacia Laboratories, Inc.
Piscataway, New Jersey

G. H. Anderson
School of Hygiene
University of Toronto
Toronto, Canada

John W. Andreoli, Jr.
Extracorporeal Medical
    Specialties, Inc.
King of Prussia, Pennsylvania

Robert K. Ausman
Travenol Laboratories
Morton Grove, Illinois

Heiner Beisbarth
J. Pfrimmer & Co.
Erlangen, West Germany

Wilbur M. Benson
USV Pharmaceutical
    Corporation
Tuckahoe, New York

Louis Bernard
Department of Surgery
Meharry Medical College
Nashville, Tennessee

John Border
Department of Surgery
State University of New York
Buffalo, New York

Helen Bratcher
Meharry Medical College
Nashville, Tennessee

James L. Breeling
Council on Scientific
    Activities
American Medical
    Association
Chicago, Illinois

Joseph Brochetti
Eaton Laboratories
Norwich, New York

J. Leo Brueggeman
Medical University of
    South Carolina
Charleston, South Carolina

C. E. Butterworth, Jr.
School of Medicine
University of Alabama
    in Birmingham
Birmingham, Alabama

Michael Caldwell
Department of Physiology
Vanderbilt University
    School of Medicine
Nashville, Tennessee

John E. Canham
Letterman Army Institute
    of Research
Letterman Army Medical
    Center
Presidio of San Francisco,
    California

Pierre-Em Carlo
9, Place Vauban
Paris, France

James P. Carter
Department of Biochemistry
Vanderbilt University
  School of Medicine
Nashville, Tennessee

William J. Darby
The Nutrition Foundation,
  Inc.
New York, New York

Richard Dean
Department of Surgery
Vanderbilt University
  School of Medicine
Nashville, Tennessee

Fred H. Deindoerfer
American Hospital
  Supply Corporation
Evanston, Illinois

Dan Dillon
Vanderbilt University
  School of Medicine
Nashville, Tennessee

Eugene A. Dolanski
Department of Pediatrics
Vanderbilt University
  School of Medicine
Nashville, Tennessee

John M. Driscoll, Jr.
Department of Pediatrics
College of Physicians &
  Surgeons of
  Columbia University
New York, New York

Richard J. Duma
Division of Immunology and
  Infectious Diseases
Medical College of Virginia
Richmond, Virginia

C. B. Edewaard
Doctor's Clinic
Vero Beach, Florida

Werner Fekl
J. Pfrimmer & Co.
Erlangen, West Germany

Herbert L. Flack
Pharmacy Service
Hospital of the
  University of Pennsylvania
Philadelphia, Pennsylvania

Allan L. Forbes
Health Protection Branch
Department of National
  Health and Welfare
Ottawa, Canada

Donald E. Francke
Drug Intelligence and
  Clinical Pharmacy
Washington, D.C.

John G. Friend
Travenol Laboratories
Morton Grove, Illinois

Thomas A. Garrett
Travenol Laboratories
Morton Grove, Illinois

Leonard G. Ginger
Travenol Laboratories
Morton Grove, Illinois

Alan M. Grant
Abbott Laboratories
North Chicago, Illinois

Richard Hardie
Cutter Laboratories, Inc.
Berkeley, California

William C. Heird
Department of Pediatrics
College of Physicians &
  Surgeons of
  Columbia University
New York, New York

Edward G. High
Department of Biochemistry
    and Nutrition
Meharry Medical College
Nashville, Tennessee

Robert E. Hodges
School of Medicine
University of California
Davis, California

Ralph T. Holman
The Hormel Institute
University of Minnesota
Austin, Minnesota

Verne L. Hoshal, Jr.
St. Joseph's Mercy Hospital
Ann Arbor, Michigan

Lyn Howard
Department of Nutrition
Albany Medical Center
Albany, New York

Robert M. Kark
Department of Medicine
Presbyterian-St. Luke's
    Hospital
Chicago, Illinois

Nicholas Kartinos
Travenol Laboratories
Morton Grove, Illinois

W. Dean Kirkland
Cutter Laboratories, Inc.
Berkeley, California

Roger Klotz
Pharmacy Service
The Children's Memorial
    Hospital
Chicago, Illinois

J. E. Knipfel
Nutrition Research Division
Department of National
    Health and Welfare
Ottawa, Ontario

Carlos L. Krumdieck
School of Medicine
University of Alabama
Birmingham, Alabama

David H. Law
Department of Medicine
Veterans Hospital
Albuquerque, New Mexico

Karl Mayer
Naperville
Illinois

Robert McCormick
Abbott Laboratories
North Chicago, Illinois

James E. McDavid
Cutter Laboratories, Inc.
Berkeley, California

Douglas B. McGill
Mayo Medical School
Rochester, Minnesota

Don C. McLeod
Duke University
Durham, North Carolina

Kas Mohammed
Johnson & Johnson
    Research Center
New Brunswick, New Jersey

Gerry Moore
San Antonio, Texas

Harry Morelli
Presbyterian Hospital
New York, New York

J. A. Muhlenpoh
Three M Company
St. Paul, Minnesota

Margarita Nagy
Nutrition Advisory
    Group on TPN
American Medical
    Association
Chicago, Illinois

476

R. Howard Nay
New York, New York

Ralph A. Nelson
Graduate School of Nutrition
University of Minnesota
Rochester, Minnesota

Alfred J. Newman
Nutrition Division
University of Alabama
Birmingham, Alabama

Robert Nicora
McGaw Laboratories
Glendale, California

C. Donald Olson
Baxter Laboratories
Deerfield, Illinois

Joe W. O'Neal
Vanderbilt University
   Hospital Pharmacy
Nashville, Tennessee

H. Biemann Othersen
Medical University of
   South Carolina
Charleston, South Carolina

Albert Otten
Vanderbilt University
   School of Medicine
Nashville, Tennessee

Joseph H. Oyama
Department of Medicine
Presbyterian-St. Luke's
   Hospital
Chicago, Illinois

Eugene A. Parker
Abbott Laboratories
North Chicago, Illinois

Hugh Paterson
Toronto, Ontario

Robert Ravin
St. Joseph's Mercy Hospital
Ann Arbor, Michigan

Jonathan E. Rhoads
School of Medicine
University of Pennsylvania
Philadelphia, Pennsylvania

Lawrence R. Rose
Bureau of Health Services
   Research
Health Resources
   Administration
Rockville, Maryland

Stanley E. Serlick
Abbott Laboratories
North Chicago, Illinois

Robert Sheffield
Bureau of Drugs
Food and Drug
   Administration
Rockville, Maryland

Ronald Simpson
Department of Nutrition
University of California
Davis, California

Don Spyrison
Travenol Laboratories
Morton Grove, Illinois

Mildred Stahlman
Vanderbilt University
   School of Medicine
Nashville, Tennessee

Lewis D. Stegink
University of Iowa
Iowa City, Iowa

Ralph Stone
Vanderbilt University
   School of Medicine
Nashville, Tennessee

Charles Styron
Duke University
Raleigh, North Carolina

Charles R. Thompson
Cutter Laboratories, Inc.
Berkeley, California

Ira D. Thompson
Department of Surgery
Meharry Medical College
Nashville, Tennessee

William Thrasher
Travenol Laboratories
Morton Grove, Illinois

Parker Vanamee
Memorial Hospital for
    Cancer and Allied Diseases
Cornell University
    Medical College
New York, New York

Lars H. Victorin
University of Gothenburg
Gothenburg, Sweden

Matthew Walker
Department of Surgery
Meharry Medical College
Nashville, Tennessee

Thomas L. Westman
McGaw Laboratories
Glendale, California

Raymond E. Weston
Beverly Hills, California

Philip L. White
Council on Foods
    and Nutrition
American Medical
    Association
Chicago, Illinois

E. Whitman
Miami, Florida

Norman N. Yoshimura
McGaw Laboratories
Glendale, California

Eleanor Anne Young
Health Science Center of
    San Antonio
The University of Texas
San Antonio, Texas